Current Issues in Healthcare Policy and Practice

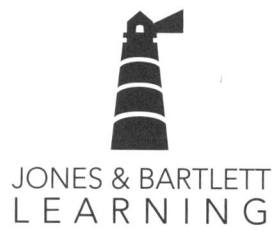

JONES & BARTLETT
LEARNING

World Headquarters
Jones & Bartlett Learning
40 Tall Pine Drive
Sudbury, MA 01776
978-443-5000
info@jblearning.com
www.jblearning.com

Jones & Bartlett Learning Canada
6339 Ormindale Way
Mississauga, Ontario L5V 1J2
Canada

Jones & Bartlett Learning International
Barb House, Barb Mews
London W6 7PA
United Kingdom

Jones & Bartlett Learning books and products are available through most bookstores and online booksellers. To contact Jones & Bartlett Learning directly, call 800-832-0034, fax 978-443-8000, or visit our website, www.jblearning.com.

Substantial discounts on bulk quantities of Jones & Bartlett Learning publications are available to corporations, professional associations, and other qualified organizations. For details and specific discount information, contact the special sales department at Jones & Bartlett Learning via the above contact information or send an email to specialsales@jblearning.com.

This publication is designed to provide accurate and authoritative information in regard to the subject matter covered. It is sold with the understanding that the publisher is not engaged in rendering legal, accounting, or other professional service. If legal advice or other expert assistance is required, the service of a competent professional person should be sought.

Production Credits
Publisher: Michael Brown
Associate Editor: Catie Heverling
Editorial Assistant: Teresa Reilly
Production Director: Amy Rose
Associate Production Editor: Tina Chen
Senior Marketing Manager: Sophie Fleck
Manufacturing and Inventory Control Supervisor: Amy Bacus
Composition: Publishers' Design and Production Services, Inc.
Cover Design: John Garland
Cover Images: Clockwise, from top: © Monkey Business Images/Dreamstime.com; © Photos.com; © Creatas/Jupiterimages;
   © Monkey Business Images/Shutterstock, Inc. Back cover: © Monkey Business Images/Dreamstime.com.
Printing and Binding: Malloy, Inc.
Cover Printing: Malloy, Inc.

ISBN 978-1-4496-1327-3

6048

Printed in the United States of America
14 13 12 11 10   10 9 8 7 6 5 4 3 2 1

Contents

Chapter 3   Health Policy **95**

Leiyu Shi, DrPH, MBA, MPA, and Douglas A. Singh, PhD, MBA

Chapter 4   The Future of Health Services Delivery **123**

Leiyu Shi, DrPH, MBA, MPA, and Douglas A. Singh, PhD, MBA

Chapter 5   Overview of Long-Term Care. **157**

Douglas A. Singh, PhD, MBA

Chapter 6   Long-Term Care Policy: Past, Present, and Future 179
Douglas A. Singh, PhD, MBA

Chapter 7   The Long-Term Care Industry. 201
Douglas A. Singh, PhD, MBA

Chapter 8   Internal Environment and Culture Change 229
Douglas A. Singh, PhD, MBA

Chapter 1

Leiyu Shi, DrPH, MBA, MPA, and Douglas A. Singh, PhD, MBA

Inpatient Facilities and Services

Learning Objectives

- To get a functional perspective on the evolution of hospitals
- To survey the factors that contributed to the growth of hospitals prior to the 1980s
- To understand the reasons for the subsequent decline of hospitals and their utilization
- To learn some key measures pertaining to hospital operations and inpatient utilization
- To differentiate between various types of hospitals
- To differentiate between nonprofit and for-profit hospitals and understand some of the issues surrounding the nonprofit status of voluntary hospitals
- To comprehend some basic concepts in hospital governance
- To get a perspective on some key ethical issues and the erosion of public trust

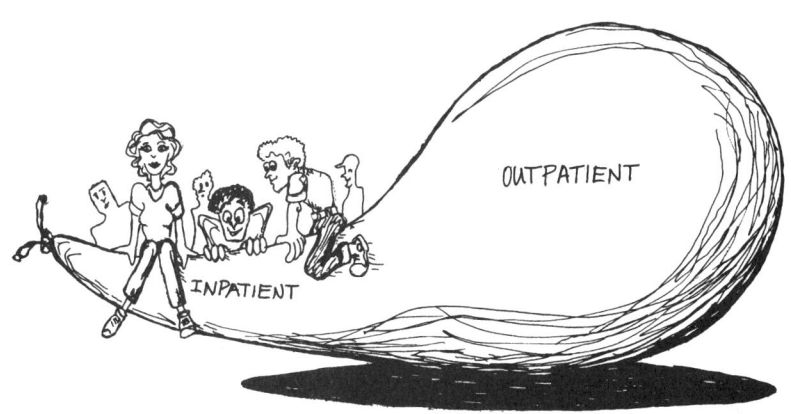

"We have the inpatient sector under control."

1

Introduction

The term *inpatient* is used in conjunction with an overnight stay in a health care facility, such as a hospital. On the other hand, outpatient refers to services provided while the patient is not lodged in a health care facility. Although the primary function of hospitals is to deliver inpatient acute care services, many hospitals have expanded their scope of services to include non-acute and outpatient care.

According to the American Hospital Association (AHA), a *hospital* is an institution with at least six beds whose primary function is "to deliver patient services, diagnostic and therapeutic, for particular or general medical conditions" (AHA 1994). In addition, a hospital must be licensed, it must have an organized physician staff, and it must provide continuous nursing services under the supervision of registered nurses. Other characteristics of a hospital include an identifiable governing body that is legally responsible for the conduct of the hospital, a chief executive with continuous responsibility for the operation of the hospital, maintenance of medical records on each patient, pharmacy services maintained in the institution and supervised by a registered pharmacist, and food service operations to meet the nutritional and therapeutic requirements of the patients (Health Forum 2001). The construction and operation of the modern hospital is governed by federal laws; state health department regulations; city ordinances; standards of the Joint Commission on Accreditation of Healthcare Organizations (Joint Commission); and national codes for building, fire protection, and sanitation.

In the past 200 years or so, hospitals have gradually evolved from ordinary institutions of refuge for the homeless and poor to ultramodern facilities providing the latest medical services to the critically ill and injured. The term "medical center" is used by some hospitals, reflecting their high level of specialization and wide scope of services, which may include teaching and research. Growth of multihospital chains, especially those providing a variety of health care services, has led to the nomenclature "hospital system" or "health system."

Hospital care consumes the biggest share of national health care spending. Hence, the hospital inpatient sector was the first to be targeted by prospective reimbursement methods during the 1980s. Subsequently, as new technologies emerged to treat patients outside the hospital setting, outpatient services for various types of medical procedures and treatments mushroomed. Managed care also played a significant role in curtailing inpatient utilization.

This chapter describes institutional care delivery with specific reference to acute care—mostly characterized by secondary and tertiary levels of care—in community hospitals. It also discusses various ways to classify hospitals and points out important trends and critical issues that will continue to shape the delivery of inpatient services.

Transformation of the Hospital in the United States

Generally speaking, from about 1840 to 1900, hospitals underwent a drastic change in purpose, function, and number. From supplying merely food, shelter, and meager medical care to the pauper sick, to armies, to those infected with contagious diseases, to the insane, and to those requiring emergency treatment, they began to provide skilled medical and surgical attention and nursing care to all people (Raffel 1980, 241). Subsequently, hospitals became centers of medical training and research. More recent transformations are mainly organizational in nature, as hospitals have consolidated into medical systems delivering a broad range of health care services. Medical technology also continues to transform the delivery of health care; in recent years, it has been a significant factor in shaping the organizational structures within the health care industry. These transformations can be neatly categorized according to five dominant functions in the evolution of hospitals:

1. Primitive institutions of social welfare
2. Distinct institutions of care for the sick
3. Organized institutions of medical practice
4. Advanced institutions of medical training and research
5. Consolidated systems of health services delivery

Primitive Institutions of Social Welfare

Except for a few hospitals that were located in some of the major US cities, municipal almshouses (or poorhouses) and pesthouses existed during the 1800s to provide food and shelter to the destitute. Financed through charitable gifts and local government funds, these institutions essentially served a social welfare function. Medical care, or more properly, nursing care, was only secondary and was quite primitive. Some almshouses had adjoining infirmaries where the sick were isolated. People generally stayed in these institutions for months rather than days.

Pesthouses were used to quarantine people who were sick with contagious diseases so the rest of the community would be protected. Later hospitals evolved from these almshouses and pesthouses, but even after hospitals developed, people generally did not want to be admitted to these establishments for treatment because a hospital could do little for them. Most illnesses were treated at home, using folk medicine or the services of physicians who made home visits.

Distinct Institutions of Care for the Sick

Not until the late 1800s did the infirmaries or hospital departments of city poorhouses break away to become independent medical care institutions. These were the first public hospitals (Haglund and Dowling 1993), in this case operated by local governments. For example, the Kings County Almshouse and Infirmary, organized in Brooklyn in 1830, later became the Kings County Hospital (Raffel 1980, 221), but such hospitals still served mainly the poor. A few hospitals serving all classes of society and built specifically to care for the sick also emerged during the 19th century. These hospitals were voluntary or nongovernment.

The founding of *voluntary hospitals*—community hospitals financed through local philanthropy as opposed to taxes—was often inspired by influential physicians with the financial backing of local donors and philanthropists. These hospitals accepted both indigent and paying patients, but to cover their operating expenses they required charitable contributions from private citizens.

In the United States, most voluntary hospitals had private rather than religious or government sponsorship. In Europe, by contrast, the first hospitals were established predominantly by religious orders. Nurses, who were primarily monks and nuns, attended to the physical as well as the spiritual needs of the patients. Later, many of these hospitals became tax-financed public institutions as less church money became available for hospitals and monasteries. In England, the "royal hospitals" were supported by private donations and taxes. Later hospitals in Britain were voluntary hospitals, which served as a model for such hospitals in the United States (Raffel and Raffel 1994, 108, 110).

The first voluntary hospital in the United States established specifically to care for the sick was the Pennsylvania Hospital in Philadelphia, opened in 1752. It was patterned after the British voluntary hospitals. The city already had an almshouse. Similar to other seaports, Philadelphia also had pest-houses to isolate people with contagious diseases, such as smallpox and yellow fever. However, Dr. Thomas Bond, a London-trained physician, brought to prominence the need for a hospital to care for the sick poor of the city. Benjamin Franklin, who was a friend and advisor of Dr. Bond, was instrumental in promoting the idea and in raising voluntary subscriptions. According to the charter, the contributors had the right to make all laws and regulations relating to the hospital's operation. The contributors also elected members to form the governing board or the *board of trustees*. Thus, the control of voluntary hospitals was in the hands of influential community laypeople rather than physicians (Raffel and Raffel 1994, 110–111). The tradition of the voluntary hospital following this early model has continued to this day, as the majority of hospitals in the United States have private nonprofit status.

Other prominent voluntary hospitals included the New York Hospital in New York, which was completed in 1775, but, due to the Revolutionary War, was not opened to civilian patients until 1791. The Massachusetts General Hospital in Boston was incorporated in 1812 and opened in 1821. During this period, the almshouses continued to serve an important function by receiving overflow patients who could not be admitted to the hospitals because of the unavailability of beds or who had to be discharged from hospitals because they were declared incurable (Raffel and Raffel 1994, 115–116). Later hospitals in the United States were modeled after Pennsylvania, New York, and Massachusetts General.

Organized Institutions of Medical Practice

Social and demographic change, but above all, the advance of medical science, transformed hospitals into institutions of medical practice. From the latter half of the 19th century, technological progress led to the development of advanced equipment, facilities, and personnel training, which became centered in the hospital. Medicine was revolutionized as investigators discovered the causes of disease and developed technological devices for diagnosis and treatment (Raffel 1980, 235). Most notable in terms of their impact on hospitals were (1) the discovery of anesthesia, which aided significantly in advancing new surgical techniques, (2) development of the germ theory of disease, which led to the subsequent discovery of antiseptic and sterilization techniques, and (3) X-ray for diagnostic imaging. Use of antiseptic procedures, and later, introduction of sulfa drugs and penicillin in the mid-20th century produced significant reductions in mortality from infections (Snook 1981). The application of medical science and technology in hospitals also made it necessary for physicians to receive their training and to practice medicine in hospitals.

Drastic improvements in the environmental conditions and the practice of medicine in hospitals made them more acceptable to the middle and upper classes. Hospitals actually began to attract affluent patients who could afford to pay privately. Hospitals also came to be regarded as a necessity because the superior medical services and surgical procedures could not be obtained at home. Thus, the hospital was transformed from a charitable institution into one that could generate a profit. In many instances, physicians started opening small hospitals, financed by wealthy and powerful sponsors. These facilities were the first proprietary hospitals.

In the early 20th century, the field of hospital administration became a discipline in its own right. Administrators with expertise in financial management and organizational skills were needed to manage hospitals. The administrative structure of the hospital was organized into departments, such as food service, pharmacy, X-ray, and laboratory. It became necessary to employ professional staff to manage the delivery of services. Efficiency began to emerge as an important element in the management of hospitals. The term was defined broadly, encompassing not only economy but also quality and breadth of services, as well as access to care. This early emphasis on efficiency foreshadowed two main issues that affect health policy and hospital management to this day: the pressure on hospitals to introduce new technology while containing cost, and the assumption that hospitals should act like businesses (Arndt and Bigelow 2006). With greater pressure for cost containment, hospitals began to limit care to the more acute periods of illness, rather than the full course of a disease.

Advanced Institutions of Medical Training and Research

The hospital had a profound influence on medical education in the United States. With the advance of medical science, hospitals became important centers for the dissemination of biomedical knowledge. Hospitals provided the desirable venue for clinical studies. The vast number of clinical records and a large array of medical conditions among patients seeking care in major hospitals provide a wealth of data to conduct investigative studies to advance medical knowledge.

Recognition of the critical role hospitals played in medical education led to collaborations between hospitals and universities. The Pennsylvania Hospital, for example, taught courses required by the College of Philadelphia's medical school, which later became the University of Pennsylvania School of Medicine. Similarly, New York Hospital served as a teaching hospital for medical students of Columbia Medical School, and Massachusetts General Hospital provided practical clinical instruction for Harvard Medical School (Raffel and Raffel 1994, 113–116). In affiliation with university based medical schools, many hospitals became centers of medical research where new discoveries were made, and the findings were disseminated through publications in medical journals.

The Johns Hopkins Hospital (opened in 1889), with its adjoining medical school (opened in 1893), inaugurated a new era in combining clinical practice with teaching and the promotion of scientific inquiry in medicine. Patterned after the great European hospitals connected with medical schools, the hospital was to teach students the best methods then known of caring for the sick, and to serve as a great laboratory to advance the knowledge of the causes, processes, and treatment of disease (Raffel 1980, 245). From the 1920s, the hospital's teaching role became even more prominent as specialization in medicine led to a proliferation of internships and residencies (Haglund and Dowling 1993).

More recently, the increasing use of non-institutional settings has shifted some aspects of medical education from inpatient to outpatient sectors and to other delivery settings such as nursing homes, hospices, and community health centers. Nevertheless, the hospital continues to play a central role in the training of physicians. Nursing education has also evolved largely around hospitals as the role of nursing has become more technically complex. The same is true of many other health care professions (Williams 1995, 56, 57). For both the training and the subsequent employment of virtually the whole spectrum of health professionals, hospitals play a significant role.

Consolidated Systems of Health Services Delivery

In the late 20th century, the major impact of radical changes in the health care delivery system has been experienced by hospitals because they constitute the institutional nucleus of health care delivery. The most profound changes are seen in the drastic reductions in the length of inpatient stays brought about by prospective and capitated payment methods and aggressive utilization review practices. The declining utilization of acute care beds had left most hospitals with excess capacity in the form of empty beds. Hence, consolidation

of hospitals was particularly intense during the mid-1990s mainly because of economic necessity. As the acute inpatient care sector of health care delivery has become less profitable, hospitals have diversified into nonacute services, such as outpatient centers, home health care, long-term care, subacute care, assisted living, and inpatient and outpatient rehabilitation. Local market pressures have also prompted many hospitals to merge or enter into formal affiliations with other hospitals. The three main types of consolidations have occurred through mergers and acquisitions, vertical integration, and participation in networks through contractual arrangements. These strategies have offered patients increased access to care across a continuum of services. However, intense consolidation in certain hospital markets has also diluted competition. Research suggests that hospital consolidation in the 1990s raised prices by at least 5 percent as competition eroded. Evidence also suggests that increasing hospital concentration may also lower quality, but the findings are not robust (Vogt and Town 2006).

The Expansion Phase: Late 1800s to Mid-1980s

Hospitals grew in numbers when they became a necessary local adjunct of medical practice. Growth in the volume of surgical work especially provided the basis for expansion of hospital beds. The expansion in surgical practice coincided with biomedical discoveries and growth of medical technology.

Profits from surgery enabled physicians to build small hospitals without upper-class sponsorship. The number of hospitals grew from 178 (35,604 beds) in 1872 to 4,359

(421,065 beds) in 1909. By 1929, 6,665 hospitals provided 907,133 beds (Haglund and Dowling 1993). As new beds were built, their availability almost ensured that they would be used. This phenomenon led Milton Roemer (1916–2001) to proclaim, "a built bed is a filled bed," known popularly as Roemer's Law (Roemer 1961).

Haglund and Dowling (1993) pointed to six significant factors in the growth of hospitals: advances in medical science, development of specialized technology, advances in medical education, development of professional nursing, growth of health insurance, and the role of government. The first three factors were discussed in the previous section; this section covers the last three.

Development of Professional Nursing

During the latter half of the 19th century, Florence Nightingale was instrumental in transforming nursing into a recognized profession in Britain. Following the founding of the Nightingale School of Nursing in England, nursing schools in the United States were established at Bellevue Hospital (New York City), New Haven Hospital (New Haven, Connecticut), and Massachusetts General Hospital (Boston). The benefits of having trained nurses in hospitals became apparent as increased efficacy of treatment and hygiene improved patient recovery (Haglund and Dowling 1993). As a result of these advances, hospitals increasingly came to be regarded as places of healing and found acceptance with the middle and upper classes.

Growth of Private Health Insurance

During and after the Great Depression of the 1930s, many hospitals were forced to close, and the financial solvency of many more was threatened. Thus, the number of hospitals in the United States dropped from 6,852 in 1928 to 6,189 in 1937. Subsequently, the growth of private health insurance became a vehicle for enabling people to pay for hospital services, and the flow of insurance funds helped revive the financial stability of hospitals. Insurance also contributed to the increased demand for health services. Historically, insurance plans provided generous coverage for inpatient care. Consequently, there were few restrictions on patients and physicians opting for more expensive hospital services (Feldstein 1971). Note that private health insurance in the United States first began as a hospital insurance plan.

Role of Government

Government funding for hospital construction perhaps played the most important role in the expansion of hospitals. Subsequently, Medicare and Medicaid provided indirect funding to the hospital industry by vastly expanding public-sector health insurance.

The Hill-Burton Act

Relatively little hospital construction took place during the Great Depression and World War II, so by the end of the war, the nation was severely short of hospitals. The Hospital Survey and Construction Act of 1946, commonly referred to as the Hill-Burton Act, provided federal grants to states for the construction of new community hospital beds; however, the hospitals would not be under federal control. This legislation required that each state develop and upgrade annually a plan for health facility construction—based on bed-to-population ratios—that would serve as a basis for allocation of federal construction grants (Raffel 1980, 588).

In 1946, after the war, 3.2 community hospital beds were available per 1,000 civilian population. The objective of Hill-Burton was to reach 4.5 beds per 1,000 population (Teisberg et al. 1991). The Hill-Burton program assisted in the construction of nearly 40 percent of the beds in the nation's short-stay general hospitals and was the greatest single factor that increase in the nation's bed supply during the 1950s and 1960s (Haglund and Dowling 1993). Hill-Burton made it possible for even small, remote communities to have their own hospitals (Wolfson and Hopes 1994). By 1980, the United States had reached its goal of 4.5 community hospital beds per 1,000 civilian population (DHHS 2002) even though the Hill-Burton program terminated in 1974.

Hill-Burton was also instrumental in promoting the growth of non-profit community hospitals because it had required that hospitals constructed with federal funds must provide a certain amount of uncompensated care. Competition from these new hospitals led to the closure of many smaller proprietary for-profit hospitals. Most of the remaining proprietary hospitals began delivering free or discounted services to those who could not afford to pay (Muller 2003). Thanks to Hill-Burton, nonprofit community hospitals in the United States far outnumber all other types of hospitals.

Public Health Insurance

The creation of Medicare and Medicaid programs in the mid-1960s also had a significant, although indirect, impact on the increase in the number of hospital beds and their utilization (Feldstein 1993, 215) as government-funded health insurance became available to a large number of elderly and poor Americans. Between 1965 and 1980, the number of community hospitals in the United States increased from 5,736 (741,000 beds) to 5,830 (988,000 beds); total admissions per 1,000 population increased from 130 to 154; and total inpatient days per 1,000 population increased from 1,007 to 1,159. The percentage occupancy also remained relatively stable at around 76 percent (AHA 1990). Figure 1–1 shows trends from 1940 to 2004 in the number of beds per 1,000 resident population.

Figure 1–1   Trends in the Number of Community Hospital Beds per 1,000 Resident Population.

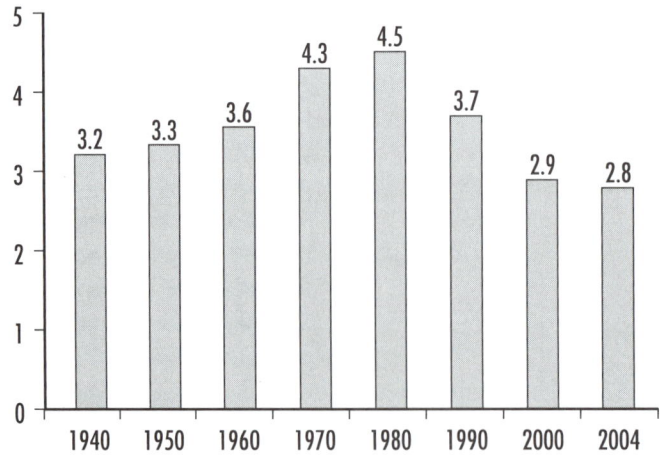

Source: Data from *Health United States, 2002*, p. 281; *Health United States, 2006*, p. 366; National Center for Health Statistics.

The Downsizing Phase: Mid-1980s Onward

The mid-1980s marked a turning point in the growth and use of hospital beds. After a sharp decline in 1985, the number of community hospitals and the total number of beds have declined fairly consistently (Figure 1–2). A sharper decline in the number of hospitals compared to hospital beds illustrates the closure of smaller hospitals, particularly in rural areas. At the same time, the average bed capacity per hospital declined from 196 beds in 1980 to 166 beds in 2004 (DHHS 2006, 364).

Even as the number of hospitals and capacity have contracted, further declines have occurred in the actual utilization of the shrunken capacity. Occupancy rates (percentage of beds occupied) in community hospitals declined from 75.6 percent in 1980 to around 64 percent in 2000. Since then, occupancy rates have increased slightly (67 percent in 2004) mainly because capacity (number of available beds) has steadily declined, from 823,560 total community hospital beds in 2000 to 808,127 in 2004. Similarly, the average length of stay (ALOS) in community hospitals has declined from 7.5 days in 1980 to 4.8 days in 2004 (DHHS 2006, 339, 364).

Within hospitals, a tremendous shift from inpatient to outpatient utilization occurred, as illustrated in Figure 1–3 in the form of increasing ratios between hospital outpatient visits and inpatient days. Along with this shift in the use of hospital services, the share of national expenditures on hospital care has also consistently declined (Table 1–1). It does not appear that hospitals were able to recoup the loss of inpatient revenues

Figure 1–2 The Decline in the Number of Community Hospitals and Beds.

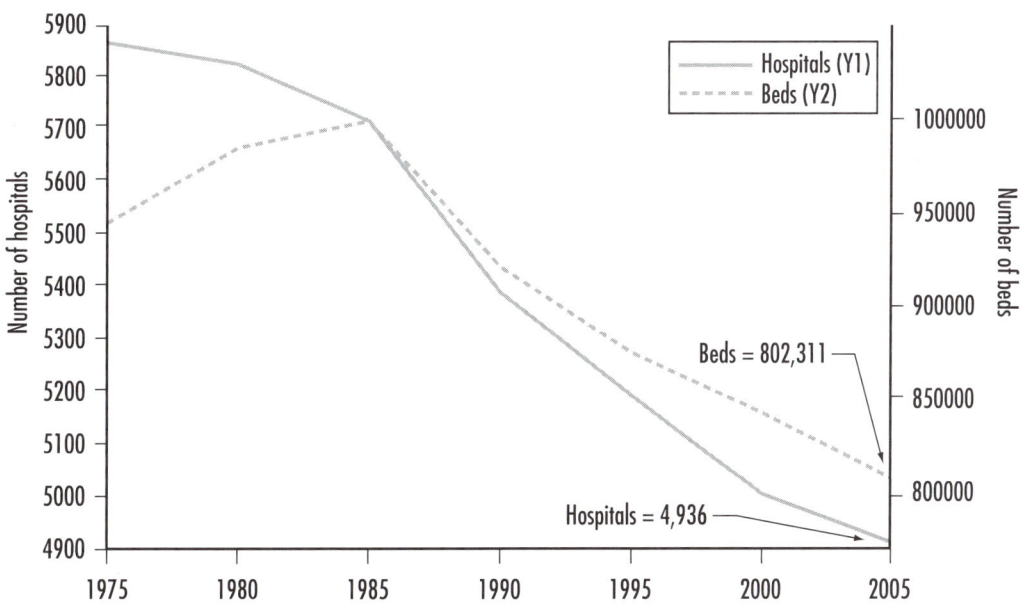

Source: Data from *Health United States, 2002*, p. 279; AHA Hospital Statistics, 2007, Health Forum LLC.

Figure 1–3   Ratio of Hospital Outpatient Visits to Inpatient Days (all hospitals), 1980–2004.

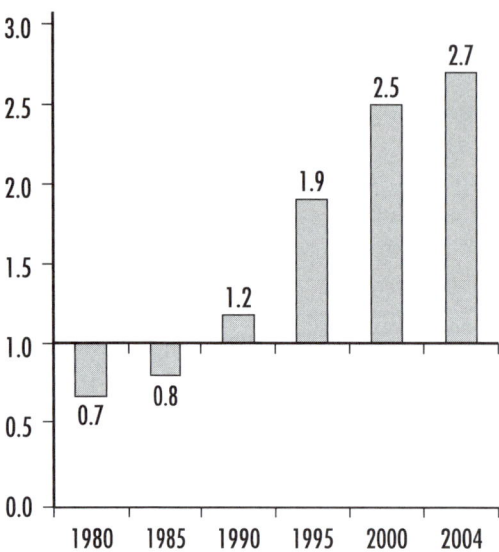

Source: Data from *Statistical Abstract of the United States, 2002,* p. 110; *Statistical Abstract of the United States, 2007,* p. 114; US Census Bureau.

by developing outpatient services. This is mainly due to the development of, and increased competition from, new outpatient services that are not affiliated with hospitals. In the future, however, we can expect to see a pick-up in hospital inpatient use as the US population continues to age. Aging is a key driver of hospital inpatient utilization.

The downward pressures on hospital utilization have been exerted by three main forces: changes in hospital reimbursement, closure of small rural hospitals, and the impact of managed care. Of these three, hospital reimbursement had the most dramatic effect on hospitals.

Changes in Reimbursement

The Tax Equity and Fiscal Responsibility Act (TEFRA) of 1982 was implemented in 1983. This legislation authorized the conversion of hospital Medicare reimbursement from cost-plus to a prospective payment system (PPS) based on DRGs. PPS marked a major change in the way hospitals were paid for inpatient services. Following Medicare's lead, several states adopted prospective methods to reimburse hospitals for services provided to their Medicaid enrollees. Private payers also resorted to competitive pricing and discounted fees, and closely monitored when patients would be hospitalized and for how long. The effect of PPS on hospitals was dramatic. In the 1980s, 550 hospitals

Table 1–1   Share of National Expenditures for Hospital Care

	1980	1990	1995	2000	2005
National health expenditures (NHE)	$245.8	$696.0	$990.3	$1299.5	1,987.7
Expenditures — hospital care	$101.5	$253.9	$343.6	$412.1	611.6
Hospital expenditures as a percent of NHE	41.3%	36.5%	34.7%	31.7%	30.8%

Source: Data from *Health United States, 2002,* p. 291, National Center for Health Statistics; Catlin, A. et al. 2007. National Health Spending in 2005: The Slowdown Continues. *Health Affairs* 26, no. 1: 142–153.

closed and 159 mergers and acquisitions occurred (Balotsky 2005).

Rural Hospital Closures

During the 1990s, many small rural hospitals had to close because of economic constraints. Hospitals of all sizes throughout the country had to close entire wings or convert those beds for alternative uses, such as psychiatric care or long-term care. To rescue many of the remaining small hospitals from closure, in 1983, the then Health Care Financing Administration (HCFA) initiated a swing bed program for rural hospitals. *Swing beds* were authorized under the Omnibus Reconciliation Act of 1980 (Public Law 96499). The program created additional revenues for small rural hospitals by allowing them to switch the use of hospitals beds between acute-care and long-term care skilled nursing facility (SNF) as needed. However, in July 2002, the Centers for Medicare and Medicaid Services (formerly called HCFA) brought hospital swing beds under the existing SNF PPS reimbursement, which created further financial pressures for these hospitals.

Impact of Managed Care

In the 1990s, managed care became a growing force transforming the delivery of health services. Managed care has emphasized cost containment and the efficient delivery of services. Because inpatient care, especially in acute care hospitals, is costly, managed care has emphasized alternative delivery settings, such as outpatient treatments, home health care, and the use of nursing homes whenever appropriate. Such measures have had a tremendous impact on

curtailing the utilization of inpatient services and on the downsizing of individual hospitals. It has been demonstrated that Health Maintenance Organizations' (HMO) penetration in health care markets has played a significant role in lowering hospital profitability (Clement and Grazier 2001). Hospitals, on the other hand, have employed consolidation strategies in an effort to cope with such external pressures.

Some Key Utilization Measures and Operational Concepts

Discharges

The total number of patient discharges per 1,000 population is one indicator of access to hospital inpatient services and of the extent of utilization. Because babies born in the hospital are not included in admissions, discharges provide a more accurate count of the inpatients served by a hospital. *Discharge* refers to the total number of patients discharged from a hospital's acute care beds in a given period. Deaths in hospitals are counted as discharges. Discharge rates per 1,000 population (Table 1–2) are important because all other inpatient use patterns depend on them. Discharges per 1,000 population from community hospitals declined from 122.3 in 1990 to 119.2 in 2004 (DHHS 2006, 339), reflecting a lower rate of inpatient hospital utilization.

Inpatient Days

An *inpatient day* (also called a patient day or a hospital day) is a night spent in the hospital by a patient. The cumulative number of patient days over a certain period is known as *days of care*. Days of care per 1,000 population over one year generally reflect access to inpatient services and their utilization. When days of care are compared according to demographic characteristics, some interesting facts about access and utilization emerge (Table 1–2). There is a direct relationship between age and days of care in hospitals (with the exception of children between birth and 4 years of age—not shown in Table 1–2). Older people spend more time in hospitals than younger people. In general, females incur higher use of hospital services than men do. However, roughly 27 percent of all discharges and 12.5 percent of

Table 1–2 Discharges, Days of Care, and Average Length of Stay per 1,000 Population in Nonfederal Short-Stay Hospitals, 2004

Characteristics	Discharges	Days of Care	Average Length of Stay
Total	119.2	574.1	4.8
Age			
Under 18 years	43.0	193.2	4.5
18–44 years	91.1	334.9	3.7
45–54 years	99.7	491.1	4.9
55–64 years	143.6	735.2	5.1
65–74 years	259.2	1,405.2	5.4
75+ years	470.2	2,714.9	5.8
Gender[1]			
Male	102.6	541.1	5.3
Male (18+ years)[2]	123.2	659.5	5.4
Female	134.9	599.6	4.4
Female (18+ years after factoring out child-birth-related utilization)[2]	129.0	639.3	5.0
Race[1]			
White	89.0	431.0	4.8
Black	110.0	597.0	5.4
Geographic Region[1]			
Northeast	128.8	687.6	5.3
Midwest	114.4	498.7	4.4
South	125.6	614.2	4.9
West	101.2	457.5	4.5

[1]Age adjusted.

[2]Author's estimate based on 2004 data from the National Center for Health Statistics and US Census Bureau.

Source: Data from *Health, United States, 2006,* pp. 339, 340, US Department of Health and Human Services, National Center for Health Statistics; Statistical Abstract of the United States, 2007, p. 117. US Census Bureau.

all days of care among women 18 years of age and older are childbirth-related. After factoring out childbirth-related use, in the 18+ age category, women still incur a higher discharge rate than men, but have 3 percent fewer population-adjusted days of care, and have a shorter average length of stay (see Table 1–2). Hospitalization is higher among blacks than whites. Generally, hospital use is higher among people of lower socioeconomic status than the more affluent because poorer population groups generally have less access to routine primary care, and there are other factors involved. Consequently, poorer population groups in the United States are more likely to suffer from acute conditions, incurring more frequent hospitalization and also longer stays once admitted. In the western United States, hospital utilization is much lower than in other parts of the country. A high rate of managed care penetration is believed to be primarily responsible for the lower utilization. The utilization patterns also suggest that overall hospital use is higher among Medicare and Medicaid recipients than among the rest of the population.

Average Length of Stay

Average length of stay (ALOS) is calculated by dividing the total days of care by the total number of discharges. It provides a measure of how many days a patient, on average, spends in the hospital. Hence, this measure, when applied to individuals or specific groups of patients, is an indicator of severity of illness. It also indicates the average inpatient resources used for specific categories of patients, under the assumption that medical resources are used in conjunction with each day a patient spends in a hospital bed. In 2003, the ALOS for community hospitals in the United States dropped to 4.8 days, the lowest ever recorded (it remained the same in 2004). Table 1–2 shows ALOS based on several patient characteristics (discussed in the previous section). Figure 1–4 shows trends in ALOS by type of hospital ownership. Federal hospitals mainly include those in the Veterans Health Administration system, which serve a population that is getting older. State and local government hospitals disproportionately serve the poor and uninsured. For 2004, the ALOS in voluntary and proprietary hospitals are similar. Figure 1–5 illustrates the downward trend in ALOS from 1970 to 2004. First, the PPS had a marked influence on the decline in the ALOS during the mid-1980s. This was followed by the influence of managed care during the 1990s. The sharp decline in average length of hospital stay during the 1990s became possible with the growth of alternative services, such as home health and subacute long-term care, which enabled people to be discharged earlier. Thanks to the development of these substitute sites of care and better technology, no evidence has emerged that quicker discharges of patients from hospitals under PPS or managed care payment systems resulted in medical harm to patients.

Capacity

The number of beds set up and staffed for inpatient use determines the size or capacity of a hospital. Eighty-four percent of all community hospitals in the United States have fewer than 300 beds (Figure 1–6). The average size of a community hospital is approximately 165 beds, which has remained relatively constant since 1995. Nationally, a typical rural hospital has 65 beds, and an

Figure 1–4   Average Lengths of Stay by Hospital Ownership: 1990–2004.

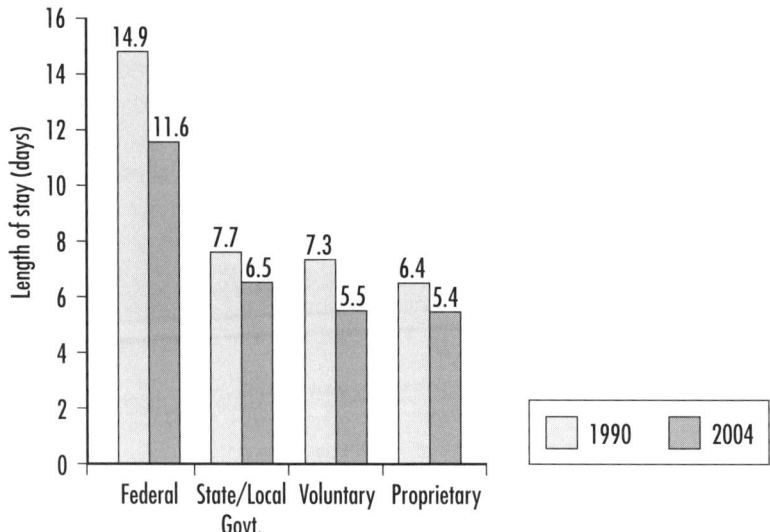

Source: Data from *Health United States, 2006*, p. 350, US Department of Health and Human Services.

Figure 1–5   Change in Average Length of Stay in All US Community Hospitals, 1970–2004.

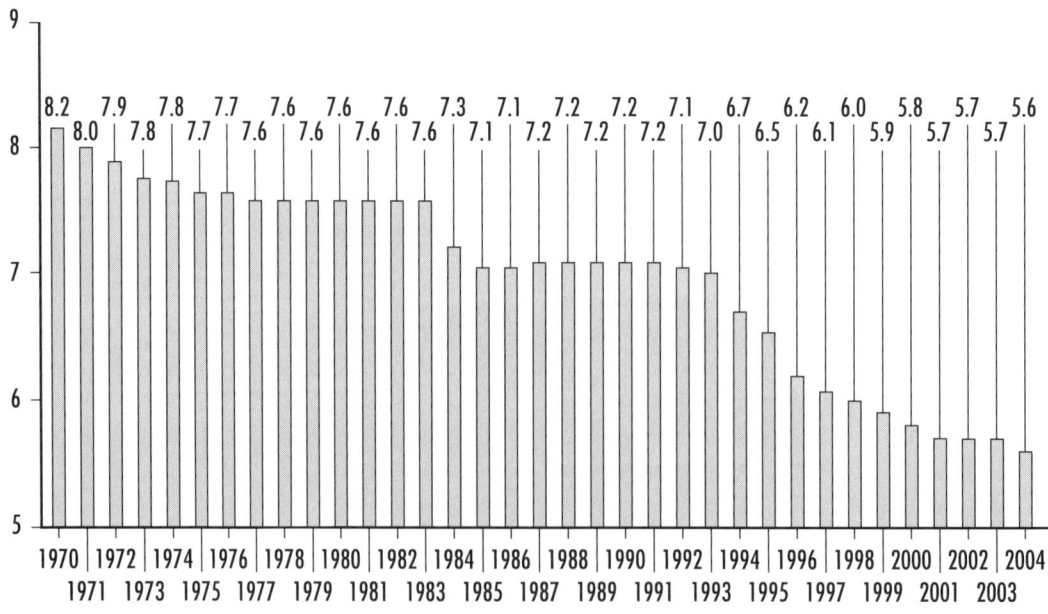

Source: Data from *Hospital Statistics, 1999*, p. 2, © American Hospital Association; *Hospital Statistics 2002*, p. 4, Health Forum; *Health United States, 2003*, p. 285; *Health United States, 2006*, p. 350, National Center for Health Statistics.

Figure 1–6 Breakdown of Community Hospitals by Size, 2004.

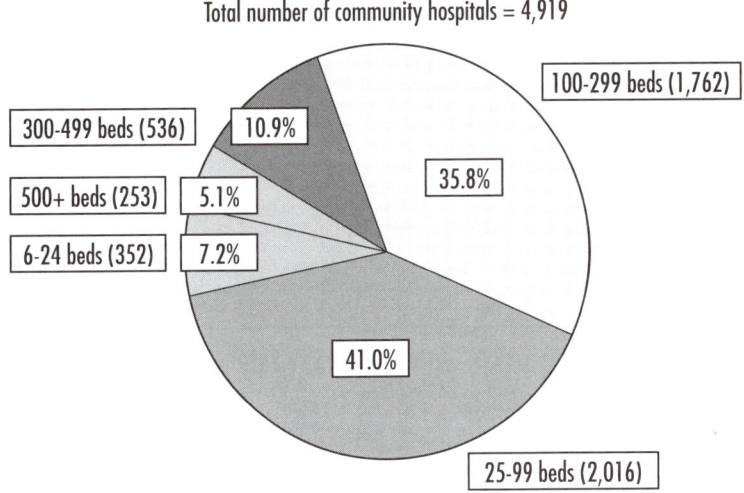

Total number of community hospitals = 4,919

300-499 beds (536) 10.9%

500+ beds (253) 5.1%

6-24 beds (352) 7.2%

100-299 beds (1,762)

35.8%

41.0%

25-99 beds (2,016)

Source: Data from *Health United States, 2006*, p. 364, National Center for Health Statistics, US Department of Health and Human Services.

urban hospital has 231 beds (Anonymous 2002).

Average Daily Census

The average number of beds occupied each day in a hospital is referred to as *average daily census*. Hence, it is one of the common measures used to define occupancy of inpatient beds in a hospital. The total inpatient days during a given period (days of care) are divided by the number of days in that period to arrive at the average daily census. For example, if the number of total inpatient days for July is 3,131, then the average daily census for July is 101 (3,131/31).

Occupancy Rate

The *occupancy rate* for a given period is derived by dividing the average daily census for that period by the number of available beds (capacity). The fraction is expressed as a percentage (percent of beds occupied). It indicates the proportion of a hospital's total inpatient capacity that is actually utilized. Occupancy rate is also commonly used for other types of inpatient facilities, such as nursing homes, and is often used as a measure of performance. Figure 1–7 shows the change in aggregate occupancy rates for US community hospitals from 1960 to 2004. Since hospitals are able to increase or decrease capacity (number of beds that are set up and staffed), trends in occupancy over time may not indicate much. However, individual hospitals can compare their own occupancy rates against the industry. In a competitive environment, facilities with higher occupancy rates are considered more successful than those with lower occupancy rates.

Figure 1–7   Change in Occupancy Rates (percent of beds occupied) in Community Hospitals, 1960–2004 (selected years).

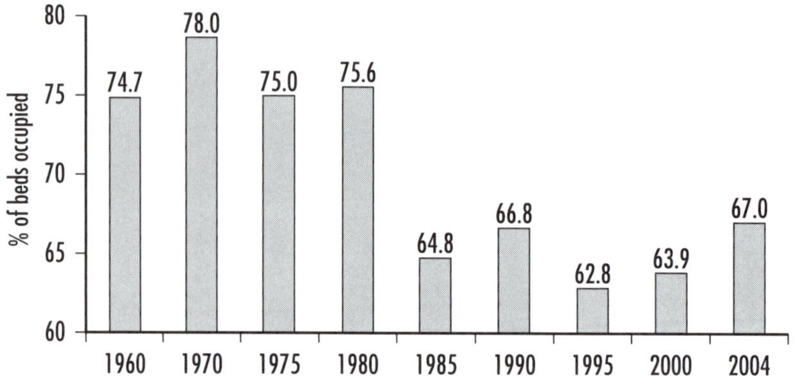

Source: Data from *Health United States, 1995,* p. 231; *Health United States, 1996–7,* p. 243, *Health United States, 2006,* p. 364, National Center for Health Statistics.

Hospital Employment

Employment in hospitals declined by 2.3 percent, to about 4 million workers over the 1983 to 1986 period. Staff cuts, hiring freezes, and the increased use of contract services were part of a belt-tightening effort in response to declining inpatient admissions (Kahl and Clark 1986). But, as hospitals chased more liberal reimbursement in outpatient markets, employment in hospitals in 1989 rose to 4.3 million workers, an increase of 6.9 percent from 1986 (Anderson and Wootton 1991). This trend has continued as hospitals have been employing an increasing number of personnel. In 2003, America's hospitals employed the full-time equivalent of 4.7 million people (Iglehart 2006). Hospital employment constitutes roughly 4 percent of all service-providing jobs in the United States.

Staffing ratios per occupied bed increased substantially between 1995 and 2000, but have moderated since then. Table 1–3 pre-

Table 1–3 Full-Time Equivalent (FTE) Staffing Per Occupied Bed

	Multihospital Systems			Independent Hospitals		
	1995	2000	2005	1995	2000	2005
Staff and resident physicians	0.48	0.63	0.54	0.75	0.92	0.65
RNs and LPNs	2.19	2.54	2.45	2.30	3.07	3.16
Ratio of RN to LPN	4.6	4.5	4.6	3.0	2.9	3.1
Other personnel	5.09	5.89	5.75	5.54	8.00	8.04
Total staff	7.76	9.06	8.74	8.59	11.99	11.85

Sources: Data from *Managed Care Digest Series: Institutional Digest,* 1998, Hoechst Marion Roussel; SMG Marketing-Verispan LLC, 2002, available at www.managedcaredigest.com; Hospitals/Systems Digest, © 2007, Sanofi-Aventis.

sents full-time equivalent staffing data per occupied bed by selected staff categories for facilities affiliated with multihospital systems (a chain of two or more hospitals) and for independent facilities. Compared to other developed nations, American hospitals are much more heavily staffed. Paradoxically, despite more resource-intensive treatments given to patients in US hospitals, quality outcomes are not appreciably greater (Reinhardt 2002).

Types of Hospitals

Instead of a centralized system of hospitals under state ownership, the United States has a variety of institutional forms, with both private and government-owned institutions under independent management. Most hospitals are voluntary, nonprofit, short-stay, general hospitals. State and local government-owned hospitals are next in predominance. Then come the for-profit (investor-owned) hospitals and, finally, federal hospitals. Figure 1–8 shows the distribution of hospitals, and Figure 1–9 shows the distribution of beds among various hospital types.

The endless variations in hospital characteristics defy any simple classification. The following classification arrangements have been commonly used to differentiate between the various types of hospitals. It is important to keep in mind, however, that these classifications are not mutually exclusive.

Figure 1–8   Proportion of Total US Hospitals by Type of Hospital, 2004.

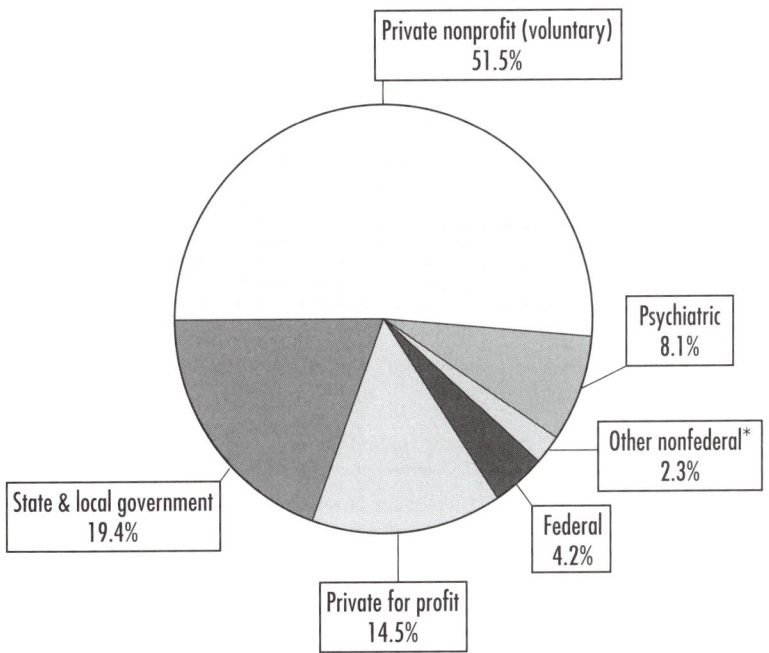

* Mainly nonfederal long-term hospitals.

Source: Data from *Statistical Abstract of the United States, 2007*, p.114, US Census Bureau.

Figure 1–9   Proportion of Total US Hospital Beds by Type of Hospital, 2004.

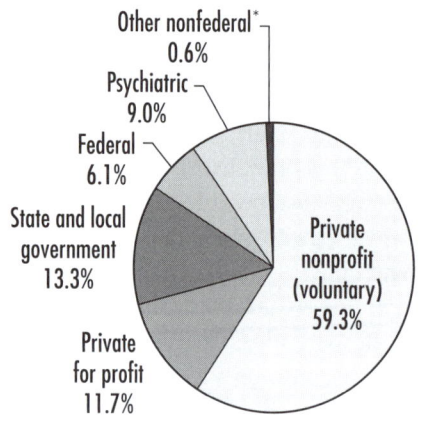

*Mainly nonfederal long-term hospitals

Source: Data from *Statistical Abstract of the United States, 2007*, p. 114. US Census Bureau.

Classification by Ownership

Public Hospitals

Generally speaking, public hospitals were the first to appear when almshouses and pesthouses evolved into hospitals providing medical services. **Public hospitals** are owned by agencies of federal, state, or local governments. It should be noted that in health care the word "public" does not carry its ordinary meaning. A public hospital, for instance, is not necessarily a hospital that is open to the general public. In business, a public corporation is one whose stock is publicly traded to attract private investors. In health care, particularly in the United States, the word "public" connotes government ownership.

Federal hospitals are maintained primarily for special groups of federal beneficiaries, such as Native Americans, military personnel, and veterans. As a general rule, federal hospitals do not serve the common public. Veterans Affairs (VA) hospitals constitute the largest group among federal hospitals.

State governments have generally limited themselves to the operation of mental and tuberculosis hospitals, reflecting government's early role in protecting communities by isolating the mentally ill and persons with contagious diseases. During the past several years, the number of state psychiatric hospitals has decreased considerably because of policies favoring deinstitutionalization of mentally ill patients, not only in the United States but also in Europe, Canada, and Australia.

Local governments, such as counties and cities, operate hospitals that are open to the general public. Many of these hospitals are located in large urban areas where they serve mainly the inner city indigent and disadvantaged populations. Medicare, Medicaid, and state and local tax dollars pay for almost 80 percent of the services these hospitals provide (Safety net in shreds 2002). Because of increasing financial pressures, many public hospitals had to privatize or close. Between 1980 and 2004, the number of state and local government-owned community hospitals declined by 37 percent, from 1,778 in 1980 to 1,117 in 2004. Most hospitals operated by city and county governments are small to moderate size. Some large public hospitals are affiliated with medical schools; they play a significant role in training physicians and other health care professionals.

Compared to voluntary and proprietary hospitals, public hospitals incur higher utilization, at least in terms of ALOS (see Figure 1–4). ALOS is the highest in federal hospitals (11.6 days), and veterans are the biggest users of these hospitals. At present, about 43 percent of the veteran population is over 65 (compared to 13 percent of the general US population) and it is aging rapidly. The proportion of veterans over the age of 65 is expected to rise to 51 percent by 2010 (Zeber et al. 2004).

Voluntary Hospitals

Voluntary hospitals are nongovernmental, and therefore, privately-owned hospitals that are operated on a nonprofit basis. They are owned and operated by community associations or other nongovernment organizations. These hospitals are called voluntary because the development and financial backing of the institutions is done voluntarily by citizens without government involvement (Raffel and Raffel 1994, 130). Their primary mission is to benefit the community in which they are located. Their operating expenses are covered from patient fees, third-party reimbursement, donations, and endowments. The private nonprofit sector constitutes the largest group of hospitals (Figure 1–8). In 2004, the private nonprofit sector accounted for over 51 percent of all hospitals and almost 60 percent of all beds with an average capacity of 191 beds per hospital (DHHS 2006, 364).

Proprietary Hospitals

For-profit *proprietary hospitals*—also referred to as *investor-owned hospitals*—are owned by individuals, partnerships, or corporations. They are operated for the financial benefit of the entity that owns the institution, that is, the stockholders. At the beginning of the 20th century, more than half of the nation's hospitals were proprietary. Most of these hospitals were small and were established by physicians who wanted a place to hospitalize their own patients (Stewart 1973). Later, most of these institutions were closed or acquired by community or-

ganizations or hospital corporations because of population shifts, increased costs, and the necessities of modern clinical practice (Raffel and Raffel 1994, 133). Even though the nonprofit hospital sector has maintained its market dominance, during the past decade, the for-profit sector has gained market share (Table 1–4). However, compared to other types of ownership, proprietary hospitals continue to have the lowest occupancy rates (60.5 percent in 2004 compared to 67 percent for all community hospitals) [DHHS 2006, 364].

Classification by Multiunit Affiliation

Hospitals are part of a multihospital chain (sometimes referred to as a multihospital system—MHS) when two or more hospitals are owned, leased, sponsored, or contractually managed by a central organization (AHA 1994). In recent years, MHSs have gained a

Table 1–4 Changes in Number of Community Hospitals, Beds, Average Size, and Occupancy Rates

	1995	2004	Change
Nonprofit Sector			
Number of hospitals	3,092	2,967	−4.0%
Number of beds	609,729	567,863	−6.9%
Average size	197	191	−2.9%
Occupancy rate	64.5%	68.3%	5.9%
For-Profit Sector			
Number of hospitals	752	835	11.0%
Number of beds	105,737	112,693	6.6%
Average size	141	135	−4.0%
Occupancy rate	51.8%	60.5%	16.8%

Source: Data from *Health, United States, 2006*, p. 364, National Center for Health Statistics.

larger share of all hospitals by acquiring facilities confronting financial problems. Acquired hospitals are more likely to be located in markets with higher numbers of health maintenance organizations (HMOs). They also tend to have lower occupancy rates and older facilities (Harrison et al. 2003). Table 1–5 lists the largest of the multihospital chains according to size. MHSs accounted for 49 percent of all hospitals nationwide in 2005, up from 46 percent five years earlier

(Sanofi-Aventis 2007). Despite inroads made by investor-owned groups into MHSs, most such systems are operated by nonprofit corporations (Table 1–6). Some of the advantages of multihospital chain affiliation include economies of scale with administrative overhead, the ability to provide a wide spectrum of care, ability to reach a variety of markets, increased access to capital markets, and access to management resources and expertise.

Table 1–5 The Largest US Multihospital Chains, 2004 (ranked by Staffed Beds)

Name of Hospital System (Location)	Number of Owned Hospitals	Number of Staffed Beds	Average Occupancy %	ALOS
Nonprofit Chains				
Ascension Health (St. Louis, MO)	44	9,966	57.8%	4.8
Catholic Health Initiatives (Denver, CO)	60	9,964	50.2%	4.8
Catholic Healthcare West (San Francisco, CA)	36	8,953	57.6%	5.1
Kaiser Permanente (Oakland, CA)	31	7,234	64.1%	4.1
Catholic Health East (Newtown, PA)	22	7,036	61.2%	5.3
Trinity Health (Novi, MI)	25	5,690	60.4%	4.4
Adventist Health System (Winter Park, FL)	27	5,463	57.3%	4.6
Christus Health (Irving, TX)	22	4,973	61.7%	5.9
Catholic Healthcare Partners (Cincinnati, OH)	21	3,753	63.5%	5.6
SSM Health Care System (St. Louis, MO)	14	3,192	62.1%	4.7
For-Profit Chains				
HCA (Nashville, TN)	171	35,335	58.5%	4.7
Tenet Health System (Dallas, TX)	71	16,182	60.7%	5.2
Community Health Systems (Brentwood, TN)	69	7,292	46.6%	4.8
Health Mgmt. Associates (Naples, FL)	51	6,972	53.1%	4.5
Universal Health Services (King of Prussia, PA)	22	4,157	65.1%	4.9
State and Local Government-Owned Chains				
New York City Health and Hospitals Corporation (New York, NY)	11	4,746	86.7%	6.6
Los Angeles County Department of Health Services (Los Angeles, CA)	5	3,054	47.3%	7.6
University of California (Oakland, CA)	6	2,493	55.1%	5.6
University of Texas Systems (Austin, TX)	3	1,336	71.5%	6.8
North Broward Hospital District (Fort Lauderdale, FL)	4	1,294	69.8%	5.3

Source: Data from *Managed Care Digest Series: Hospital/Systems Digest,* Sanofi-Aventis, 2006, Bridgewater, NJ: Sanofi-Aventis.

Table 1–6 Multihospital Health Care Systems: Number of Hospitals and Beds, 2005
(Includes owned, leased, sponsored and contract-managed hospitals)

Type of Control	Number of Systems	Hospitals	Beds	% Beds*
Catholic church related	42	555	108,538	18.6
Other church related	13	108	21,699	3.7
Total church related	**55**	**663**	**130,237**	**22.3**
Other nonprofit	244	1,210	262,051	44.8
Total nonprofit	**299**	**1,873**	**392,288**	**67.1**
Investor owned	65	1,241	146,541	25.1
Federal government owned	5	223	46,095	7.9
Total	**369**	**3,337**	**584,924**	**100.0**

*As a percentage of all systems

Source: Data from *AHA Hospital Statistics, 2007*, p. 197, © Health Forum.

The VA operates the single largest hospital system in the country, with 163 medical centers, owned by the federal government. In fiscal year 2000, the Veterans' Health System treated 3.3 million veterans and had over 600,000 hospital discharges. The overall ALOS for a veteran admitted to the hospital was 12.5 days (Pfizer Inc. 2003).

Classification by Length of Stay

A ***short-stay hospital*** is one in which the average length of stay is less than 25 days; that is, most hospitals. Patients admitted to these hospitals suffer from acute conditions. Hospitals with average stays of more than 25 days are long-stay hospitals. These include state-run as well as private psychiatric hospitals, long-term care hospitals (LTCHs) providing subacute care, tuberculosis hospitals, and chronic disease hospitals.

A ***long-term care hospital*** (LTCH) is a special type of long-stay hospital described in section 1886(d)(1)(B)(iv) of the Social Security Act. LTCHs must meet Medicare's conditions of participation for acute (short-stay) hospitals, and must have an ALOS greater than 25 days. LTCHs serve patients who have complex medical needs and may suffer from multiple chronic problems requiring long-term hospitalization. Many LTCH patients are admitted directly from short-stay hospital intensive care units with respiratory/ventilator-dependent or other complex medical conditions. The number of LTCHs has grown rapidly from 105 facilities in 1993 to 318 in 2003 (MedPAC 2004). The demand for other types of long-stay hospitals has generally declined over the years. The number of tuberculosis hospitals, for example, has declined from 103 in 1970 to 4 (US Census Bureau 2007, 114), mainly because the disease has been largely eradicated or controlled with modern drugs.

Classification by Type of Service

General Hospitals

A ***general hospital*** provides a variety of services, including general and specialized medicine, general and specialized surgery, and obstetrics, to meet the general medical needs of the community it serves. It provides diagnostic, treatment, and surgical services for patients with a variety of medical conditions. Most hospitals in the United States are general hospitals.

It is important to note that the term "general hospital" does not imply that these hospitals are less specialized or that their care is inferior to that of specialty hospitals. The difference lies in the nature of services, not their quality. General hospitals provide a broader range of services for a larger variety of conditions; whereas specialty hospitals provide a narrow range of services for specific medical conditions or patient populations.

Specialty Hospitals

According to the North American Industry Classification System of the US Census Bureau, *specialty hospitals* are establishments that primarily engage in providing diagnostic and medical treatment to inpatients with a specific type of disease or medical condition, except services for psychiatric care or substance abuse. Specialty hospitals forge a distinct service niche. Traditionally, the two most common specialty hospitals have been rehabilitation hospitals and children's hospitals. With increasing competition, however, other types of specialty hospitals have emerged to provide treatments that are also available in many general hospitals. Examples include orthopedic hospitals, cardiac hospitals, cancer (oncology) hospitals, and women's hospitals. Physicians find such specialized hospitals more efficient, and in many instances, physicians are full or part owners of these hospitals. Affiliation with such hospitals gives physicians control over hospital operations, flexibility with their time, and opportunity to enhance their incomes. However, physician-owned facilities raise legal and ethical issues with regard to self-referrals without full disclosure. Stark Laws that prohibit self-referrals do not apply when physicians self refer to a "whole hospital." Under this exception, physicians may refer patients to a facility if their ownership interest is in the whole hospital, rather than a smaller entity (Guterman 2006). Also, in 2003, Congress amended the Stark Laws to impose an 18-month moratorium during which physician-investors in new specialty hospitals could not refer Medicare patients to those hospitals (Zimmerman 2006). Although, the moratorium had effectively stifled the development of new specialty hospitals, the development boom has reignited as the moratorium ended in 2006. Currently, the Centers for Medicare and Medicaid Services (CMS) has proposed changes in hospital reimbursement with the intent of making private investments in specialty hospitals less lucrative.

Another issue, emergency care, is at the heart of the controversy between specialty hospitals and community general hospitals. Administrators of general hospitals argue that specialty hospitals are cream-skimming insured patients and leaving costly emergency and uncompensated cases to general hospitals (Snyder 2003). Recent studies also suggest that compared to community hospitals, physician-owned specialty hospitals seem to treat less complex and more profitable cases (Guterman 2006).

Psychiatric Hospitals

The primary function of a psychiatric inpatient facility is to provide diagnostic and treatment services for patients who have psychiatric-related illnesses. Specifically, such an institution must have facilities to provide psychiatric, psychological, and social work services. A psychiatric hospital must also have a written agreement with a general hospital for the transfer of patients who may require medical, obstetrics, or surgical services (Health Forum 2001, A3).

Historically, state governments have taken the primary responsibility for establishing facilities for the care of the mentally ill. Trends during the 1970s and 1980s resulted in significant deinstitutionalization of the inpatient population that resided in state mental hospitals. As a result, the responsibility for much psychiatric care shifted to psychiatric units in general hospitals, private psychiatric hospitals, other types of residential facilities, and community care programs (Mechanic 1998). However, state mental institutions continue to provide long-term treatment to people with severe and persistent mental illness (Patrick et al. 2006). In 2004, the United States had 466 psychiatric hospitals (US Census Bureau 2007, 114).

Rehabilitation Hospitals

Rehabilitation hospitals specialize in therapeutic services to restore the maximum level of functioning in patients who have suffered recent disability due to an episode of illness or an accident. These hospitals serve patients who generally cannot be cured but whose functioning can be improved. According to Medicare rules, to be classified as a rehabilitation hospital, 75 percent of a hospital's inpatients must require intensive rehabilitation services for the treatment of stroke, spinal cord injury, major multiple trauma, brain injury, and other specific conditions (Grimaldi 2002). Rehabilitation hospitals also serve amputees and victims of accident or sports injuries. Patients often transfer to these facilities after orthopedic surgery in a general hospital. Facilities and

staff are available to provide physical therapy, occupational therapy, and speech and language pathology. Most rehabilitation hospitals have special arrangements for psychological, social work, and vocational services, and are required to have written arrangements with a general hospital for the transfer of patients who need medical, obstetrical, or surgical care not available at the institution (Health Forum 2001, A3).

Children's Hospitals

Children's hospitals are community hospitals that typically have specialized facilities to deal mainly with complex, severe, or chronic illnesses among children. Nearly all children's hospitals provide neonatal intensive care units, pediatric intensive care units, trauma centers, and transplant services. Thus, these hospitals provide a wide range of high-intensity services for children, such as pediatric surgery, cardiology, orthopedic surgery, cancer treatment, HIV/AIDS treatment, and rehabilitation services (DelliFraine 2006).

There are 45 freestanding children's hospitals in the United States. They have an average capacity of 124 beds. All of these hospitals are nonprofit, and are located in major metropolitan areas. Many are affiliated with medical schools and academic medical centers. However, many large communities do not have specialty children's hospitals. In these communities, general acute-care hospitals serve as de facto children's hospitals by providing the same services and treating the same types of patients (DelliFraine 2006).

Classification by Public Access

Most people are familiar with the community hospital. A *community hospital* is a nonfederal short-stay hospital whose facilities and services are available to the general public. Its primary mission is to serve the general community. These hospitals are not restricted to serving a certain category of people. A community hospital may be proprietary, voluntary, or owned by the state or local government (but not by the federal government). It may be a general hospital or a specialty hospital. Generally speaking, the larger the community served, the larger the hospital, range of specialties, and range of supporting equipment and services (Raffel and Raffel 1994, 131). Noncommunity hospitals include hospitals operated by the federal government, such as VA hospitals to serve veterans; hospital units of institutions, such as prisons and infirmaries in colleges and universities; and long-stay hospitals.

In 2004, of the 5,759 US hospitals, 4,919 (over 85 percent) were community hospitals (DHHS 2006, 364). Figure 8–10 shows the breakdown of community hospitals by ownership type.

Classification by Location

Based on location, hospitals can be classified as urban or rural. ***Urban hospitals*** are located in a county that is part of a metropolitan statistical area (MSA). The US Bureau of Census has defined an MSA as a geographical area that includes at least (1) one city with a population of 50,000 or more or (2) an urbanized area of at least 50,000 inhabitants and a total MSA population of at least 100,000. ***Rural hospitals*** are located in a county that is not part of an MSA. It is estimated that rural hospitals deliver health care to 54 million Americans, including 9 million Medicare beneficiaries (Slusky 2006).

From an operational standpoint, compared to rural hospitals, urban hospitals have higher costs because they typically pay higher salaries in more competitive markets, offer a broader scope of more sophisticated services, and generally treat patients requiring more complex care. Urban hospitals are located either in inner cities or in the suburbs. Because suburbs of metropolitan areas are generally more affluent than inner cities or rural areas, both inner city urban hospitals and rural hospitals treat a patient mix that is disproportionately poor and elderly compared to suburban hospital patients (HCIA Inc. and Deloitte & Touche 1997, 64). Because of the disproportionate numbers of the elderly and poor in rural areas, rural community hospitals often find themselves in financial trouble. Conversion to a facility that provides nonacute health care services, such as a primary care clinic, a long-term care facility, or a specialty hospital, is sometimes a viable alternative when these hospitals are threatened with closure.

Figure 1–10   Breakdown of Community Hospitals by Types of Ownership, 2004.

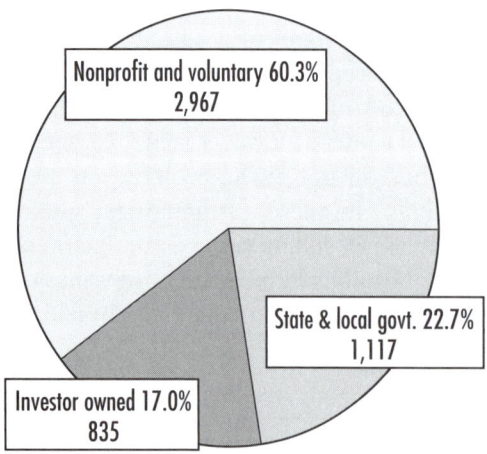

Source: Data from *Health United States, 2006*, p. 364, National Center for Health Statistics.

For example, adoption of long-term care strategies has demonstrated to improve profitability of rural hospitals (Stuart et al. 2006).

The plight of rural hospitals was discussed earlier. To save some of the very small rural hospitals, the Balanced Budget Act of 1997 created the Medicare Rural Hospital Flexibility Program (MRHFP). Under this program, certain rural hospitals can be classified as *Critical Access Hospitals* (CAH) if they have no more than 25 acute care beds and if they provide emergency medical services. Although CAH status is not necessarily the best alternative for all small rural hospitals, the number of such hospitals jumped from 850 in 2003 to 1,050 at the end of 2004 (Mantone 2005). If a hospital elects CAH status, and meets the criteria for CAH designation, it can receive cost-plus reimbursement under Medicare Part A. Since cost-plus reimbursement allows inclusion of capital costs, these hospitals have now access to capital for new construction and renovations. The CAH program has provided the financial stability that many small rural hospitals need.

Classification by Size

There is no standard way to classify hospitals by size. According to one classification scheme, hospitals with fewer than 100 beds would be classified as small, those with 100 to 500 beds as medium, and those with 500-plus beds as large. Others may classify by size a little differently. Just a little over half (52 percent) of all hospitals in the United States have 100 beds or more (US Census Bureau 2007, 114).

Figure 1–11 illustrates expenses per inpatient day by hospital size. Experience in the manufacturing and retail sectors of the

Figure 1–11　Expenses per Inpatient Day by Hospital Size, Community Hospitals, 2004.

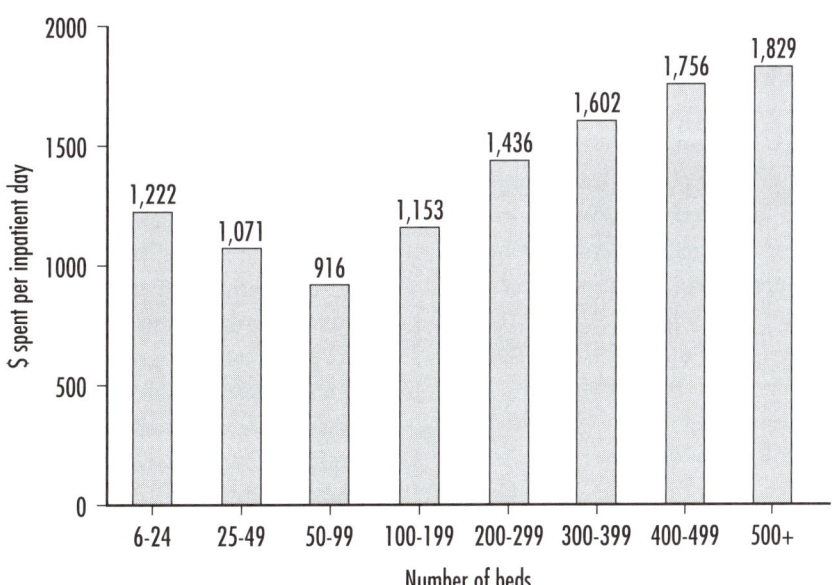

Source: Data from *Health United States, 2006,* p. 392, National Center for Health Statistics.

economy suggests that large enterprises should realize economies of scale. The reason is that certain overhead costs are fixed or semi-fixed—they do not increase proportionally as the size of the enterprise increases. Examples are administrative costs and plant maintenance costs. In the hospital industry, economies of scale seem to evaporate when the size exceeds 100 beds or so. Higher costs in larger hospitals are mainly attributable to a more extensive array of specialized and resource-intensive services that these hospitals must be equipped to provide. Such services require sophisticated technology and personnel with advanced training. Large teaching hospitals incur the additional costs of residency training and medical research.

Other Types of Hospitals

Teaching Hospitals

To be designated as a ***teaching hospital***, a hospital must have one or more graduate residency programs approved by the American Medical Association (AMA). The mere presence of nursing programs or training affiliations for other health professionals, such as therapists and dietitians, does not make an institution a teaching hospital.

The term ***academic medical center*** is commonly used when a hospital or health system is organized around a medical school. Apart from the training of physicians, research activities and clinical investigations become an important undertaking.

Among the largest and most prestigious teaching hospitals are the members of the Council of Teaching Hospitals and Health Systems (COTH). They usually have substantial teaching and research programs and are affiliated with medical schools of large

universities. The approximately 400 COTH member institutions train about three-quarters of the physician residents in the United States (AAMC 2003).

Three main traits separate teaching and nonteaching hospitals. First, teaching hospitals provide medical training to physicians, research opportunities to health services researchers, and specialized care to patients. They incur certain costs directly associated with medical education programs, the largest category being the salary and benefits expense for interns and residents. Medicare reimburses the additional costs of graduate medical education in teaching hospitals separately, in addition to the prospective DRG rates (Dalton 1995). Secondly, teaching hospitals have a broader and more complex scope of services than nonteaching hospitals. Teaching hospitals often operate several intensive care units, possess the latest medical technologies, and attract a diverse group of physicians representing most specialties and many subspecialties. Major teaching hospitals also offer many unique tertiary care services not generally found in other institutions, such as burn care, trauma care, and organ transplantation. Because more specialized services are available, teaching hospitals attract patients who frequently have more complicated diagnoses or need more complex procedures. Because of the greater case-mix complexity of teaching hospitals, greater resources are required for treatment. Third, many of the major teaching hospitals are located in economically depressed, older inner city areas, and are generally owned by state or local governments. Consequently, these hospitals often provide disproportional amounts of uncompensated care to uninsured patients (HCIA Inc. and Deloitte & Touche 1997, 66).

Church-Affiliated Hospitals

Various churches established hospitals mainly during the latter half of the 19th and the early 20th centuries. The first church-sponsored hospitals in the United States were established by various Catholic sisterhoods. Later, protestant denominations organized hospitals in accord with their missions of service, and Jewish philanthropic organizations opened hospitals so that Jewish patients could observe their dietary laws more faithfully and Jewish physicians could more easily find sites for training and work opportunities (Raffel 1980, 241).

Church-affiliated hospitals are often community general hospitals. They may be large or small, teaching or nonteaching. Affiliation with a medical school may also vary. They are different only in that they are owned or heavily influenced by the church groups that sponsor them. Church hospitals do not discriminate in rendering care; however, they are generally sensitive to the sponsoring denomination's special spiritual and/or dietary emphasis (Raffel and Raffel 1994, 131–132).

Osteopathic Hospitals

For all practical purposes, osteopathic hospitals are community general hospitals. In 1970, osteopathic hospitals became eligible to apply for registration with the AHA (AHA 1994). Approximately 200 osteopathic hospitals operate in the United States.

Osteopathic medicine represents an approach to medical practice employing all the methods traditionally associated with allopathic medicine, such as pharmaceuticals, laboratory tests, X-ray diagnostics, and surgery. ***Osteopathic medicine***, however, takes a holistic approach and goes a step further in advocating treatment that involves correction of the position of the joints or tissues, and in emphasizing diet and environment as factors that might influence natural resistance. For many years after osteopathy was established as a separate branch of medicine in 1874, osteopaths had to develop their own hospitals because of antagonism from the established allopathic medical practitioners. Both groups have now inspected each other's medical schools and satisfied themselves that each is worth associating with, and that each could serve on the other's faculties and practice side by side in the same hospitals (Raffel and Raffel 1994, 45).

Due to the emphasis on preventive care and less invasive solutions to medical problems, one would expect that osteopathic hospitals would deliver cost-efficient care. However, results of one study show that osteopathic hospitals are more costly and less productive in comparison to their counterparts. Inefficient production of outpatient services and high cost of medical education are two reasons for their poor performance (Sinay 2005).

What Makes a Hospital Nonprofit?

Laypeople make a common assumption that nonprofit (sometimes called not-for-profit) health care corporations are driven by the mission to meet the health care needs of patients regardless of their ability to pay. It is further assumed that these corporations do not make a profit. The fact is that every corporation, regardless of whether it is for profit or nonprofit, has to make a profit (surplus of revenues over expenses) to survive over the long term. No business can survive for long if it continually spends more than it takes in. That is true for both the nonprofit and the for-profit sectors (Nudelman and Andrews 1996).

The Internal Revenue Code, Section 501(c)(3), grants tax-exempt status to nonprofit organizations. As such, these institutions are exempt from federal, state, and local taxes, such as income taxes, sales taxes, and property taxes. In general, these organizations must (1) provide some defined public good, such as service, education, or community welfare, and (2) not distribute any profits to any individuals. A major goal for a for-profit corporation, on the other hand, is to provide its shareholders with a return on their investment, but it achieves this goal primarily by excelling at its basic mission. For any health services provider the basic mission is to deliver the highest quality care at the most reasonable price possible.

Community hospitals owned by various groups, such as local citizens, fraternal orders, churches, and the government, have traditionally been classified as nonprofit. Among all private (non-government) hospitals in the United States, nearly 80 percent (84 percent of beds) are nonprofit. These hospitals receive substantial tax subsidies. Current rules for tax-exempt hospitals require them to provide charity care as well as community benefits. The latter broadly refer to services that the government would otherwise have to undertake (Owens 2005). Also, Section 4958 of the IRS code prohibits executive compensation that may be deemed unreasonable for tax-exempt organizations. Under current scrutiny, nonprofit hospitals have to be prepared to demonstrate not only that they are paying salaries within some reasonable range of industry standards, but also that executives are bringing measurable value in key areas of operations, including community

benefits (Appleby 2004). Hence, it is recommended that some portion of hospital chief executive officers' salaries should directly hinge on his or her performance in two critical areas: (1) organizational effectiveness (financial performance, market share, quality, daily operations, and achievement of strategic objectives), and (2) community health (charitable care, health promotion and education, and overall state of the community's health) (Newman et al. 2001).

The problem is that nonprofit hospitals, in many instances, compete head-on with for-profit hospitals. For example, nonprofit hospitals frequently engage in the same kinds of aggressive marketplace behaviors that for-profit hospitals pursue. Institutional theory actually predicts such behavior. When for-profit and nonprofit organizations face similar regulatory, legal, and professional constraints, they will imitate each other, according to institutional theory (O'Connell and Brown 2003). In the hospital industry, competition commonly occurs in the same communities, for the same patients, with revenues coming from the same public and private third-party sources, and often involving the same physician providers who have admitting privileges at more than one hospital.

The empirical evidence indicates that, in general, for-profit and nonprofit hospitals provide similar levels of charity and uncompensated care (Thorpe et al. 2000). Their quality of care and the adoption of new technology are also similar (Sloan 1998). Generally, conversion of nonprofit to for-profit status does not adversely affect the provision of uncompensated care. However, some reduction in uncompensated care may occur particularly when public hospitals are acquired by for-profit owners (Thorpe et al. 2000).

Whether nonprofit hospitals are indeed charitable institutions remains controversial, and there is continued scrutiny of nonprofit hospitals by Congress to determine whether nonprofit hospitals provide sufficient services to warrant their exemption from taxes. The Internal Revenue Service now monitors how well nonprofit hospitals are complying with federal law that requires them to provide social benefits, such as free or low-cost health care for the poor. The viability of nonprofit hospitals will continue to be challenged until they produce decisive evidence of tangible value to their communities beyond that produced by their for-profit counterparts. Nonprofit hospitals could play a unique role if they can refocus on maintaining the delicate balance between market justice and social justice orientations. This balance will be jeopardized if nonprofit organizations continue to emulate profit-seeking, investor-owned providers.

Many nonprofit hospitals are in fact engaged in various community outreach programs that directly or indirectly impact the health of their communities. Many hospitals across the nation are engaged in community health assessments, educational activities, support groups, and wellness programs. Some outreach activities even go beyond the hospital's core competencies of delivering health care, extending into improving the social and economic environments or influencing lifestyle behaviors to promote better health and well-being. For example, St. Bernard Hospital and Health Care Center in Chicago has been involved in developing an affordable housing project in its economically depressed neighborhood (Robbins 2002).

The question can arise as to whether nonprofit hospitals merely have a legal obligation to provide community benefits or whether the hospitals could also derive tangible benefits by providing community benefits which cost the hospitals money. A study

of a sample of nonprofit hospitals in Massachusetts found a significant positive association between corporate citizenship, such as providing unmet health needs in the community, and financial performance of the hospitals (Longest and Lin 2005).

Some Management Concepts

From a management standpoint, hospitals are complex organizations. Compared to other business enterprises of similar size, both external and internal environments of hospitals are more complex. A hospital is generally responsible to numerous stakeholders in its external environment. These stakeholders include the community, the government, insurers, managed care organizations, and accreditation agencies. Internally, hospital governance involves three major sources of power whose motivations are sometimes at odds. A hospital's organizational structure (Figure 1–12) also differs substantially from that of other large organizations. The CEO receives delegated authority from the board and is responsible for managing the organization with the help of senior managers. In large hospitals, these senior managers often carry the title of senior vice president or vice president for various key service areas, such as nursing services, restorative (rehabilitation) services, human resources, finance, and so forth. The medical staff constitute a separate organizational structure parallel to the administrative structure. Such a dual structure is rarely seen in other businesses and presents numerous opportunities for conflict between the CEO and the medical staff. Matters are further complicated when the lines of authority cross between the two structures. For example, nursing service, pharmacists,

Figure 1–12 Hospitals Governance and Operational Structures.

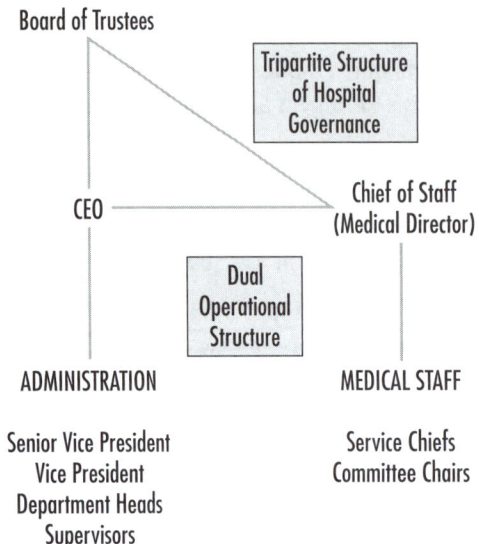

Board of Trustees

Tripartite Structure of Hospital Governance

CEO

Chief of Staff (Medical Director)

Dual Operational Structure

ADMINISTRATION

MEDICAL STAFF

Senior Vice President
Vice President
Department Heads
Supervisors

Service Chiefs
Committee Chairs

diagnostic technicians, and dietitians are administratively accountable to the CEO (via the vertical chain of command) but professionally accountable to the medical staff (Raffel and Raffel 1994, 139). The medical staff generally are not paid employees of the hospital, yet they play a significant role in its success. It requires special skills on the part of the CEO to manage this dual structure to achieve the organization's overall objectives.

Hospital Governance

Hospital governance has traditionally followed a tripartite structure. The three major sources of authority are the CEO, the board of trustees, and the chief of staff (medical director), as illustrated in Figure 1–12. In earlier periods, when physicians operated their own hospitals, the hospitals were dominated by the trustees. Trustees were often the source of capital investment, and their influence in the community brought prestige to the hospital. Later, as voluntary hospitals increased

in number, the balance of power shifted into the hands of physicians because they played a critical role in bringing patients to the hospitals. Changes in the health care environment over the last two decades have made the management of hospitals more complex; administrators now wield considerable power.

Board of Trustees

The **board of trustees** (also referred to as the governing body or board of directors) consists of influential business and community leaders. The board is legally responsible for the operations of the hospital. It is also responsible for defining the hospital's mission and long-term direction. It also sets policy guidelines that establish the overall framework for day-to-day operations. It approves long-range plans and annual budgets, and monitors performance against plans and budgets (Griffith 1995). The CEO is generally a member of the board. One or more physicians also sit on the board as voting members. One of the most important responsibilities of the board is to appoint and evaluate the performance of the CEO, who is charged with providing the board timely reports on the institution's progress in achieving its mission and objectives. The board has the power to remove the CEO. In most hospitals, the board also approves the appointment of physicians and other professionals to the hospital's medical staff.

Boards often function through committees. Standing committees usually include executive, medical staff, human resources, finance, planning, quality improvement, and ethics. Special, or ad hoc, committees are established as needed. The two most important committees from a governance standpoint are the executive committee and the medical staff committee. The **executive committee** has continuing monitoring responsibility and authority over the hospital. Usually, it receives reports from other committees, monitors policy implementation, and makes recommendations. The *medical staff committee* is charged with medical staff relations. For example, it reviews admitting privileges and the performance of the medical staff. There is also increased emphasis on the legal and ethical obligations of the hospital regarding patient safety, quality improvement, and patient satisfaction.

Chief Executive Officer

Formerly, the titles of "superintendent" and later "administrator" were commonly used for a hospital's chief executive. Now, "chief executive officer" and "president" are the common titles used. The CEO's job is to accomplish the organization's mission and objectives through leadership within the organization. He or she has the ultimate responsibility for day-to-day operations.

Medical Staff

The hospital's medical staff is an organized body of physicians who provide medical services to the hospital's patients and perform related clinical duties. The physicians, in most hospitals, are in private practice outside the hospital. The hospital grants them admitting privileges that enable them to admit and care for their patients in the hospital. Other clinicians, such as dentists and podiatrists, may also be granted admitting privileges. Appointment to the medical staff is a formal process outlined in the hospital's medical staff bylaws. The medical staff use a framework of self-governance, which represents the strong tradition of physician independence. The medical staff are formally accountable to the board. Lines of communication to the CEO and the board of trustees

are established through various committee representations.

A medical director or *chief of staff* heads the medical staff. In all but the smallest hospitals, medical staff are organizationally divided by major specialties into departments, such as anesthesiology, internal medicine, obstetrics and gynecology, orthopedic surgery, pathology, cardiology, and radiology. A *chief of service*, such as chief of cardiology, heads each specialty.

The medical staff generally have their own executive committee that sets general policies and is the main decision-making body in medical matters. Other medical staff committees, such as the following, are common to most hospitals. The *credentials committee* grants and reviews admitting privileges for those already credentialed and for new doctors whose skills are yet untested. The *medical records committee* ensures that accurate documentation is maintained on the entire regimen of care given to each patient. This committee also oversees confidentiality issues related to medical records. The *utilization review committee* performs routine checks to ensure that inpatient placements, as well as the length of stay, are clinically appropriate. The *infection control committee* is responsible for reviewing policies and procedures for minimizing infections in the hospital (Griffith 1995; Rakich et al. 1992). The *quality improvement committee* is responsible for overseeing the program for continuous quality improvement.

Licensure, Certification, and Accreditation

A license to operate a certain number of hospital beds is a basic regulatory requirement. State governments oversee the *licensure* of health care facilities, and each state sets its own standards for licensure. All facilities must be licensed to operate, but they do not have to be certified or accredited. Licensure is generally carried out by a state's department of health. State licensure standards strongly emphasize the physical plant's compliance with building codes, fire safety, climate control, space allocations, and sanitation. Minimum standards are also established for equipment and personnel. Generally, state licensure is not directly tied to the quality of care a health care facility actually delivers.

Certification entitles a hospital to participate in Medicare and Medicaid. Legislation in 1972 mandated federal oversight of hospitals if they wished to admit Medicare and Medicaid patients. The Department of Health and Human Services (DHHS) developed standards called *conditions of participation*. The purpose of the hospital conditions of participation is to protect patient health and safety and help assure that quality care is furnished to all hospital patients. Hospitals must meet the conditions of participation in order to participate in Medicare or Medicaid. Conditions, as currently revised, are intended to focus primarily on the actual quality of care furnished to patients and the outcomes of that care. Actual compliance with the standards is verified through periodic inspections by each state's department of health.

In contrast with licensure and certification, which are government regulatory mechanisms, *accreditation* is a private mechanism designed to assure that accredited health care facilities meet certain basic standards. Seeking accreditation is voluntary, but the passage of Medicare in 1965 specified that accredited facilities were eligible for purposes of Medicare reimbursement. Accreditation of a hospital by the Joint Commission on Accreditation of Healthcare Organizations (JCAHO) con-

fers *deemed status* on the hospital, meaning the hospital has deemed to have met Medicare and Medicaid certification standards. Thus, an accredited hospital does not need to go through the certification process. Private organizations that have been approved by the Centers for Medicare and Medicaid Services to confer deemed status are said to have "deeming authority." In addition to JCAHO, the American Osteopathic Association also has deeming authority to accredit hospitals.

The American College of Surgeons (ACS) began surveying hospitals in 1918 and established the hospital standardization program after it was recommended that a system of standardization of hospital equipment and hospital wards be developed. Until 1951, the ACS single-handedly worked to improve hospital-based medical practice. This effort evolved into the formation of the Joint Commission on Accreditation of Hospitals, a private nonprofit body formed in 1951 by joint effort of the ACS, the American College of Physicians, the AHA, and the AMA. The organization changed its name in 1987 to the Joint Commission on Accreditation of Healthcare Organizations (JCAHO), which more accurately describes the variety of health facilities it accredits.

The Joint Commission sets standards and accredits most of the nation's hospitals, as well as many of the long-term care facilities, psychiatric hospitals, substance abuse programs, outpatient surgery centers, urgent care clinics, group practices, community health centers, hospices, and home health agencies. Other private organizations also have deeming authority for some of these facilities. Different sets of standards apply to each category of health care organization. Some facilities, such as nursing homes, do not receive deemed status as a result of accreditation, and must also be certified by DHHS to receive Medicare and Medicaid reimbursement. Over the years, JCAHO has refined its accreditation standards and process of verifying compliance. In 2006, JCAHO has moved from scheduled to unannounced inspections with the objective that hospitals will attempt to be in compliance with all the standards all the time.

Ethical and Legal Issues in Patient Care

Ethical issues arise in all types of health services organizations, but the most significant ones occur in acute-care hospitals. Increasing levels of technology create situations requiring decision making under complex circumstances. For example, life-sustaining therapies in intensive care and dealing with life and death issues commonly raise ethical concerns. Ethical issues also arise in health care research and in experimental medicine. In management, ethical conduct becomes important when competition is intense or when cost cutting becomes necessary to save an organization from bankruptcy.

Ethics Principles

Ethics requires judgment. Clear-cut rules are often not available. Hence, medical practitioners and managers generally have to rely on certain well-established principles as guides to ethical decision making.

Four important principles of ethics are respect for others, beneficence, nonmaleficence, and justice. The principle of respect for others has four elements: autonomy, truth-telling, confidentiality, and fidelity.

Autonomy allows people to govern themselves by choosing and pursuing a course of action without external coercion. In health care delivery, it refers to patient empowerment: obtain consent for treatment, explain the various treatment alternatives, allow the patient to participate in decision making and selection of treatment options, and treat the patient with respect and dignity. Constant tension exists between autonomy and paternalism, the view that someone else must direct what the patient must undergo without the patient's involvement. Truth-telling requires a caregiver to be honest. This principle often needs to be balanced with nonmaleficence because a tension is created when truth-telling would result in harm to the patient. The principle of confidentiality sometimes comes into conflict when the legal system requires disclosure of patient information. Fidelity means performing one's duty, keeping one's word, and keeping promises.

In a general sense, the principle of beneficence implies that all individuals have some moral obligation to benefit others. A health services organization is ethically obligated to do all it can to alleviate suffering caused by ill health and injury. This obligation includes providing the needy with certain types of services, such as emergency department services.

The principle of nonmaleficence implies that people have a moral obligation not to harm others, but many health care interventions, including certain preventive measures, such as immunization, often carry risks. Hence, in health care, nonmaleficence requires that the potential benefits from medical treatment sufficiently outweigh the potential harm.

The principle of justice encompasses fairness and equality. It denounces discrimination in the delivery of health care.

Legal Rights

Ethical concerns are often triggered in decisions related to informed consent and continuation of life support services to terminally ill patients. One of the most critical decisions relates to patient competency and the right to refuse treatment. Although the right of competent patients to refuse medical care is well established, the desires of incompetent or comatose patients present ethical challenges. Unless such patients have expressed their wishes in advance, family members or legal guardians end up making decisions regarding sustained medical treatment, or state laws may govern such decisions. Medical and legal experts and family members may differ, often bitterly, on the controversial issue of withdrawing nutrition and other life support means for dying patients, as the case of Theresa Schiavo, which made national news in 2004, demonstrated in the state of Florida. However, certain legal mechanisms have been established to deal with the issues of patients' rights.

Bill of Rights and Informed Consent

The Patient Self-Determination Act of 1990 applies to all health care facilities participating in Medicare or Medicaid. The law requires hospitals and other facilities to provide all patients, on admission, with information on patients' rights. Most hospitals and other inpatient institutions have developed what is referred to as the *patient's bill of rights*. This document reflects the law concerning issues such as confidentiality and consent. Other rights include the right to make decisions regarding medical care, to be informed about diagnosis and treatment, to refuse treatment, and to formulate advance directives.

Based on the principle of autonomy, *informed consent* is a fundamental patient right. It refers to the patient's right to make an informed choice regarding medical treatment. The current climate in medical ethics supports honest and complete disclosure of medical information. In 1972, the Board of Trustees of the American Hospital Association affirmed a Patient's Bill of Rights, which states that the patient has the right to obtain from his physician complete current information concerning his diagnosis, treatment, and prognosis in terms the patient can be reasonably expected to understand (Rosner 2004). Informed consent is customarily obtained via a signature on preprinted forms and becomes part of the patient's medical record.

Some of these principles are being incorporated in provider mindsets and organizational culture that has been referred to as *patient-centered care*. Patients' involvement in their treatment, grounding treatment decisions in patients' preferences, and creating a caregiving environment in which staff solicit patients' inputs and patients' need for information and education collectively promote patient-centered care (Cross 2004).

Advance Directives

Advance directives refer to the patient's wishes regarding continuation or withdrawal of treatment when the patient lacks decision-making capacity. Advance directives are intended to ensure that the patient's end-of-life wishes are carried out.

Three types of advance directives are in common use: do-not-resuscitate orders, living wills, and durable powers of attorney. A *do-not-resuscitate order* directs medical caregivers not to administer any artificial means to resuscitate the person when his or her heart or breathing stops. It is based on the theory that a patient may prefer to die rather than live when strong odds are against a good quality of life after cardiopulmonary resuscitation because severe disabilities would likely remain. A *living will* communicates a patient's wishes regarding medical treatment when he or she is unable to make decisions due to terminal illness or incapacitation. The main drawback of a living will is that it is general in nature because it cannot possibly cover all possible situations. A *durable power of attorney* for health care is a written legal document in which the patient appoints another individual to act as the patient's agent for purposes of health care decision making in the event that the patient is unable or unwilling to make such decisions. Although a durable power of attorney can cover most circumstances, its main drawback is that the appointed person may not act in the same manner in which the patient would have acted had he or she remained competent.

Mechanisms for Ethical Decision Making

Many health care organizations, especially large acute care hospitals, have *ethics committees* charged with developing guidelines and standards for ethical decision making in the delivery of health care (Paris 1995). Ethics committees are also responsible for resolving issues related to medical ethics. Such committees are multidisciplinary, involving physicians, nurses, clergy, social workers, legal experts, ethicists, and administrators.

Although physicians and other caregivers have moral responsibilities on the clinical side, the health care executive who leads the health services organization must also assume the role of a moral agent. As a *moral agent*, the manager morally affects and is morally affected by actions taken. Although executives are entrusted with the fiduciary responsibility to act prudently in managing the affairs of the organization, their responsibilities to patients must take precedence. In governing the affairs of an organization, health care executives must also recognize that ethics is much more than obeying the law. The law represents only the minimum standard of morality established by society. Similarly, health care professionals who deliver care must recognize that even though they are bound by the law, they also have a higher calling, one that includes numerous positive duties to patients and society, and to each other (Darr 1991).

Hospitals and Public Trust

Well-run hospitals are generally regarded with pride by their communities. If a hospital's mission is to benefit the community, then it should be viewed as a community asset regardless of whether it is investor owned or nonprofit. When such a viewpoint is lost, and hospital governance starts placing other priorities ahead of its primary responsibility to serve the community, a breach of public trust can ensue, which sometimes can be irreparable. This balance is one of the greatest challenges hospitals have faced in recent years. As business enterprises, hospitals must respond to economic changes and must maintain their financial and operational integrity. The real danger occurs when these factors are put above a genuine concern for the welfare of the patients and the community. Because hospitals form the institutional hub of health care delivery, their integrity within the system is crucial.

At times, a relentless pursuit of profits and a disconnect from their communities may have blinded management to their institutions' primary mission. For example, a 2004 AHA-sponsored survey found that 60 percent of the people did not completely trust hospitals, and 55 percent feared that they would be harmed during a hospital stay (King 2006). In addition to people's apprehensions about quality of care and patient safety, the public's trust has been eroded by reports of fraud as a number of hospitals and multihospital systems across the country have faced charges of Medicare fraud and abuse because of questionable billing and collection practices. Several hospitals have paid heavy fines, and some hospital executives have served jail sentences for fraud. Although most hospital executives are honest, the wide negative publicity generated by such reports influences the public's perception of hospitals. Rebuilding public trust in the face of scandals and negative press can squander resources that could be used for serving the communities.

Summary

Hospitals are institutions engaged primarily in the delivery of inpatient acute care services. However, they have increasingly branched out to provide postacute and outpatient services. Hospitals developed from the almshouses and pesthouses of the 18th and 19th centuries, and early hospitals mainly served a custodial function and provided services that were more akin to social welfare than to medicine. Taking care of the sick did not develop as a main function of hospitals until the late 19th century, when many of the almshouses were replaced by public hospitals to serve the poor. Voluntary hospitals were developed to serve all classes of people. The growth of medical science and technology made it necessary for physicians to use hospitals as the main venue for the practice of medicine and for training residents. Today, hospitals are at the heart of consolidation and diversification activities that aim to develop a full continuum of health care services.

The growth of hospitals occurred in conjunction with advances in science and medical technology, advances in medical education, the development of professional nursing, and the growth of health insurance. The Hill-Burton Act of 1946 stands as the greatest single factor contributing to the increase in nation's bed supply. The government played an equally important role in reducing inpatient utilization by means of the PPS implemented in 1983. The growth of managed care has been significant in reducing inpatient utilization during the 1990s. Some of the key measures of inpatient utilization are discharges, inpatient days, ALOS, capacity, average daily census, and occupancy rates.

Hospitals can be classified in numerous ways, and the various classification schemes help differentiate one hospital from another. Performance statistics by hospital type can help executives compare their hospital to others in the same category. Although most US hospitals are general community hospitals, various specialty hospitals treat specific types of patients or conditions. Teaching hospitals and academic medical centers play a leading role in graduate medical education. Church-affiliated hospitals are mostly voluntary community hospitals, but they serve a special purpose by emphasizing the sponsoring organization's dietary and spiritual aspects of health care. Osteopathic hospitals are also community general hospitals for the most part, with an emphasis on holistic medicine. Most public and voluntary hospitals are nonprofit. As such, these institutions enjoy some tax advantages. They are expected to provide charity care that is equivalent in value to the tax subsidies received; however, many nonprofit hospitals emulate the behavior of their for-profit counterparts, which has raised some concerns in the US Congress. Some nonprofit hospitals, on the other hand, are beginning to take their mission of service seriously and are finding creative ways to serve their communities.

Hospitals are among the most complex organizations to manage because of the numerous external stakeholders who must be satisfied, and because of hospitals' complex internal governance structure. Hospital organization is represented by a triad in which authority is shared by the board of trustees, the CEO, and the medical staff. The CEO must possess exceptional skills to manage the day-to-day operations while satisfying the demands of the board, the medical staff, and the external stakeholders. Hospital administrators have been under growing pressure to handle the issues of resource allocation, cost containment, and uncompensated care.

A hospital cannot operate unless it is licensed by the state in which it is located. To participate in Medicare and Medicaid, a hospital must also be certified by the DHHS. Certification is maintained by satisfying the conditions of participation. As an alternative to certification, a hospital can voluntarily apply for accreditation by the Joint Commission. Accreditation confers deemed status on a hospital, which exempts the hospital from Medicare and Medicaid certification.

Ethical decision making has been a special area of concern for hospitals. From a medical standpoint, ethical issues often pertain to patient privacy, confidentiality, informed consent, and end-of-life treatment. Bills of rights and advance directives are two of the legal means to address these issues. Active ethics committees must continually address the development of policies and standards for clinicians and administrators. These same multidisciplinary committees also deal with ethical problems as they arise.

Communities usually trust their hospitals, but the behavior of some institutions has called this trust into question. When hospitals fail to be accountable to their communities and when insurance fraud and abuse emerge, the negative repercussions tend to last for years.

Test Your Understanding

Terminology

academic medical center	credentials committee	infection control committee
accreditation	Critical Access Hospital	informed consent
advance directives	days of care	inpatient
average daily census	deemed status	inpatient day
average length of stay	discharge	investor-owned hospital
board of trustees	do-not-resuscitate orders	licensure
certification	durable power of attorney	living will
chief of service	ethics committee	long-term care hospital
chief of staff	executive committee	medical records committee
community hospital	general hospital	medical staff committee
conditions of participation	hospital	moral agent

occupancy rate	*quality improvement*	*swing bed*
osteopathic medicine	*committee*	*teaching hospital*
patient-centered care	*rehabilitation hospital*	*urban hospital*
patient's bill of rights	*rural hospital*	*utilization review*
proprietary hospital	*short-stay hospital*	*committee*
public hospital	*specialty hospital*	*voluntary hospital*

Review Questions

1. What is the difference between inpatient and outpatient services?

2. As hospitals evolved from rudimentary custodial and quarantine facilities to their current state, how did they change in their purpose and function?

3. What were the main factors responsible for the growth of hospitals until the latter part of the 20th century?

4. Name the three main forces that have been responsible for hospital downsizing. How has each of these forces been responsible for the decline in inpatient hospital utilization?

5. What is a voluntary hospital? Explain. How did voluntary hospitals evolve in the United States?

6. Discuss the role of government in the growth as well as the decline of hospitals in the United States.

7. What are inpatient days? What is the significance of this measure?

8. How does hospital utilization vary according to a person's age, gender, and race?

9. Discuss the different types of public hospitals and the roles they play in the delivery of health care services in the United States.

10. What are some of the differences between voluntary and investor-owned hospitals?

11. What is a long-term care hospital (LTCH)? What role does it play in health care delivery in the United States?

12. The table below gives some operational statistics for two hospitals located in the same community. Answer the questions following the table.

Calendar Year 2006	Nonprofit Community Hospital (A)	Proprietary Community Hospital (B)
Number of beds in operation	320	240
Total discharges	12,051	9,230
Medicare	5,130	3,876
Medicaid	3,565	2,118
Private insurance	3,356	3,236

Calendar Year 2006	Nonprofit Community Hospital (A)	Proprietary Community Hospital (B)
Total hospital days	72,421	51,684
Medicare	36,935	26,359
Medicaid	23,175	12,921
Private insurance	12,311	12,404
Total inpatient revenues	$45,755,000	$35,800,000
Dollar value of charity care	$5,000,000	$3,500,000

(a) Calculate the following measures for each hospital (wherever appropriate, calculate the measure for each pay type). Discuss the meaning and significance of each measure, and point out the differences between the two hospitals.

(1) Hospital capacity

(2) ALOS

(3) Occupancy rate

(b) Operationally, which hospital is performing better? Why?

(c) Do you think the nonprofit hospital is meeting its service obligations to the community in exchange for its tax-exempt status? Please give reasons for your answer.

(d) Do you think the hospitals have a problem with excess capacity? If so, what would you recommend?

13. Why have physicians developed their own specialty hospitals? What legal issues can likely arise when physicians have an ownership interest in a hospital?

14. What criteria does Medicare use to classify a hospital as a rehabilitation hospital?

15. How do you differentiate between a community hospital and a non-community hospital?

16. What is a Critical Access Hospital (CAH)? Why was this designation created?

17. What are some of the main differences between teaching and nonteaching hospitals?

18. Can church-affiliated hospitals be classified as voluntary hospitals? Please explain.

19. Discuss some of the issues relative to the tax-exempt status of nonprofit hospitals. If you were a member of the board of trustees of a nonprofit hospital, what would you recommend such a hospital do to justify its nonprofit status?

20. Why are hospitals among the most complex organizations to manage?

21. Discuss the governance of a modern hospital.

22. In the context of hospitals, what is the difference between licensure, certification, and accreditation?

23. What can a hospital do to address some of the difficult ethical problems relative to end-of-life treatment?

24. What can hospitals do to maintain the public's trust?

REFERENCES

American Hospital Association. 1990. *Hospital statistics 1990–1991 edition*. Chicago.

American Hospital Association. 1994. *AHA guide to the health care field 1994 edition*. Chicago.

Anderson, K., and B. Wootton. 1991. Changes in hospital staffing patterns. *Monthly Labor Review* 114, no. 3: 3–9.

Anonymous. 2002. Nearly half of US public hospitals had negative margins in 2000. *Healthcare Financial Management* 56, no. 9: 22–23.

Appleby, J. 2004. IRS looking closely at what non-profits pay. *USA Today*, September 30, 2004, p. 02b.

Arndt, M., and B. Bigelow. 2006. Toward the creation of an institutional logic for the management of hospitals: Efficiency in the early nineteen hundreds. *Medical Care Research and Review* 63, no. 3: 369–394.

Association of American Medical Colleges (AAMC). 2003. *Teaching hospitals*. *http://www.aamc.org/teachinghospitals.htm*.

Balotsky, E.R. 2005. Is it resources, habit or both: interpreting twenty years of hospital strategic response to prospective payment. *Health Care Management Review* 30, no. 4: 337–346.

Bazzoli, G.J. et al. 2006. Construction activity in US hospitals. *Health Affairs* 25, no. 3: 783–791.

Bresnohan, J.F., and J.F. Drane. 1986. A challenge to examine the meaning of living and dying. *Health Progress* 67: 32–37, 98.

Clement, J.P., and K.L. Grazier. 2001. HMO penetration: Has it hurt public hospitals? *Journal of Health Care Finance* 28, no. 1: 25–38.

Cross, G.M. 2004. What does patient-centered care mean for the VA? *Forum* (November 2004), Academy Health.

Dalton, M.J. 1995. Inpatient hospital reimbursement. In *Health care administration: Principles, practices, structure, and delivery*. 2nd ed., ed. L.F. Wolper, 166–191. Gaithersburg, MD: Aspen Publishers, Inc.

Darr, K. 1991. *Ethics in health services management*. 2nd ed. Baltimore, MD: Health Professions Press.

D'Cruz, M.J., and T.L. Welter. 2005. No small change: Payment trends call for big preparations for 2006. *Healthcare Financial Management* 59, no. 12: 50–60.

DelliFraine, J.L. 2006. Communities with and without children's hospitals: Where do the sickest children receive care? *Hospital Topics* 84, no. 3: 19–26.

Department of Health and Human Services (DHHS). 1999. *Health, United States, 1999*. Hyattsville, MD.

Department of Health and Human Services (DHHS). 2002. *Health, United States, 2002*. Hyattsville, MD.

Department of Health and Human Services (DHHS). 2006. *Health, United States, 2006*. Hyattsville, MD.

Feldstein, M. 1971. *The rising cost of hospital care*. Washington, DC: Information Resource Press.

Feldstein, P.J. 1993. *Health care economics*. 4th ed. Albany, NY: Delmar Publishers.

Griffith, J.R. 1995. *The well-managed health care organization*. Ann Arbor, MI: AUPHA Press/Health Administration Press.

Grimaldi, P.L. 2002. Inpatient rehabilitation facilities are now paid prospective rates. *Journal of Health Care Finance* 28, no. 3: 32–48.

Guterman, S. 2006. Specialty hospitals: A problem or a symptom? *Health Affairs* 25, no. 1: 95–105.

Haglund, C.L., and W.L. Dowling. 1993. The hospital. In *Introduction to health services*. 4th ed., eds. S.J. Williams and P.R. Torrens, 135–176. Albany, NY: Delmar Publishers.

Harrison, J.P. et al. 2003. A profile of hospital acquisitions. *Journal of Healthcare Management* 48, no. 3: 156–170.

HCIA Inc. and Deloitte & Touche. 1997. *The comparative performance of US hospitals: The sourcebook*. Baltimore, MD: HCIA Inc.

Health Forum. 2001. *AHA guide to the health care field. 2001–2002 edition*. Chicago: Health Forum.

Hoechst Marion Roussel. 1999. *Managed care digest series 1999: Institutional digest*. Kansas City, MO: Hoechst Marion Roussel, Inc.

Iglehart, J.K. 2006. U.S. hospitals: Examining their fraying social contract. *Health Affairs* 25, no. 1: 8–9.

Kahl, A., and D.E. Clark. 1986. Employment in health services: Long-term trends and projections. *Monthly Labor Review*, August, 28.

King, J.G. 2006. Strong public trust is the key to a successful future for every hospital. *AHA News* 42, no. 11: 4–5.

Longest, B.B., and C.J. Lin. 2005. Can nonprofit hospitals do both well and good? *Health Care Management Review* 30, no. 1: 62–68.

Mantone, J. 2005. Critical time at rural hospitals. *Modern Healthcare* 35, no. 10: 22.

Mechanic, D. 1998. Emerging trends in mental health policy and practice. *Health Affairs* 17, no. 6: 82–98.

MedPAC (Medicare Payment Advisory Commission). 2004. *New Approaches in Medicare : Report to the Congress*. Washington DC: Medicare Payment Advisory Commission.

Muller, R.W. 2003. The changing American hospital in the twenty-first century. *Policy Brief No. 26/2003*. Syracuse, NY: Center for Policy Research, Syracuse University.

Newman, J.F. et al. 2001. CEO performance appraisal: Review and recommendations. *Journal of Healthcare Management* 46, no. 1: 21–37.

Nudelman, P.M., and L.M. Andrews. 1996. The "value added" or not-for-profit health plans. *New England Journal of Medicine* 334, no. 16: 1057–1059.

O'Connell, L., and S.L. Brown. 2003. Do nonprofit HMOs eliminate racial disparities in cardiac care? *Journal of Healthcare Finance* 30, no. 2: 84–94.

Owens, B. 2005. The plight of the not-for-profit. *Journal of Healthcare Management* 50, no. 4: 237–250.

Paris, M. 1995. The medical staff. In *Health care administration: Principles, practices, structure, and delivery*. 2nd ed., ed. L.F. Wolper, 32–46. Gaithersburg, MD: Aspen Publishers, Inc.

Patrick, V. et al. 2006. Facilitating discharge in state psychiatric institutions: A group intervention strategy. *Psychiatric Rehabilitation Journal* 29, no. 3: 183–188.

Pfizer Inc. 2003. *Utilization of Veterans Affairs Medical Care Services by United States Veterans.* New York, NY: Pfizer Inc.

Raffel, M.W. 1980. *The US health system: Origins and functions.* New York: John Wiley and Sons.

Raffel, M.W., and N.K. Raffel. 1994. *The US health system: Origins and functions.* 4th ed. Albany, NY: Delmar Publishers.

Rakich, J.S. et al. 1992. *Managing health services organizations.* 3rd ed. Baltimore, MD: Health Professions Press.

Reinhardt, U.E. et al. 2002. Cross-national comparisons of health systems using OECD data, 1999. *Health Affairs* 21, no. 3: 169–181.

Robbins, J.V. 2002. Beyond the walls. *Hospitals & Health Networks* 76, no. 7: 28.

Roemer, M.I. 1961. Bed supply and hospital utilization: A natural experiment. *Hospitals* 35, no. 21: 36–42.

Rosner, F. 2004. Informing the patient about a fatal disease: From paternalism to autonomy—The Jewish view. *Cancer Investigation* 22, no. 6: 949–953.

Safety net in shreds. 2002. *Trustee* (Oct 2002) 55, no. 9: 3.

Sanofi-Aventis. 2007. *Managed care digest series, 2007: Hospital/systems digest.* Bridgewater, NJ: Sanofi-Aventis US, LLC.

Sinay, T. 2005. Cost structure of osteopathic hospitals and their local counterparts in the USA: Are they any different? *Social Science and Medicine* 60, no. 8: 1805–1814.

Sloan, F.A. 1998. Commercialism in nonprofit hospitals. *Journal of Policy Analysis and Management* 17, no. 2: 234–252.

Slusky, R. 2006. An investment in rural hospitals is an investment in healthier communities. *AHA News* 42, no. 5: 4–5.

Snook, I.D. 1981. *Hospitals: What they are and how they work.* Rockville, MD: Aspen Systems Corporation.

Snyder, J. 2003. Specialty hospitals on rise: Facilities source of controversy. *The Arizona Republic*, February 23, 2003.

Stewart, D.A. 1973. The history and status of proprietary hospitals. *Blue Cross Reports—Research Series 9.* Chicago: Blue Cross Association.

Strunk, B.C. et al. 2006. The effect of population aging on future hospital demand. *Health Affairs* 25, no. 3: w141–149.

Stuart, B. et al. 2006. Financial consequences of rural hospital long-term care strategies. *Health Care Management Review* 31, no. 2: 145–155.

Teisberg, E.D. et al. 1991. *The hospital sector in 1992.* Boston: Harvard Business School.

Thorpe, K.E. et al. 2000. Hospital conversions, margins, and the provision of uncompensated care. *Health Affairs* 19, no. 6: 187–194.

US Census Bureau. 2002. *Statistical abstract of the United States, 2002.*

US Census Bureau. 2007. *Statistical abstract of the United States, 2007.*

Vogt, W.B., and R. Town. 2006. *How has hospital consolidation affected the price and quality of hospital care?* Princeton, NJ: The Robert Wood Johnson Foundation.

Williams, S.J. 1995. *Essentials of health services.* Albany, NY: Delmar Publishers.

Wilson, F.A., and D. Neuhauser. 1985. *Health services in the United States.* 2nd ed. Cambridge, MA: Ballinger Publishing Co.

Wolfson, J., and S.L. Hopes. 1994. What makes tax-exempt hospitals special? *Healthcare Financial Management*, July, 56–60.

Zeber, J.E. et al. 2004. Serious mental illness and aging with the veteran population. http://www.hsrd.research.va.gov/meetings/2003/abstracts/2004.htm

Zimmerman, E. 2006. The implications of reimbursement changes for specialty hospitals. *Healthcare Financial Management* 60, no. 7: 42–45.

Chapter 2

Leiyu Shi, DrPH, MBA, MPA, and Douglas A. Singh, PhD, MBA

Cost, Access, and Quality

Learning Objectives

- To understand the meaning of health care costs and review recent trends
- To examine the factors that have led to cost escalations in the past
- To become familiar with both regulatory and market-oriented approaches to contain costs
- To understand why some regulatory cost-containment approaches were unsuccessful
- To appreciate the framework and various dimensions of access to care
- To learn about access indicators and measurement
- To understand the nature, scope, and dimensions of quality
- To understand the difference between quality assurance and quality assessment

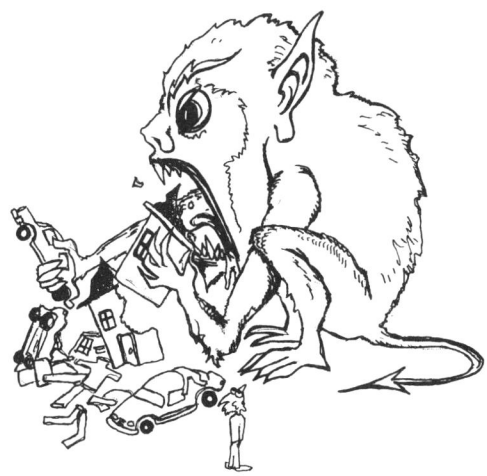

The health care sector of the economy is like a monster with a voracious appetite that needs to be controlled.

Introduction

Cost, access, and quality are three major cornerstones of health care delivery (Al-Assaf 1993a). For many years, employers and third-party payers in the United States have been preoccupied with controlling the growth of health care expenditures. One reason past attempts to bring universal access into the United States have failed is the concern that such a move would be extremely costly in terms of national health care expenditures. This fear is founded on the premise that cost and access go hand in hand. Although cost and access have remained the primary concerns within the US health care delivery system, quality of health care is increasingly taking center stage. At the same time, rising systemwide costs will remain the focus of attention for a long time to come.

The cost of health care, people's ability to obtain health care when needed, and the quality of services are interactively related. From a macro perspective, costs of health care are commonly viewed in terms of national expenditures for health care. A widely used measure of national health care expenditures is the proportion of the gross domestic product (GDP) a country spends on the delivery of health care services. In simple terms, it refers to the proportion of its national income a country spends on health care. From a micro perspective, health care expenditures refer to costs incurred by employers to purchase health insurance and out of pocket costs incurred by individuals when they receive health care services. Improving access to health care and equal access to quality health care are contingent on expenditures at both the macro and micro levels. High-quality care is also the most cost-effective care. Hence, cost is an important factor in the evaluation of quality. On the other hand, quality is achieved when accessible services are provided in an efficient, cost-effective, and acceptable manner (Al-Assaf 1993a).

This chapter discusses some major reasons for the dramatic rise in health care expenditures. Costs are compared with those in other countries, and the impact of cost-containment measures is examined. A considerable proportion of the US population is not assured basic access, and that is a serious problem. The government has played a significant role in cost containment and quality improvement, but extension of universal access to all Americans has remained an elusive dream.

Cost of Health Care

The term "cost" can carry different meanings in the delivery of health care. The meaning of health care costs depends on one's perspective. It has three different meanings: (1) When consumers and financiers speak of the "cost" of health care, they usually mean the "price" of health care. This could refer to the physician's bill, the price of a prescription, or the premiums employers pay to purchase health insurance for their employees. (2) From a national perspective, health care costs refer to how much a nation spends on health care services. In this context, health care costs are also commonly referred to as health care expenditures or health care spending. They primarily reflect the consumption of economic resources in the delivery of health care. The economic resources include health insurance, the skills of health care professionals, organizations and institutions of health care delivery, pharmaceuticals, medical equipment and supplies, public health functions, and new medical discoveries. Since expenditures (E) equals price (P) times quantity (Q), growth in health care spending can be accounted for by growth in prices charged by the providers of health services and by increases in the utilization of services. (3) A third perspective is that of the providers. For these suppliers of health care, the notion of cost refers to the cost of producing health care services. Staff salaries, capital costs for buildings and equipment, rental of space, purchase of supplies, etc. constitute the costs of production.

Trends in National Health Expenditures

Health care spending spiraled upward at double digit rates during the 1970s. This was right after the Medicare and Medicaid programs created a massive growth in access in 1965. By 1970, government expenditures for health care services and supplies had grown by 140%, from $7.9 to $18.9 billion (DHHS 1996). During much of the 1980s, average annual growth in national health spending continued in the double digits, but the rate of increase slowed down considerably (Figure 2–1). In the 1990s, medical inflation was finally brought under control, down to a single digit rate of growth, mainly due to control over medical care costs and utilization through managed care. Recently, the rate of growth has started to accelerate, but at a relatively slow pace (Table 2–1).

Trends in national health expenditures are commonly evaluated in two different ways. One is to compare medical inflation to general inflation in the economy, which is measured by annual changes in the consumer price index (CPI). Except for a brief period

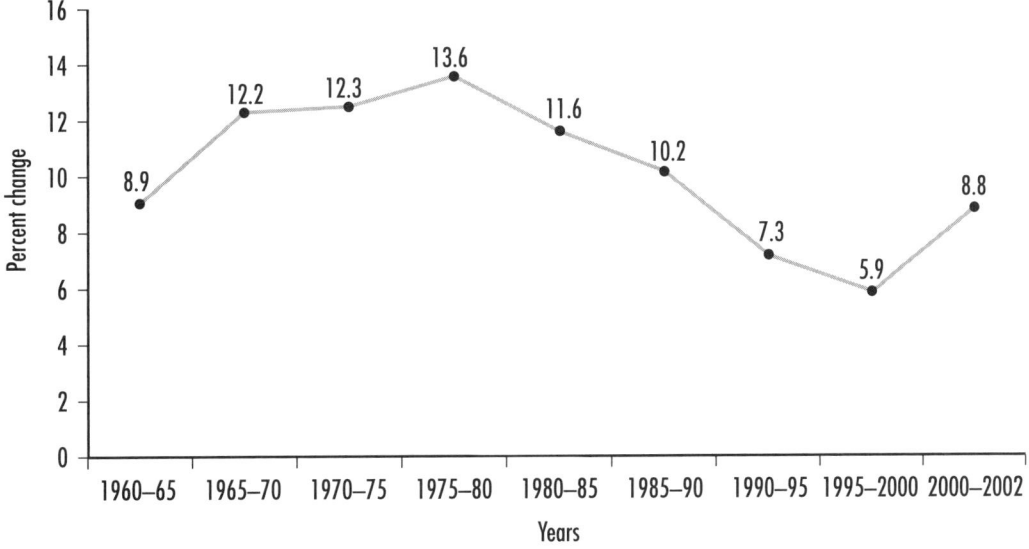

Figure 2–1 Average Annual Percentage Growth in National Health Care Spending During Five-Year Periods, 1960–2002.

Sources: Data from *Health, United States, 1995*, p. 244; *Health, United States, 2002*, p. 291; *Health, United States, 2006*, p. 377, Department of Health and Human Services.

Table 2–1 Average Annual Percentage Increase in National Health Care Spending, 1975–2004

Periods	% Increase	Periods	% Increase
1975–1980	13.6	1990–1995	7.2
1975–1976	14.7	1990–1991	9.2
1976–1977	13.7	1991–1992	9.5
1977–1978	11.9	1992–1993	6.9
1978–1979	12.9	1993–1994	5.1
1979–1980	14.8	1994–1995	4.9
1980–1985	11.6	1995–2000	5.5
1980–1981	16.1	1995–1996	4.6
1981–1982	12.5	1996–1997	4.7
1982–1983	10.0	1997–1998	5.4
1983–1984	9.7	1998–1999	5.7
1984–1985	9.9	1999–2000	6.9
1985–1990	10.2	2000–2004	8.3
1985–1986	7.6	2000–2001	8.7
1986–1987	8.5	2002–2003	8.2
1987–1988	11.9	2003–2004	7.9
1988–1989	11.2		
1989–1990	12.1		

Sources: Data from *Health, United States, 1996–97*, p. 249, 1997; *Health, United States, 1995*, p. 243; National Center for Health Statistics, *1996–97, Health, United States, 1999*, p. 284; *Health, United States, 2000*, p. 322; *Health, United States, 2002*, p. 288; *Health, United States, 2006*, p. 374; and K. Levit et al., Trends in US health care spending, 2003. *Health Affairs*, Vol. 22, no. 1: 154–164.

between 1978 and 1981 when the US economy was experiencing hyperinflation, the rates of change in medical inflation have remained consistently above the rates of change in the CPI (Figure 2–2). The second method compares changes in national health spending to those in the GDP. With only isolated exceptions (in 1983 to 1984, after DRG implementation for payment to hospitals; and in 1995 to 1998, after significant managed care penetration), health care spending growth rates have consistently surpassed growth rates in the general economy (Figure 2–3). When spending on health care grows at a faster rate than GDP, it means that health care consumes a larger share of the total economic output. Put another way, a growing share of total economic resources is devoted to the delivery of health care.

Compared to other nations, the United States uses a larger share of its economic resources for health care (Table 2–2). In

Figure 2–2 Annual Percentage Change in CPI and Medical Inflation, 1975–2005.

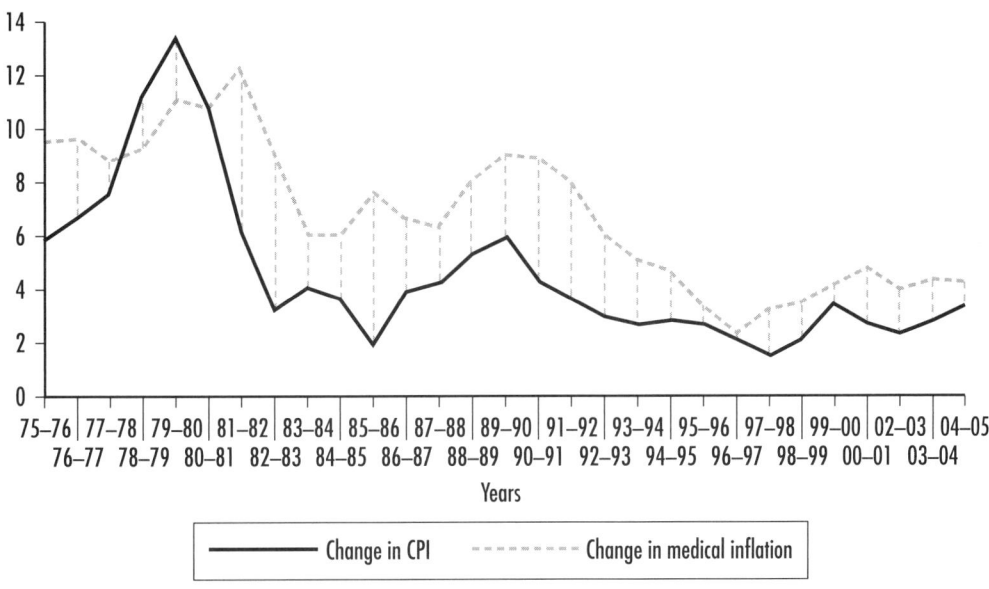

Sources: Data from *Health, United States, 1995,* p. 241; *Health, United States, 1996–97,* p. 251; *Health, United States, 2002,* p. 289; and *Health, United States, 2006,* p. 375.

Figure 2–3 Annual Percentage Change in US National Health Care Expenditures and GDP, 1980–2004.

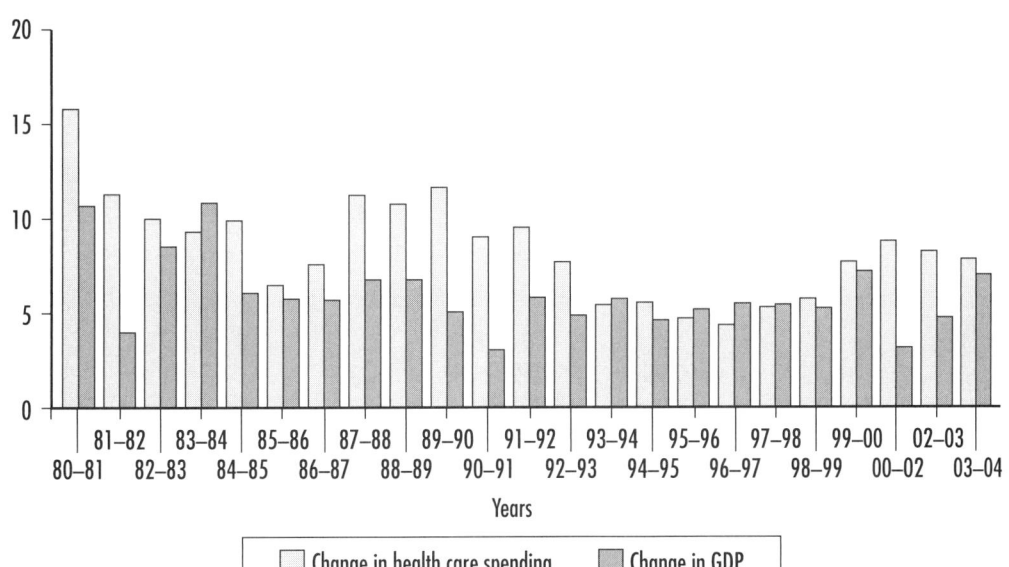

Sources: Data from *Health, United States, 1996–97,* p. 249; *Health, United States, 2002,* p. 288; *Health, United States, 2006,* p. 374; and National Center for Health Statistics, 2002.

Table 2–2 Total Health Care Expenditures as a Proportion of GDP and Per Capita Health Care Expenditures (Selected Years, Selected OECD Countries; Per Capita Expenditures in US Dollars)

	1990	1995	2000	2002
Australia	7.8 $1,307	8.2 $1,745	9.0 $2,220	9.3 $2,521
Austria	7.0 $1,338	8.0 $1,870	7.6 $2,184	7.6 $2,280
Belgium	7.4 $1,345	8.4 $1,820	8.7 $2,279	9.1 $2,607
Canada	9.0 $1,737	9.2 $2,051	8.9 $2,503	9.6 $2,845
Denmark	8.5 $1,567	8.2 $1,848	8.4 $2,382	8.8 $2,655
Finland	7.8 $1,422	7.5 $1,433	6.7 $1,718	7.2 $2,013
France	8.6 $1,568	9.5 $2,033	9.3 $2,456	9.7 $2,762
Germany	8.5 $1,748	10.6 $2,276	10.6 $2,761	10.7 $2,916
Italy	7.9 $1,391	7.3 $1,535	8.1 $2,049	8.4 $2,248
Japan	5.9 $1,115	6.8 $1,538	7.6 $1,971	7.9 $2,139
Netherlands	8.0 $1,438	8.4 $1,826	8.3 $2,259	9.3 $2,775
Sweden	8.4 $1,579	8.1 $1,738	8.4 $2,273	9.2 $2,594
United Kingdom	6.0 $986	7.0 $1,374	7.3 $1,833	7.7 $2,231
United States	11.9 $2,738	13.3 $3,654	13.1 $4,539	13.8 $5,287

[1]Proportion of GDP.

[2]Per capita expenditures adjusted to US dollars using GDP purchasing power parities.

Sources: Data from *Health, United States, 2006*, p. 373.

addition, the United States has outpaced the growth in health care spending in other countries (Figure 2–4). Numerous reasons have been given for the growth of health care expenditures, and several different measures have been undertaken over the years to prevent these costs from mushrooming to previously projected levels. These topics are discussed a little later in the chapter.

The rate of growth in health spending came down to its lowest levels in four decades (5.7% average annual growth) between 1993 and 2000 as managed care proliferated (Levit et al. 2003). However, the good news ended as the year 2001 recorded the fastest annual growth (8.7%) since 1991 (see Table 2–1). In 2004, the average annual percentage increase in national health care spending declined slightly to 7.9%. The main culprits for this recent rise in expenditures are hospital services, prescription drugs, and physician services (Levit et al. 2003). Once again, the US health care delivery system has

come to a crossroads, which will require some difficult decisions in the near future. The rise in private health insurance premiums, coupled with growing Medicare and Medicaid expenditures, will force private employers and the government to take some drastic steps to prevent any uncontrolled rise in health care costs. Current trends may force a restructuring of managed care plans toward more tightly managed models.

In 2005, the United States spent $2 trillion on health care. This amounted to a per capita spending of $6,697 and consumed 16% of the GDP (Catlin et al. 2007). According to current projections, national health care expenditures will grow to 20% of GDP by 2015 (Borger 2006). These forecasts portend that the health care sector will remain one of the fastest growing components of the US economy. Increased demand for services will expand job opportunities, including those for health services administrators. On the other hand, we can expect to see policy

Figure 2–4 Health Care Spending as a Percentage of GDP for Selected OECD Countries, 1985 and 2000.

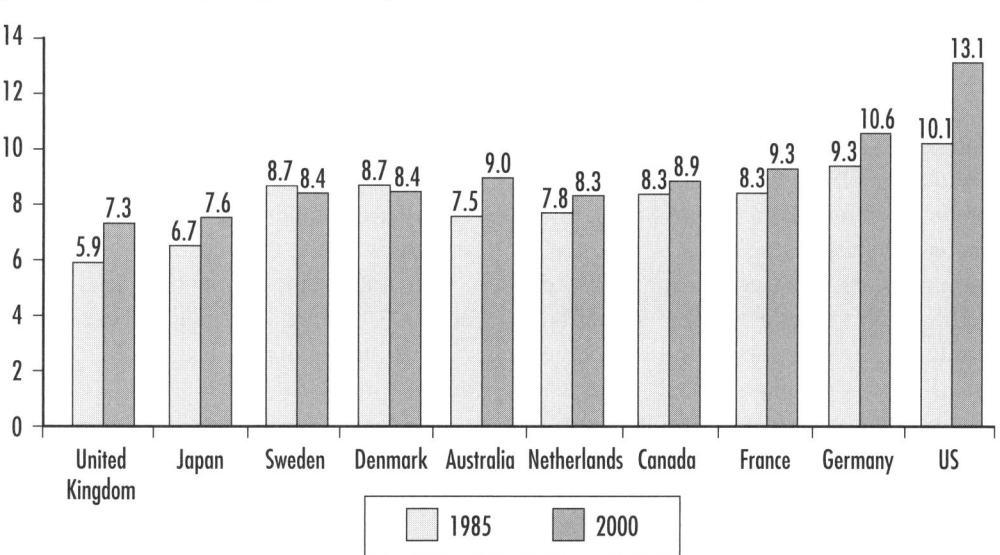

Source: Data from *Health, United States, 2002,* p. 287; *Health, United States, 2006,* p. 373; and National Center for Health Statistics.

debates and new initiatives to keep costs from getting out of control.

Do Health Care Costs Need to Be Contained?

Americans view growth in expenditures in other sectors of the economy, such as manufacturing, much more favorably than expenditures on medical care. Increased medical expenditures create new health care jobs, do not pollute the air, save rather than destroy lives, and alleviate pain and suffering. Why shouldn't society be pleased that more resources are flowing into a sector that cares for the aged and the sick? It would seem to be a more appropriate use of a society's resources than spending those same funds on faster cars, fancy clothes, or other consumable items. Yet, increased expenditures on these other industries do not cause the concern that arises when medical expenditures increase (Feldstein 1994, 12).

Even though rising health care expenditures may seem innocuous to some, they need to be controlled for several reasons. First, rising health care costs consume greater portions of the total economic output. Because economic resources are limited, rising health care costs mean that Americans have to forgo other goods and services when more is spent on health care. Second, limited economic resources should be directed to their highest valued uses, but consumers decide how much should be spent to purchase a product or service based on their perception of the value they expect to receive, knowing that an expenditure on one good means forgoing other goods and services (Feldstein 1994, 13). Health care delivery does not follow the principles of free markets. In the United States, individual patients want maximum expenditures incurred while receiving health care because out-of-pocket payments amount to only a small fraction of the costs of services. They want to get the maximum returns out of prepaid expenditures or health insurance benefits. In countries with national health insurance, patients want to get the maximum in return for the taxes they have paid toward their health coverage. Hence, in either system, unless deliberate attempts are made to control costs, the total health care expenditures will far exceed what they would be under free market conditions.

In the United States, employer-financed health benefits represent a substantial cost of doing business (operating cost). These costs are believed to be the third highest expense category in US corporations after salaries and raw materials (Loubeau and Maher 1996). In 2004, the costs of employer-sponsored coverage was about $575.5 billion. Of this, the employer paid about 77% ($443.2 billion) and employees and retirees paid about 23% ($132.3 billion) (Sheils and Haught 2004). For a business to stay profitable, these costs must be incorporated into the pricing structure and passed on to consumers in higher prices. Some observers think that health care costs are placing businesses at a competitive disadvantage in the international market. To compete internationally, US businesses must reduce costs, including health care costs.

In addition to cost control in the private sector, Medicare and Medicaid expenditures need to be restrained at a level close to the growth in the GDP. Otherwise, health care puts a greater burden on the economy, which increases pressure on the federal and state governments to raise taxes. From time to time, serious concerns have been expressed regarding the long-term solvency of the Medicare Hospital Insurance Trust Fund that finances Part A benefits. The Balanced Budget Act of 1997 was intended to slow down the rapid rise in Medicare spending. According to the latest estimates based on the most probable economic and demographic assumptions, Medicare trustees project that the trust fund will be depleted by 2018 (Van de Water 2006). In past years, these projections have shifted significantly. The conclusion, however, is that at some point the Medicare trust fund will not have adequate funds to pay for the growing health care needs of an aging population, unless steps are taken now to address this issue. According to Representative David Obey, a member of the House Budget Committee, Medicare will absolutely have to be cut in a few years. "When the time comes, there is no way out of it." That time will come as baby boomers move into the system (Tucker 1997). The same is true for countries that have national health care programs. Governments cannot continue to raise taxes indefinitely. Various mechanisms must therefore be employed to contain ever-rising health care costs. One proposal already floated in the US Congress is to raise the eligibility age for Medicare from 65 years to 67 or higher. The downside is that it would leave many elderly uninsured.

Reasons for Cost Escalation

Numerous factors have been attributed to rising health care expenditures. They interact in complex ways. Hence, one cannot just point to one or two main causes. General inflation in the economy is a more visible cause of health care spending because it affects the cost of producing health care services through higher wages, cost of supplies, etc. But, apart from the effects of general inflation, medical cost inflation is influenced by the following factors:

- third-party payment
- imperfect market
- growth of technology
- increase in elderly population
- medical model of health care delivery
- multipayer system and administrative costs
- defensive medicine
- waste and abuse
- practice variations

Third-Party Payment

Health care is among the few services for which a third party, not the consumer, pays for most services used. Whether payment is made by the government or by a private insurance company, individual patients pay a price far lower than the actual cost of the service (Altman and Wallack 1996). Since they have to bear only a fraction of the financial burden out of pocket, the patients are not too concerned about the cost of care. The patient has no incentive to be cost conscious when someone else is paying the bill. Introduction of prospective payment methods and capitation have, to a large extent, minimized provider-induced demand. However, the backlash against managed care from consumers and providers alike has, in a sense, kept the door open to overuse of high-cost technologies and other services. Also, fee-for-service reimbursement and its discounted fee variation are still widely used. Hence, provider-induced demand has not been expunged from the system.

The number of persons with health insurance jumped dramatically after World War II, and so did the spending for health care services. The passage of Medicare and Medicaid in 1965 added third-party protection for an additional 50 million elderly and poor Americans (Altman and Wallack 1996). The Rand Health Insurance Experiment empirically demonstrated the theoretical connection between health insurance and costs. The most comprehensive study of its type, the experiment ran from 1974 through 1981. It enrolled more than 7,000 people into one of 14 different health plans. They included a free plan carrying no deductible or co-payments. The other plans involved varying degrees of cost sharing. It was found that cost sharing resulted in lower costs compared to the free plan. Coinsurance rates of 25% resulted in a 19% decline in expenditures because out of pocket costs reduced health care utilization. Increased coinsurance rates resulted in further declines in utilization and expenditures. Another important finding of the Rand Experiment was that lower utilization due to cost sharing did not affect most measures of health status. People enrolled in the free plan did better in three areas: vision, blood pressure, and dental health, but the average appraised mortality risk for people on the free plan was close to the risk for those with cost sharing (Feldstein 1993, 93–95).

Imperfect Market

Prices charged by providers for health care services are likely to be much closer to the cost of producing the services in a highly regulated or highly competitive market (Altman and Wallack 1996). The US health care market is neither. Because the US health care delivery system does not consist of a national health care program, it is not highly regulated as are the single-payer systems in other countries. Health care delivery in the United States also does not represent a highly competitive market because of various market imperfections. In an imperfect market, utilization of health care is driven by need rather than economic demand, the quantity of health care services produced and delivered is likely to be much higher than in a competitive market, and the prices charged for health care services will be permanently higher than the true economic costs of production (Altman and Wallack 1996). Because $E = Q \times P$, it is not difficult to see why an unregulated quasi-market would result in increased health care expenditures because both Q and P remain unchecked. One reason for an imperfect market is the existence of third-party payments. Third-party payments insulate patients from higher prices and higher utilization. This and other market imperfections also insulate providers against the possibility of facing lower demand from higher prices. In other words, because of the imperfect nature of the health care market, demand is not sensitive to changes in prices, as it would be under free-market conditions*.

Growth of Technology

The United States has been characterized as following an early-start-fast-growth pattern

---

*Chiropractic care and outpatient mental health services are more sensitive to prices than overall medical and dental care. Access to free chiropractic care among health maintenance organization (HMO) enrollees increased chiropractic use ninefold compared with a contemporaneous sample of HMO enrollees who faced 95% cost sharing. When patients have to share 25% or more of the cost, they decrease their chiropractic expenses by one half. (P.G. Shekelle, W.H. Rogers, and J.P. Newhouse. 1996. The effect of cost sharing on the use of chiropractic services. *Medical Care* 34, 9: 863–872.)

in the adoption and diffusion of intensive procedures (TECH Research Network 2001). Growth and intensive use of technology have a direct impact on the escalation of health care costs. New technology is expensive to develop, and costs incurred in research and development (R&D) are included in the total health care expenditures. One reason Canada and European nations, compared to the United States, have incurred lower costs is because they have proportionally invested far less in R&D. They have been able to buy or duplicate American breakthroughs (Easterbrook 1987).

Once technology is developed, it drives up demand for its use. Compared to other nations, the overall diffusion and utilization of technology is greater in the United States, although countries like Japan, Austria, and Switzerland have more magnetic resonance imagers (MRIs) and computed tomography (CT) scanners (Reinhardt et al. 2002). Development of new technology raises the expectations of consumers about what medical science can do to diagnose and treat diseases and prolong life.

Technology has been at least partly responsible for the surplus of specialists in the United States. Specialty services are more technology intensive and, consequently, more expensive than primary care services. Since disease prevalence is too low to support all the specialists, many high-tech procedures are overused.

Technology has substantially increased diagnosis and treatment and improved quality of life, but it is also used simply to keep people alive with little or no chance of recovery. Third-party insurance has generally paid for almost all diagnostic tests and procedures with few questions asked. Attempts to limit diffusion of certain expensive technologies in the United States have been largely unsuccessful. Hence, many more cost-increasing technologies have been developed than cost-reducing technologies (Weisbrod 1991).

Increase in Elderly Population

Since the early part of the 20th century, life expectancy in the United States has consistently risen (see Figure 2–5). Life expectancy at birth increased by over 30 years from 47.3 years in 1900 to 77.5 years in 2003 (National Center for Health Statistics 2006). Consequently, the United States and other industrialized nations are also experiencing an aging boom. Growth in the US elderly population has outpaced growth in the nonelderly population since 1900. Figure 2–6 shows changes in the makeup of the US population from 1970 to 2004. Most remarkable is the growth in the age group 85 years and older while the youngest age group is shrinking. Growth of the elderly population is projected to continue through the middle of the 21st century. Between 2000 and 2030, the proportion of the US population that is 65 years of age and older is expected to rise from 12.4% to 20%, or one in five. The number in the 85-and-older category is projected to more than double. The swelling of the elderly population will result from the aging of the baby-boom generation of roughly 77 million Americans born between 1946 and 1964. The youngest of the baby boomers will be 66 years old in 2030.

Elderly people consume more health care than younger people. In 2003, the average medical expenses for people 65 years of age and older was $8,209 per person compared to $2,837 per person for those under the age of 65 (National Center for Health Statistics 2006). In other words, health care

Figure 2–5 Life Expectancy of Americans at Birth, Age 65, and Age 75, Selected Years 1900–2003.

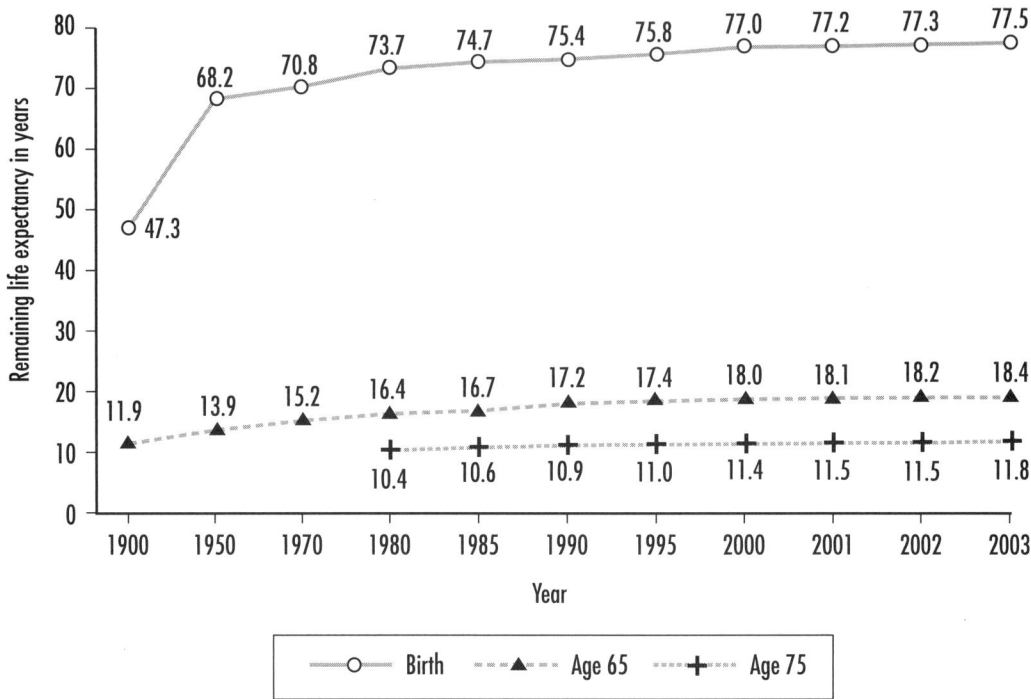

Sources: Data from *Health, United States, 2002*, p. 116 and *Health, United States, 2006*, p. 176.

costs for the elderly are nearly three times more than those for the nonelderly. Total Medicare expenditures are projected to increase from 2.7% of GDP in 2005 to 9% of GDP in 2050 (Van de Water 2006). A growing elderly population and expansion of Medicare by adding prescription drug coverage will seriously affect future health care expenditures.

Medical Model of Health Care Delivery

The medical model emphasizes medical interventions after a person has become sick and plays down prevention and lifestyle behavior changes to promote health. Although health promotion and disease prevention are not the answer to every health problem, these principles have not been accorded their rightful place in the US health care delivery system. Consequently, more costly health care resources must be deployed to treat health problems that could have been prevented. For example, smoking-related illnesses are estimated to cost the United States $75.5 billion annually for direct medical care and an additional $167 billion in lost productivity (CDC 2005). However, evidence suggests the costs of smoking cessation programs pose a minimal burden to insurers and employers with potential for significant cost savings in subsequent years (Levy 2006). Although the prevalence of cigarette smoking has been slowly declining, in 2004, 23% of American adult males and 18.7% of women were smokers (National Center for Health Statistics 2006).

Figure 2–6 Change in US Population Mix between 1970 and 2000, and Projections for 2030.

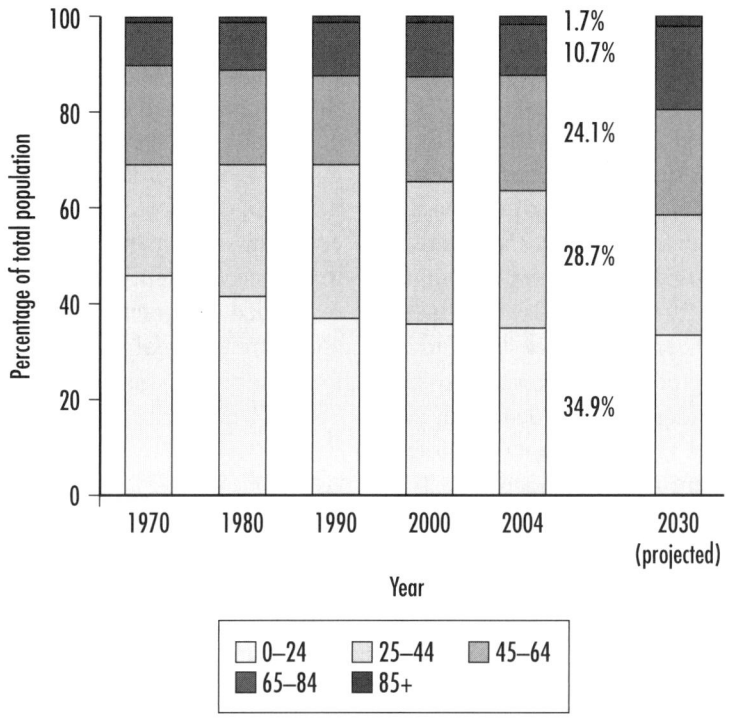

Sources: Data from *Health, United States, 2006*, p. 127, National Center for Health Statistics; *Census 2000*, US Census Bureau; *Projections of the Total Resident Population by 5-Year Age Groups, and Sex with Special Age Categories: Middle Series, 2025 to 2045*, US Census Bureau.

Overweight conditions and obesity have reached alarming rates in the United States and in many other developed nations. In 2004, 66% of Americans age 20 and over were overweight with 31.4% obese (National Center for Health Statistics 2006). Overweight and obesity substantially elevates the risk of heart disease, diabetes, some types of cancers, musculoskeletal disorders, and gallbladder problems.

Consequently, overweight and obesity are contributing to the nation's health care spending at a growing rate. Recent estimates suggest that of the total medical spending in the United States, 9.1% could be attributed to overweight and obesity, rivaling that attributable to smoking. Total health care ex-

penditures attributable to overweight and obesity may be as high as $92.6 billion in 2002 dollars. Both Medicare and Medicaid spend a disproportionate share to treat overweight- and obesity-related health problems (Finkelstein et al. 2003). Even though considerable preventive efforts have been targeted at smoking cessation, to date very little has been done to combat overweight and obesity among both children and adults.

Multipayer System and Administrative Costs

Administrative costs are associated with the management of the financing, insurance, delivery, and payment functions. They include management of the enrollment process, setting up contracts with providers, claims processing, utilization monitoring, denials and appeals, and marketing and promotional expenses. The enrollment process in private employer-financed health plans and in publicly financed Medicaid and Medicare programs includes determination of eligibility, enrollment, and disenrollment. Each activity has associated costs. Insurers and managed care organizations (MCOs) also incur enrollment and disenrollment costs, in addition to marketing costs to promote and sell their plans. Providers have to deal with numerous plans in which the extent of benefits and reimbursement are not standardized. It is difficult and costly to remain current with the numerous and frequently changing rules and regulations. Denials of payment result in appeals and follow-up. Utilization monitoring has become commonplace in the delivery of health care services. Review and authorization of care incur additional costs for payers. They also incur additional costs for providers, who must provide the required information to payers. Denial of hospitalization and specialist referrals may result in appeals, which again create additional costs.

Due to the complexity of a multi-payer system, costs are often duplicated. It is estimated that administrative costs associated with the delivery of health care in the United States may be as high as 24% to 25% of total health care expenditures. A single-payer health care system might cut health care administrative costs by one-half (Hellander et al. 1994).

Defensive Medicine

The US health care delivery system is characterized by legal risks for providers, which promote defensive medicine. The practice of *defensive medicine* leads to tests and services that are not medically justified but are performed by physicians to protect themselves against potential malpractice lawsuits. Induction of labor and cesarean sections are commonly overused procedures in the United States. Fear of legal liability is one of the main reasons for carrying out unnecessary cesarean sections because it makes it easier to defend a potential birth injury case. Unrestrained malpractice awards by the courts and increased malpractice insurance premiums for physicians add significantly to the cost of health care.

Waste and Abuse

The previous discussions pinpoint some of the inefficiencies in the US health care delivery system. These inefficiencies are wasteful. Another type of waste is fraud and abuse within the system. In general terms, *fraud* involves a knowing disregard of the truth. Fraudulent activities are both illegal and immoral. Fraud generally occurs when billing claims or cost reports are intentionally falsified. A mere oversight or an inadvertent error will not rise to the level of fraud; however, a pattern of oversights or errors may be tantamount to fraud (Lovitky 1997). Health care fraud has been identified as a major problem in the Medicare and Medicaid programs.

Fraud may also occur when more services are provided than are medically necessary or when unprovided services are billed. The latter practice may include billing for a higher priced service when a lower priced service is actually delivered. In the managed care sector, some providers may not deliver necessary services even though they are included in the capitated fees. Another type of fraud involves misallocation of costs to increase Medicaid and/or Medicare reimbursement. As some services still continue to be reimbursed on a cost-plus basis, disguising a nonallowable cost as an allowable cost to increase reimbursement is fraudulent.

It is illegal to provide any remuneration to any individual or entity in exchange for a referral for services to be paid by the Medicare or Medicaid program. Knowingly providing such financial inducements amounts to a federal crime punishable by imprisonment. Under the Anti-Kickback Act, several physicians have been prosecuted for accepting payments from hospitals to which the doctors referred Medicare patients. Similar types of prosecutions have occurred with respect to illegal payments to nursing homes and home health agencies made by durable medical equipment suppliers. The Stark Law prohibits physician self-referral for laboratory or other designated health services. This law prevents physicians from referring a patient to laboratories in which they or members of their immediate families have a financial interest (Lovitky 1997).

Practice Variations

The work of John Wennberg and others brought to the fore a disturbing aspect of physician behavior accounting for wide variations in treatment patterns for similar patients. Numerous studies, in the United States and abroad, have documented notable differences in utilization rates for hospital admissions and surgical procedures among different communities as well as for the same specialties (Feldstein 1993, 204). These practice variations are referred to as *small area variations* (SAV) because the differences in practice patterns have only been associated with geographic areas of the country. For example, in earlier studies, variations in the rate

of tonsillectomies in New England counties could not be explained by differences in the demographics or other characteristics of the populations studied (Wennberg and Gittelsohn 1973); the overall inpatient hospital utilization by an aged population in East Boston was higher than that by an equivalent population in New Haven, after controlling for several variables (Wennberg et al. 1987). More recent investigations on regional differences in Medicare spending demonstrated that higher rates of inpatient-based care and specialist services were associated with higher costs but not with improved quality of care, health outcomes, access to services, or satisfaction with care (Fisher et al. 2003a; Fisher et al. 2003b). This variation, which can be as great as twofold, cannot be explained by age, gender, race, pricing variations, or health status (Baucus and Fowler 2002). Geographic variations, as discussed here, signal gross inefficiencies in the US health care delivery system because they increase costs without yielding appreciably better outcomes. This variation is also unfair because workers and Medicare beneficiaries in low-cost, more efficient regions subsidize the care of those in high-cost regions (Wennberg 2002). SAVs cannot be explained by demand inducement. For example, no incentives exist for physicians to induce demand in Canada or Britain, yet variations similar to those in the United States also exist in those countries. SAVs indicate that patients in some parts of the country are receiving too much treatment, whereas others may be receiving too little. Medical opinions often differ on the appropriateness of clinical interventions because physicians use different criteria for hospital admissions and surgical interventions (Gittelsohn and Powe 1995).

Cost Containment — Regulatory Approaches

Many attempts to control health care spending have been undertaken in the United States; however, most of these attempts have met with only limited success mainly because the United States has never been able to implement a systemwide cost-control initiative. An *all-payer system*, in which centralized controls would allow cost-containment efforts to sweep through the entire health care delivery system, has never been tried in the United States, because that would require a major overhaul of the system. Cost-containment measures have been piecemeal, affecting only certain targeted sectors of the health care delivery system at a time. So, for instance, when prices have been regulated, utilization has been left untouched; when capital expenditures have required preapprovals, operating costs of production have been exempted; when reimbursement rates have been set for inpatient services, the outpatient sector has remained free of cost-cutting regulation. In a fragmented system, it is impossible to implement cost-control measures in a systematic and global manner.

Other industrialized nations have created national regulatory mechanisms to keep their health care spending in line with their national income. Many of these countries follow what is referred to as *top-down control* over total expenditures. They establish budgets for entire sectors of the health care delivery system. Funds are distributed to providers in accordance with these global budgets. Thus, total spending remains within established budget limits. The downside to this approach is that, under fixed budgets, providers are not as responsive to patient needs, and the system provides little incentive to be efficient in the delivery of services. Once budgets are expended, providers are forced to cut back services, particularly for illnesses that are not life threatening or do not represent an emergency. This top-down approach is in sharp contrast to the "bottom-up" approach used in the United States, where each provider and MCO establishes its own fees or premiums (Altman and Wallack 1996). Competition, created by employers shopping for the best premium rates and by MCOs contracting with providers who agree to favorable fee arrangements, determines what the total expenditures will be. To some extent, the United States also uses regulatory cost control, although it is not as comprehensive as it is in countries with national health care programs.

Cost-control efforts in the United States are characterized by a combination of government regulation and market-based competition. As a result of this fragmented approach, only short-lived successes have been achieved to date. The main reason for this lack of success is cost shifting between programs and/or sectors when cost-control measures are not comprehensive. *Cost shifting* refers to the ability of providers to make up for lost revenues in one area by increasing utilization or charging higher prices in areas free of controls. For example, when regulatory controls are employed to squeeze costs out of the inpatient sector, providers experience reduced revenues from inpatient services. To make up for the lost revenues, they increase utilization of outpatient services if that sector is free of controls. In another scenario, when the government implements cost-control measures, providers may start charging higher prices to private payers. This practice is very common in the nursing home industry, in which reimbursement is restricted under Medicaid rate setting criteria. In this case, nursing home administrators make a conscious attempt to make up for the lost revenues by admitting more private-pay residents and by establishing higher private-pay charges.

Regulatory approaches to cost containment typically control the capacity of the supply-side, prices, and utilization (Exhibit 2–1). Supply-side constraints are accomplished through "health planning." Planning enables policymakers to limit the number of hospital beds and diffusion of costly technology, but regulatory limits on the health care system's capacity inevitably create monopolies on the supply-side. To make sure that these artificially created monopolies do not exploit their economic power, health planning is always coupled with stiff price and budgetary controls (Reinhardt 1994). Countries with national health care programs

Exhibit 2–1 Regulation-Based and Competition-Based Cost-Containment Strategies

Regulation-Based Cost-Containment Strategies	
Supply-side controls	Restrictions on capital expenditures (new construction, renovations, and technology diffusion)
	Example: Certificate of need
	Restrictions on supply of physicians
	Example: Entry barriers for foreign medical graduates
Price controls	Artificially determined prices
	Examples: Reimbursement formulas
	Prospective payment systems
	Diagnosis-related groups
	Resource utilization groups
	Global budgets
Utilization controls	Peer review organizations
Competition-Based Cost-Containment Strategies	
Demand-side incentives	Cost sharing
	Sharing of premium costs
	Deductibles and co-payments
Supply-side regulation	Antitrust regulation
Payer-driven competition	Competition among insurers
	Competition among providers
Utilization controls	Managed care

tightly control supply. Demand-side constraints are used in the form of utilization control. These countries also use global budgets to restrict payments to hospitals and physicians, and place limitations on total expenditures. This simultaneous and comprehensive approach cannot work in the United States due to the system's fragmentation because of multiple payers. Instead, the United States can only implement piecemeal programs.

Health Planning

Health planning refers to a government undertaking to align and distribute health care resources so that in the eyes of the government, it will achieve desired health outcomes for all people. The planning function becomes critical in a centrally controlled national health care program so that the basic health care needs of the population are met and expenditures are maintained at predetermined levels. Health planning employs supply-side constraints to control health care expenditures. The central planning function does not fit so well in a system that is largely private because of the absence of a central administrative agency to monitor the system. Instead, the system is governed by market forces, and the types of health care services, their geographic distribution, access to these services, and the prices charged by providers develop independently of any preformulated plans. Levels of expenditures cannot be predetermined, and such a system is not conducive to achieving broad social objectives. Nevertheless, the United States has tried some forms of health planning on voluntary or mandated bases, but these efforts have met with limited success.

Some of the early efforts to control health care costs in the United States took the form of voluntary health planning. The goal was to minimize duplication of services. Early forms of health planning—in the 1930s and 1940s—were primarily the result of communitywide voluntary organizations, called hospital councils, which were established by hospitals in some of the largest cities. Hospitals agreed to share or consolidate services, or they traded the closing of a service in one hospital for the expansion of another service (Williams 1995, 154). Voluntary planning worked only on a limited basis and only in instances where participating hospitals could gain an advantage through cooperative planning. Consequently, voluntary planning contributed little to overall efficiency (Gottlieb 1974).

The federal government got involved in health planning after the passage of Medicare and Medicaid in the 1960s. These programs were designed to achieve broad social objectives by extending health care access to the underprivileged, but the passage of these programs generated an explosion in health care spending. Recognizing the increasing dollars that the federal government was putting into health care, Congress believed that it had the right to control escalating costs (Williams 1995, 154). The comprehensive health planning legislation of the mid-1960s mandated the establishment of local and state health planning agencies. These agencies assessed local health care needs and advocated better coordination and distribution of resources. However, the agencies had little or no actual regulatory power and were largely ineffective (Williams 1995, 154). When these agencies were evaluated, planned and unplanned areas had the same amount of duplication of facilities and services, and the rate of increase in hospital costs was the same (May 1974). The Health Planning and Resource Development Act of 1974 was enacted to provide incentives and penalties that would encourage states to adopt *certificate-of-need* (CON) legislation (Feldstein 1993, 273) in an attempt to implement an enhanced regulatory approach.

CON statutes were state-enacted legislation whose primary purpose was to control capital expenditures by health facilities. The CON process required prior approval from a state government agency for construction of new facilities, such as hospitals and nursing homes. Similar approvals were required for the expansion of existing facilities or the acquisition of expensive equipment. Approvals were based on the demonstration of a community need for additional services. Although the reasons given for the CON legislation were better planning of resources and control of increasing expenditures, in reality, the adoption of CON was easier in states having greater competition among hospitals (Wendling and Werner 1980), indicating that hospitals supported CON legislation when it was to their own benefit. These hospitals did not want additional capital spending on new construction and equipment by their competitors. On the other hand, CON laws did not seem to lower hospital expenditures on a per patient day basis. CON also represented a conservative approach to containing the rise in hospital costs because it did not address reimbursement and provided no incentives to change utilization behavior in patients or physicians (Feldstein 1993, 273). In the case of nursing homes, however, CON regulations have been used to contain Medicaid costs. In the face of a growing demand for nursing home beds, the CON regulations have restricted the supply of nursing home beds that otherwise would have been utilized. Because Medicaid plays a significant role in financing nursing home care, the added utilization would have in-creased overall Medicaid costs. The downside is that for years CON regulations have restricted genuine competition in the nursing home industry.

In the early 1980s, the US government moved away from its commitment to health care planning. The Health Planning and Resource Development Act was repealed in 1986. Between 1983 and 1988, 11 states followed the federal government and dropped their CON programs (Altman and Wallack 1996). By 2007, 19 states no longer had CON regulation (Ross 2007). However, several states have retained their programs, and others have reactivated them as a boom in outpatient care and ambulatory surgery centers has led to fears of oversaturation.

Price Controls

In 1971, President Nixon imposed the Economic Stabilization Program (ESP) as an economywide measure to contain general inflation through wage and price controls. The ESP limited the amount by which hospitals could raise their prices from year to year (Williams and Torrens 1993). Although controls on most of the economy were dropped by the end of 1971, the special problems of health care inflation led the administration to keep tight controls on the health care sector through 1974 (Altman and Wallack 1996). The ESP controls did generate a moderating influence on price increases for most medical services; however, the program had placed no limits on the quantity of services (Altman and Eichenholz 1976). For example, the quantity of services delivered to Medicare patients increased by about 10% during the first year of the ESP and between 8% and 15%, depending on physician specialty, during the second year (Gabel and Rice 1985). Also, the costs of production remained relatively unchanged. Therefore, once controls were lifted, inflation returned to its precontrol levels (Altman and Eichenholz 1976). ESP demonstrated that, although price increases can be limited for a short period, effective controls on total spending require much more extensive limits on the costs of production as well as on the quantity of services utilized (Altman and Wallack 1996).

During 1984 and 1986, Medicare froze physician fees; however, during each year fees were frozen, per-enrollee physician expenditures increased by at least 10% (Mitchell et al. 1988) because physicians could induce demand and thus increase the quantity of services provided. Similar results from price controls have been demonstrated in other countries. Perhaps the most important effort to control prices of inpatient hospital care was the conversion of hospital

Medicare reimbursement from cost-plus to a prospective system based on diagnosis-related groups (DRGs) authorized under the Social Security Amendments of 1983. The DRG-based reimbursement significantly reduced growth in inpatient hospital spending, but had little impact on total per capita Medicare cost inflation because costs were shifted from the inpatient to the outpatient sector (Figure 2–7). Use of per capita spending data in Figure 2–7 controls for the growth in Medicare population; hence, the increased rate of spending in the outpatient sector and the corresponding decline in the inpatient sector are mainly attributable to the types of services.

Most states have also employed price-control measures to control their Medicaid expenditures. Both retrospective and prospective methods have been used to define pay-

Figure 2–7 Percent Increase in Per Capita Medicare Spending with 1970 as the Base Year.

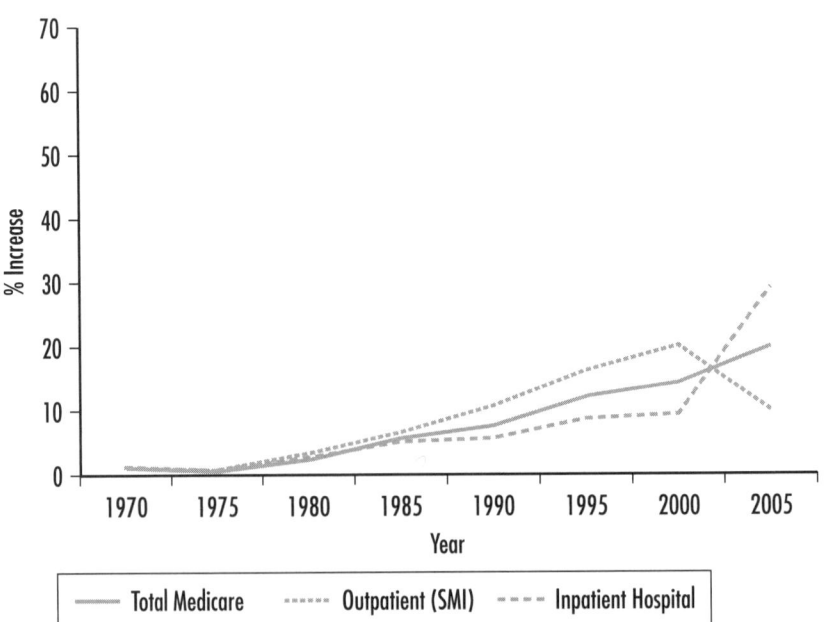

Sources: Data from *Health, United States, 1995*, p. 263; *Health, United States, 2002*, p. 322; *Health, United States, 2006*, p. 404, National Center for Health Statistics.

ment rates for hospitals and nursing homes. Often, complex formulas are used which, in essence, produce arbitrary reimbursement rates and rate ceilings. For example, two neighboring states can have sizable differences in Medicaid reimbursement for practically the same level of services.

Another rate-setting mechanism instituted the most significant change in the way Medicare pays physicians. It was the Omnibus Budget Reconciliation Act (OBRA) of 1989, which was implemented in 1992. The law authorized Medicare's Physician Payment Reform Program (MPPRP) to establish a national Medicare Fee Schedule (MFS). The MFS is based on a resource-based relative value scale (RBRVS). In other words, physicians are paid according to relative value units established for more than 7,000 covered services. A volume performance standard (VPS) was implemented to contain the annual rate of growth in Medicare physician payments. The program seems to have had some success. Between 1992 and 1997, the average annual growth in total Part B expenditures was 9.2%, compared to 6.1% for physician services. Between 1999 and 2005, total Part B expenditures increased from $82.3 to $152.4 billion (National Center for Health Statistics 2006).

The most sweeping price-control initiatives were authorized by the Balanced Budget Act (BBA) of 1997 for Medicare postacute services, namely, home health and skilled nursing facility services, which had been left untouched by the earlier prospective payment system for inpatient hospital care.

Another recent development in Medicare reimbursement is the move toward pay-for-performance. Pay-for-performance, which is receiving attention in both the private and public sectors, aims to align provider payments with the quality of care provided. In 2003, as part of the Medicare Prescription Drug, Improvement, and Modernization Act, the US Congress asked the Institute of Medicine (IOM) to assess the potential for implementing pay-for-performance in the Medicare program (IOM, 2004). Specifically, the IOM studied the performance measure set that could be used, the payment policy that could be used, and the key implementation issues involved, such as data and information technology requirements. The IOM found mixed evidence regarding the effectiveness of pay-for-performance demonstration programs, and it noted that unintended adverse consequences of pay-for-perfomance could include decreased access to care, increased disparities in care, and impediments to innovation. However, the IOM concluded that careful monitoring of pay-for-performance could minimize these adverse ·consequences. Further, the IOM argued that if Medicare payment structures were left unchanged, they would pose a barrier to improved quality of care. The IOM recommended a phased approach to implementing pay-for-performance in Medicare, consisting of small-scale implementation initially, allowing for adjustments as needed before launching large-scale changes.

The Medicare program is not alone in considering pay-for-performance strategies. At least 12 states have instituted pay-for-performance in their Medicaid programs (CMS, 2007). While these programs are in the early stages of development, the Centers for Medicare and Medicaid Services is offering technical assistance to states who are implementing and evaluating pay-for-performance.

Peer Review

The term *peer review* refers to the general process of medical review of utilization and quality when it is carried out directly or under the supervision of physicians (Wilson and Neuhauser 1985, 270). Based on this concept, the Social Security Amendments of 1972 required the establishment of professional standards review organizations (PSROs). These associations of physicians reviewed professional and institutional services provided under Medicare and Medicaid. The stated purpose was monitoring and control of cost and quality. When Congress evaluated the performance of PSROs for their cost-control effectiveness, the program had not produced any net savings. Because of their questionable effectiveness, the PSROs were replaced in 1984 by a new system of peer review organizations (PROs). *PROs* are statewide private organizations composed of practicing physicians and other health care professionals who are paid by the federal government to review the care provided to Medicare beneficiaries. Each state has a PRO. To control utilization, PROs determine whether care is reasonable, necessary, and provided in the most appropriate setting. PROs also decide whether care meets standards of quality generally accepted by the medical profession. PROs can deny payments if care is not medically necessary or not delivered in the most appropriate setting (Health Care Financing Administration [HCFA] 1996). PROs are now referred to as Quality Improvement Organizations (*QIOs*).

Cost Containment — Competitive Approaches

Competition refers to rivalry among sellers for customers (Dranove 1993). In health care delivery, it means that providers of health care services will try to attract patients who can choose among several different providers.

Although competition more commonly refers to price competition, it may also be based on technical quality, amenities, access, or other factors (Dranove 1993). Because competition is an essential element for the operation of free markets, competitive approaches are also referred to as market-oriented approaches.

During the Reagan presidency in the 1980s, competitive reforms were given preference because of growing interest in market-oriented approaches in many sectors of the economy. These reforms were accompanied by waning interest in comprehensive health care reform at the national level. Market-oriented reforms were accompanied by mounting cost-containment efforts in the private sector and the growth of managed care. Competitive reforms have been diverse and have often entailed simultaneous reforms in the regulation of health care markets (Arnould et al. 1993). Competitive strategies fall into four broad categories: demand-side incentives, supply-side regulation, payer-driven price competition, and utilization controls (Exhibit 2–1).

Demand-Side Incentives

The underlying notion of cost sharing is that if consumers pay more of the insurance cost, they will be more cost-conscious in selecting the insurance plan that best serves their needs. They will not automatically opt for the most comprehensive plan. Also, when consumers pay a larger share of the cost of health care services they use, they will consume services more judiciously. In essence, cost sharing encourages consumers to ration their own health care. By foregoing unnecessary services, health care consumers can save money. Their cost-conscious behavior then leads to lower costs within the health delivery system as unnecessary utilization is minimized and the system becomes more cost-efficient.

Findings of the Rand Health Insurance Experiment, discussed earlier, have been confirmed by more recent evidence. In addition, Wong and colleagues (2001) demonstrated that, as a result of cost sharing, people are more likely to forego professional services for minor ailments than for more serious problems. Only very high levels of cost sharing deterred the use of medical care considered appropriate and necessary.

Supply-Side Regulation

US antitrust laws prohibit business practices that stifle competition among providers. These practices include price fixing, price discrimination, exclusive contracting arrangements, and mergers the Department of Justice deems anticompetitive. The purpose of antitrust policy is to ensure the competitiveness, and thus the efficiency, of economic markets. In a competitive environment, MCOs, hospitals, and other health care organizations have to be cost-efficient to survive.

Payer-Driven Price Competition

Generally speaking, consumers drive competition. However, because health care markets are imperfect, patients are not typical consumers in the marketplace because insured patients lack the incentive to be good shoppers and because patients face information barriers that prevent them from being efficient shoppers. Despite the information boom, it is extremely difficult for individual patients or their surrogates to obtain needed information on cost and quality. Payer-driven competition in the form of managed care has overcome the drawbacks of patient-driven competition (Dranove 1993). Payer-driven competition occurs at two different points. First, employers shop for the best value in terms of the cost of premiums and the benefits package (competition among insurers). Second, MCOs shop for the best value from providers of health services (competition among providers).

Utilization Controls

Managed care also helps overcome some of the other inefficiencies of an imperfect health care market. The utilization controls in managed care have cut through some of the unnecessary or inappropriate services provided to consumers. Managed care is designed to intervene in the decisions made by care providers to ensure that they give only appropriate and necessary services, and that they provide the services efficiently. MCOs base this intervention on information that is not generally available to consumers. MCOs thus act on the consumer's behalf (Dranove 1993).

Access to Care

In broad terms, *access* to care is the ability to obtain needed, affordable, convenient, acceptable, and effective personal health services in a timely manner. Access has several key implications for health and health care delivery.

- Access to medical care is one of the key determinants of health, along with environment, lifestyle, and heredity factors.

- Access is a significant benchmark in assessing the effectiveness of the medical care delivery system. For example, access can be used to evaluate national trends against specific goals, such as those proposed in Healthy People 2010, or to evaluate the performance and accountability of health care plans and providers.

- Measures of access reflect whether or not the delivery of health care is equitable.

- Recently, with the growth of managed care and the ensuing integration of health care delivery functions (financing, insurance, delivery, and payment), access is increasingly linked to quality of care and the efficient use of needed services.

Although "access" is a familiar term often employed by popular and academic media, it can indicate several different concepts. It may refer to whether an individual has a usual source of care (such as a primary care physician), the actual use of health services (based on availability, convenience, referral, etc.), or it may reflect the acceptability of particular services (according to an individual's preferences and values). In the 1970s, it was commonly perceived that more use was better, and the policy objective was to overcome barriers to access and to increase utilization. In the 1980s, under resource constraints, this belief was seriously challenged. The beginning of DRGs and prospective reimbursement mechanisms marked the end of unlimited use.

Framework of Access

The conceptualization of access to care (see Figure 2–8) can be traced to Andersen (1968) and was later refined by Aday and Andersen (1975) and Aday and colleagues (1980). Andersen (1968) believed that in addition to need, predisposing and enabling conditions also prompt some people to use more medical services than others. Predisposing conditions include an individual's sociodemographic characteristics, such as age, sex, education, marital status, family size, race and ethnicity, and religious preference. These factors indicate a person's propensity to use medical care. For example, holding everything else constant, elderly people are more likely to use medical care than young people are. The enabling conditions are income, socioeconomic status, price of medical services, financing of medical services, and occupation. They focus on the individual's means enabling that person to use medical care. For example, holding everything else constant, those with high incomes are more likely to use medical care than those with low incomes, particularly in countries where no national health insurance is provided.

The distinction between predisposing and enabling conditions can be applied to assess the equity of a health care system (Aday et al. 1993). To the extent that significant differences in medical care utilization can be explained by need and certain predisposing characteristics (e.g., age, gender), the delivery of medical care is considered equitable. When enabling characteristics create significant differences in medical care utilization, the delivery of medical care is considered inequitable.

This access to care model has been expanded to include characteristics of health policy and the health care delivery system (Aday et al. 1980). Examples of health policy include major health care financing initiatives (Medicare, Medicaid, State Children's Health Initiative) and organization of health services delivery (Medicaid managed care, community health centers). Character-

Figure 2–8 The Expanded Behavioral Model.

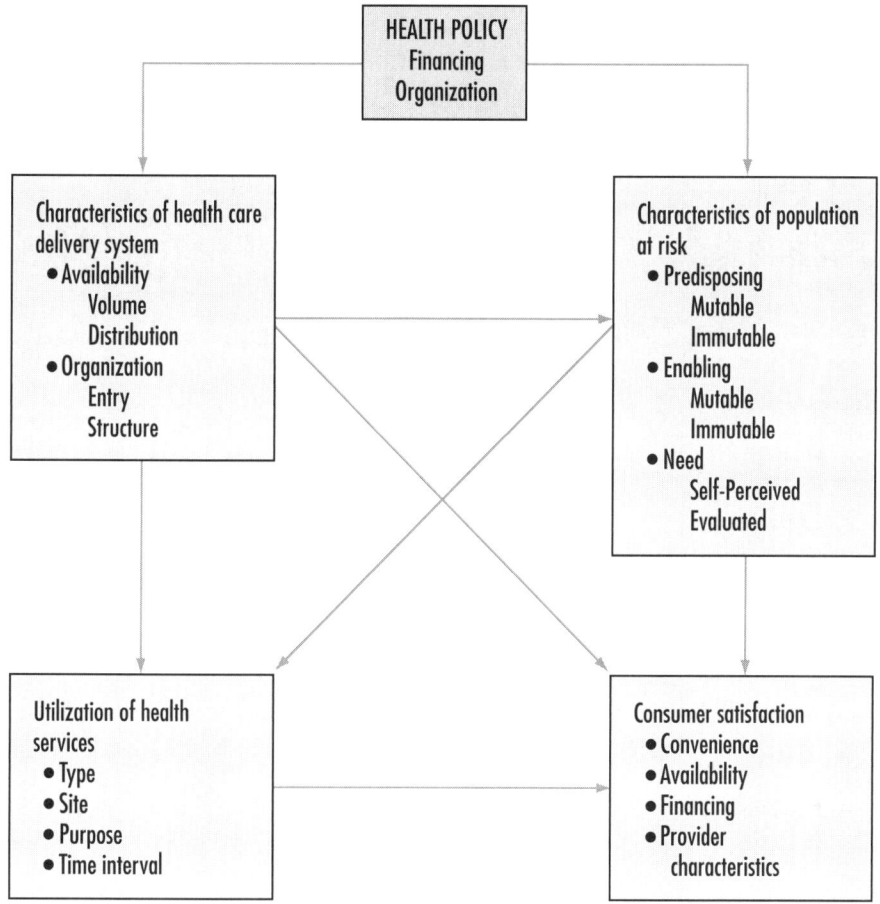

istics of the health care delivery system include availability (volume and distribution of services) and organization (mechanisms of entry into, and movement within, the system). Both health policy and the health care delivery system are aggregate components in contrast to the individual components of predisposing, enabling, and need characteristics. The expanded model recognizes the importance of systemic and structural barriers to access and is useful in comparing access to care among countries with different health policies and health care delivery systems.

Managed care's growth and the ensuing integration of the health care delivery functions represent a fundamental change in health care delivery. Accordingly, the access framework must be updated to reflect the new paradigm under managed care. Gold contributed a revised framework for access in the context of managed care (Docteur et al. 1996) (see Figure 2–9). According to this framework, access to care is a two-stage process in a managed care environment. In the first stage, individuals select among the health plans available to them, constrained

Figure 2–9 Framework for Access in the Managed Care Context.

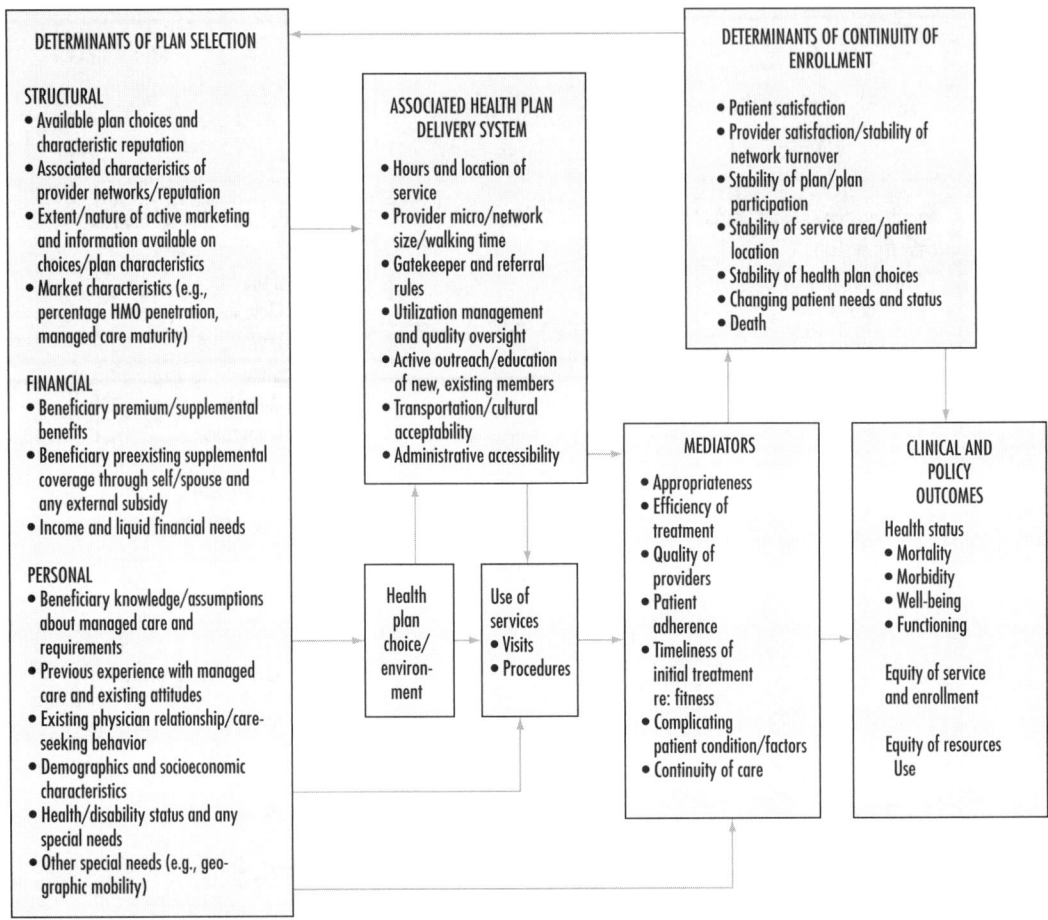

Source: Reprinted from E. Docteur and M. Gold, "Shifting the Paradigm," *Health Care Financing Review* 17, no. 4 (1996): p. 12.

by structural, financial, and personal characteristics. In the second stage, individuals seek medical care, constrained by both plan-specific and nonplan factors. The framework accounts for people enrolling and staying with the plan or disenrolling. It also links actual utilization with clinical and policy outcomes. Although comprehensive models are useful in conceptualizing access to care, they are difficult to test because of the range of variables and the differing levels of analysis they require. Empirical research is more likely to focus on specific dimensions of access.

Dimensions of Access

Penchansky and Thomas (1981) described access to care as consisting of five dimensions: availability, accessibility, accommodation, affordability, and acceptability.

Availability refers to the fit between service capacity and individuals' requirements. Availability-related issues include whether primary and preventive services are available to patients; whether enabling services, such as transportation, language, and social services, are made available by the provider;

whether the health plan has sufficient specialists to care for patients' needs; and whether access to primary care services is provided 24 hours a day, 7 days a week.

Accessibility refers to the fit between the locations of providers and patients. It is likely that individuals with different enabling conditions (e.g., transportation) may have different perceptions of accessibility. Accessibility-related issues include convenience (Can the provider be reached by public or private transportation?), design (Is the provider site designed for convenient use by disabled or elderly patients?), and payment options (Will the provider accept patients regardless of payment source, e.g., Medicare, Medicaid?).

Affordability refers to individuals' ability to pay. Even individuals with insurance often have to consider deductibles and co-payments prior to utilization. Affordability-related questions include: Are insurance premiums too high? Are deductibles and co-payments reasonable for the services covered under the plan? Are prescription prices affordable?

Accommodation refers to the fit between how resources are organized to provide services and the individual's ability to use the arrangement. Accommodation-related questions include: Can a patient schedule an appointment? Are scheduled office hours compatible with most patients' work and way of life? Can most of the urgent cases be seen within one hour? Can most patients with acute, but nonurgent, problems be seen within one day? Can most appropriate requests for routine appointments, such as preventive exams, be met within one week? Does the plan permit walk-in services?

Acceptability is based on the attitudes of patients and providers and refers to the compatibility between patients' attitudes about providers' personal and practice characteristics, and providers' attitudes toward their clients' personal characteristics and values. Acceptability issues include waiting time for scheduled appointments; whether patients are encouraged to ask questions and review their records; and whether patients and providers are accepted regardless of race, religion, or ethnic origin.

Types of Access

Andersen (1997) described four main types of access: potential access, realized access, equitable or inequitable access, and effective and efficient access.

Potential access refers to both health care system characteristics and enabling characteristics. Examples of health care system characteristics include capacity (e.g., physician–population ratio), organization (e.g., managed care penetration), and financing mechanisms (e.g., health insurance coverage). Enabling characteristics include personal (e.g., income) and community resources (e.g., residence).

Realized access refers to the type, site, and purpose of health services (Aday 1993). The type of utilization refers to the category of services rendered: physician, dentist, or other practitioners; hospital or long-term care admission; prescriptions; medical equipment; and so on. The site of utilization refers to the place where services are received (e.g., inpatient setting, such as short-stay hospital, mental institution, or nursing home; or ambulatory setting, such as hospital outpatient department, emergency department, physician's office, staff HMO, public health clinic, community health center, freestanding emergency center, or patient's home). The purpose of utilization refers to the reason medical care was sought: for health maintenance in the absence of symptoms (primary prevention), for the diagnosis or treatment of illness to return to well-being (secondary prevention or illness related), or for rehabilitation or maintenance in the case of a chronic health problem (tertiary prevention or custodial care).

Equitable access refers to the distribution of health care services according to the patient's self-perceived need (e.g., symptoms, pain, physical and functional status) or evaluated need as determined by a health professional (e.g., medical history, test results). Inequitable access refers to services distributed according to enabling characteristics (e.g., income, insured status).

Effective and efficient care links realized access to health outcomes (Institute of Medicine 1993). For example, does adequate prenatal care lead to successful birth outcomes, as measured by birth weight? Is immunization related to reduction of vaccine-preventable childhood diseases, such as diphtheria, measles, mumps, pertussis, polio, rubella, and tetanus? Are preventive services related to the early detection and diagnosis of treatable diseases? The concepts of effectiveness and efficiency link access to quality of care.

Measurement of Access

Using the conceptual models, access can be measured at three different levels: individual, health plan, and the delivery system. Access indicators at the individual level include (1) measures of medical services utilization relative to enabling and predisposing factors while controlling for need for care (Aday and Andersen, 1975) and (2) the patient's assessment of the interaction with the provider. Examples include differences in physician visits by race/ethnicity, gender, age, income, and insurance. Patients' perceived level of access is closely related to patient satisfaction with care and is part of the access framework (Aday et al. 1984).

At the health plan level, indicators include (1) plan characteristics that affect enrollment, such as cost of premium, deductibles, co-payments, coverage for preventive care, authorization of new and expensive procedures, physician referral incentives, and out-of-plan use; (2) plan practices that affect access, such as travel time to a usual source of care and waiting time to see a physician (accessibility), whether an appointment is necessary, hours of operation, language and other enabling services (accommodation), the content of encounters, including tests ordered and done, and referral to specialists (contact); and (3) plan quality as measured by the Health Plan Employer Data and Information Set (HEDIS) (discussed later) and patient satisfaction surveys.

Indicators of access at the level of the health care delivery system comprise ecological measures that affect populations rather than individuals. System indicators help study access in an environmental context; that is, how context affects the access of persons and groups. Examples of system access indicators include health policies or programs related to access, physician–population ratio, hospital beds per 1,000 population, percentage of population with insurance coverage, median household income, state per capita spending on welfare and preventive care, and percentage of population without access to primary care physicians.

Population-based surveys supported by federal statistical agencies are the major sources of data for conducting access-to-care analyses. Large national surveys, such as the National Health Interview Survey, the Medical Expenditure Panel Survey (MEPS), and the Community Tracking Survey are the leading data sources used to monitor access trends and other issues of interest. MEPS is a series of surveys that contain data on health care use and expenditures (e.g., inpatient, outpatient, and office-based care; dental care; and prescription medications), health insurance coverage, access to care, sources of payment, health status and disability, medical conditions, health care quality, and socioeconomic and demographic measures.

Other well-known national surveys include the Current Population Survey and Survey of Income and Program Participation (Bureau of the Census), which collects information on population characteristics. The Area Resource File (Bureau of Health Professions) pools information on characteristics of population and the health care delivery system. The National Health and Nutrition Examination Survey (National Center for Health Statistics [NCHS]) collects information on demographics, prevalence of selected diseases, nutrition, and behavioral risk factors. The National Hospital Discharge Survey (NCHS) provides data on short-stay hospital discharges and utilization. The Ambulatory Medical Care Survey (NCHS) provides data on ambulatory medical encounters. The National Hospital Ambulatory Medical Care Survey (NCHS) provides data on ambulatory hospital encounters. The National Nursing Home Survey (NCHS) provides data on nursing homes and utilization, nursing home residents, and nursing home staff. The Behavioral Risk Factor Survey (Centers for Disease Control and Prevention) provides data on health practices and behavioral risks of illness.

In addition, the federal government also collects data on special topics. Human immunodeficiency virus (HIV) and acquired immune deficiency syndrome (AIDS) were studied in the AIDS Cost and Services Utilization Survey 1991 to 1992 and the HIV Cost and Services Utilization Study 1994 to 1998. Managed care was studied in the Consumer Assessment of Health Plans Study 1996, and mental health is being examined in the Mental Health Care Services Study. Health care utilization by veterans, military staff, and dependents has been researched in the National Survey of Veterans 1994; the Patient Satisfaction Survey, Patient Treatment File; and AQCESS CHAMPUS. The Medicare Current Beneficiary Survey, the Medicare Statistical System, the Medicaid Data System, and the Medicaid Demonstration Projects (1983–1984, 1992–1996) have collected data relevant to Medicare and Medicaid. Other studies report on community health centers (Bureau of Common Reporting Requirement and Uniform Data System), immunization (National Immunization Survey), ambulatory surgery (National Survey of Ambulatory Surgery), home and hospice care (National Home and Hospice Care Survey), inpatient facilities (National Health Provider Inventory), aging (Longitudinal Survey on Aging), nursing homes (National Nursing Home Survey Follow-Up), insurance (National Employer Health Insurance Survey), and vital statistics (Vital Statistics of the US). The Bureau of Primary Care, Health Resources and Services Administration, collects information on vulnerable populations served by community health centers. In addition to the Uniform Data System, which collects center-specific financial, patient, and provider information, the Bureau regularly launches large-scale data collection on individual users. The Community Health Center Visit Survey, modeled after the National Ambulatory Medical Care Survey, collects information on patient visits to community health centers. The Community Health Center User Survey, modeled after the

National Health Interview Survey, collects information from users of community health centers on a wide range of topics associated with health care and health practices.

In addition to the federal government, states, associations, and research institutions also regularly collect data on topics of interest to them. Examples of state-based initiatives include state health services utilization data (all-payer hospital discharge data systems), state managed care data (managed care encounter data), and state Medicaid enrollee satisfaction data (Medicaid enrollee satisfaction surveys). Examples of association-based initiatives include data on physicians (American Medical Association's Physician Masterfile and the Periodic Survey of Physicians 1969 to present) and hospitals (American Hospital Association's Annual Survey of Hospitals 1946 to present). Examples of research institution-based initiatives include collecting data on the health care delivery system (Center for Evaluative Clinical Sciences: Dartmouth Atlas of Health Care in the US), women's health (Kaiser Family Foundation: Women's Health Survey 2004), minority health (Commonwealth Fund: Minority Health Survey 1997), family health (Urban Institute National Survey of America's Families 1997, 1999, 2002), health insurance (Commonwealth Fund Bienniel Health Insurance Survey 2005), and access to care (Robert Wood Johnson Foundation National Access Surveys).

With the growth of managed care, encounter databases have become increasingly critical in recording and evaluating access. Good encounter databases combine electronic medical records (which contain diagnostic information based on ICD-9 and CPT codes) with administrative data (which contain plan, individual, payment, and cost information). In addition to the federal government, private nonprofit research centers also collect information on managed care. Examples are the National Health Maintenance Organization Census (1977 to the present, sponsored by Interstudy) and the HEDIS (sponsored by the National Committee for Quality Assurance [NCQA]).

Access to care data for vulnerable populations is systematically collected by the Sentinel Centers Network (SCN) initiative. The SCN is a partnership among the Bureau of Primary Health Care (BPHC), HRSA, the Johns Hopkins Bloomberg School of Public Health, and Morehouse School of Medicine. They are all participants in the SCN and BPHC health center grantees. The SCN is currently composed of 37 participants located in the majority of states in the United States. Approximately 650 health care practitioners provide services to 1 million registered users within the SCN. The SCN data system is the first primary care administrative database that focuses exclusively on care delivery and outcomes for medically underserved populations.

Current Indicators of Access

In the United States, significant barriers to access still exist at both the individual and the system level. People without health insurance, minorities, low-income individuals, those with little formal education, or those with special needs defined by disability and chronic illness continue to face greater barriers to access than the rest of the population. Access is best predicted by race, income, and occupation. These three factors are interrelated. People belonging to minority groups tend to be poor, not well educated, and more likely to work in jobs that pose greater health risks.

Geographic disparities in access are also present, and individuals from rural areas face greater access barriers than those residing in urban areas. Rural Americans have higher

Table 2–3 Visits to Office-Based Physicians, 2004

Characteristic	Number of Visits (million)	Percentage Distribution	Visits per 100 Persons/Year
All visits	910.9	100.0	315.9
Age			
Under 15 years old	147.9	16.2	243.4
15–44 years old	264.9	29.1	410.3
45–64 years old	264.1	29.0	376.2
65–74 years old	113.4	12.4	622.6
75 years old and over	120.6	13.2	733.6

Source: Data from US Bureau of the Census. *Statistical Abstracts of the United States, 2007,* Washington, DC, p. 112.

mortalities and morbidities and shorter life expectancies than their urban counterparts (Cordes 1989; DeFriese and Ricketts 1989; Rowland and Lyons 1989; Sherman 1991). Rural Americans are more likely to be poor, to suffer from chronic impairment, to be uninsured if under 65 years of age and to be elderly than their urban counterparts (Norton and McManus 1989). The health care system available to address these problems, however, faces severe limitations, including maldistribution of physicians, lack of sufficient primary care services, and lack of access to care for geographic, financial, or discrimination/cultural reasons (Freeman et al. 1982; Sardell 1988). Tables 2–3 and 2–4 summarize physician contacts by categories of age, sex, race, income, and geographic location. Table 2–5 summarizes dental visits. These results are not adjusted for health need, however, and therefore are not true indicators of access. Rather, they provide utilization measures as a proxy for access.

It is society's duty to ensure that all have equitable access to an adequate level of health care. According to one view, economic scarcity is a relative measure. Scarcity in the US medical delivery system is largely the result of distributive practices that limit access for

Table 2–4 Physician Contacts, According to Selected Patient Characteristics, 1996

Characteristic	Physician Contacts per Person
Total	5.8
Sex	
Male	5.0
Female	6.5
Race and age	
White	5.8
Black	5.7
Family income	
Less than $16,000	7.5
$16,000–$24,999	5.5
$25,000–$34,999	5.6
$35,000–$44,999	5.9
$50,000 or more	5.3
Geographic region	
Northeast	5.7
Midwest	5.7
South	6.1
West	5.3
Location of residence	
Within MSA	5.8
Outside MSA	5.7

Source: Data from *Health, United States, 1999,* p. 229, National Center for Health Statistics, Division of Health Interview Statistics, 1999.

Table 2–5 Dental Visits in the Past Year among Persons 18–64 Years of Age, 2004

Characteristic	Percentage of Persons
All persons	64.0
Poverty status	
Poor	44.5
Near poor	47.6
Nonpoor	71.3
Race and Hispanic origin	
White, non-Hispanic	65.2
Black, non-Hispanic	56.9
Hispanic	49.6
Sex	
Male	60.5
Female	67.4

Source: Data from *Health, United States, 2006*, p. 329, National Center for Health Statistics.

those who are poor and those who live in rural areas. In the overall system, a surplus exists, for instance, of hospital beds and physicians practicing in urban areas. The problem is that these surpluses are not generally shifted to respond to need (Brown 1992).

There is a lack of access for the uninsured. Access, however, is also limited because of underinsurance and, for a few people, because of lifetime caps on health insurance. For years, these lifetime caps have been arbitrarily set at about $1 to $2 million. A number of otherwise insured Americans are affected by lifetime caps because of a costly catastrophic injury or illness. For example, the average lifetime cost of care for a person with a spinal cord injury who is ventilator-dependent can be more than $5 million. When the cap is reached, insurance companies stop coverage, although the need for medical care continues.

Quality of Care

One reason why the pursuit of quality in health care has trailed behind the emphasis on cost and access is the difficulty of defining and measuring quality. On the other hand, growth of managed care and the emphasis on cost containment have produced a heightened interest in quality because of the intuitive concern that control of costs may negatively impact quality. Indeed, changes occurring within the US health care delivery system in recent years have created fears of diminished quality because these changes have brought about disruptions in the way health care professionals are allowed to provide care and the way in which patients may seek care. Since the 1990s, quality has taken center stage in the delivery of health care. However, a great deal of ambiguity still exists about the definition of quality. There is still a long road ahead to specify what constitutes good quality in medical care, how to ensure it for patients, and how to reward providers and health plans whose outcomes indicate successes in quality improvement. One challenge in achieving such a goal is that patients, providers, and payers each define quality differently, which translates into different expectations of the health care delivery system and thus differing evaluations of its quality (McGlynn 1997).

The Institute of Medicine (IOM) has defined *quality* as "the degree to which health services for individuals and populations increase the likelihood of desired health outcomes and are consistent with current professional knowledge" (McGlynn 1997). The definition has several implications: (1) Quality performance occurs on a continuum, theoretically ranging from unacceptable to excellent. (2) The focus is on services provided by the health care delivery system (as opposed to individual behaviors). (3) Quality may be evaluated from the perspective of individuals and populations or communities. (4) The emphasis is on desired health outcomes. Research evidence must identify the services that improve health outcomes. (5) In the absence of scientific evidence regarding appropriateness of care, professional consensus can be used to develop criteria for the definition and measurement of quality (McGlynn 1997).

Although complete in many respects, the IOM definition leaves out the role of cost in the evaluation of quality. Even though the United States spends more of its national income on health care than other nations, Americans are not the healthiest people in the world. For example, based on comparative data on 37 countries, 27 nations had better outcomes than the United States on infant mortality rates in 2003, and 25 countries had better outcomes on life expectancy at birth for both males and females in 2002 (National Center for Health Statistics 2006). Clearly, more health care expenditures or a greater intensity of medical services does not produce better health. In other words, more is not better, and more does not represent better quality.

Another element missing from the IOM definition is the relationship between access and quality. Perhaps a key reason why the United States, despite its tremendous advances in medical technology, trails behind other industrialized nations in broad population measures of health is lack of access to basic health care for many Americans. Hence, unless access to primary care and preventive services is improved, population-based indicators of health are unlikely to improve. In other words, amelioration of the overall quality of the US health care delivery system would require universal access to basic health care.

Dimensions of Quality

Quality needs to be viewed from both micro and macro perspectives. The microview focuses on services at the point of delivery and their subsequent effects. It is associated with the performance of individual caregivers and health care organizations. The macroview looks at quality from the standpoint of populations. It reflects the performance of the entire health care delivery system.

The Microview

The micro dimension of health care quality encompasses the clinical aspects of care delivery, the interpersonal aspects of care delivery, and quality of life.

Clinical Aspects

Clinical aspects of care deal with technical quality, which evaluates the appropriateness of care according to several criteria. Some of the key criteria evaluated to determine clinical appropriateness of care are the facilities where care is delivered, the qualifications and skills of caregivers, the processes and interventions used, cost-efficiency of care, and the results or effects on patients' health.

Small area variations, discussed earlier in this chapter, compromise clinical quality. Geographic variations also indicate widespread inefficiencies. Hence, addressing the problem of clinical variations would result in improved cost as well as quality. The variability in the delivery of care cannot be blamed on physicians alone. The variations do not reflect negatively on the sincerity, honesty, or diligence of most physicians. One of the main causes of variability is that physicians often have to make decisions about phenomenally complex problems under difficult circumstances. Often, they are in the impossible position of not knowing the outcomes of different actions, but having to act anyway (Eddy 1994).

Incidents of medical errors in hospitals have been widely reported. For example, the IOM reported that 44,000 to 98,000 patients die in American hospitals each year because of medical errors, making "adverse events" the eighth leading cause of death in the United States (IOM 2000). Even though medical errors and adverse events in outpatient settings have not received as much emphasis, concerns do exist. One reason the outpatient sector has not come under the spotlight is that only a handful of states have implemented reporting systems for it (Lapetina and Armstrong 2002). Yet, evidence is slowly gathering for adverse occurrences in outpatient settings. For example, death and brain damage due to adverse anesthesia administration for children have been found to be more than twice as high in outpatient settings as in hospitals (Coté 2000). The mortality rate for lipoplasty, a cosmetic procedure for remodeling fat tissue under skin, is higher than it is for motor vehicle deaths and homicides; most of the deaths occur in outpatient settings (Minino and Smith 2001). As an increasing number of surgical procedures are now being performed in ambulatory clinics, surgi-centers, and physicians' offices, medical errors in the outpatient sector are likely to come under increased scrutiny.

Interpersonal Aspects

When quality is viewed from the patient's perspective, clinical quality remains important, but interpersonal aspects of care take on added significance. Patients generally lack technical expertise and often judge the quality of technical care indirectly by their perceptions of the practitioner's interest, concern, and demeanor during clinical encounters (Donabedian 1985). Interpersonal relations and satisfaction become even more important when placed within the holistic context of health care delivery. Positive interactions between patients and practitioners are major contributors to treatment success through greater patient compliance and return for care (Svarstad 1986). Expressions of love, hope, and compassion can enhance the healing effects of medical treatments. Without these elements, the quality of health care remains incomplete.

Interpersonal aspects of quality are also important from the standpoint of organizational management. Consumers—that is, patients and their surrogates—gain lasting impressions of organizational quality from the way they are treated by an organization's employees. Such employee–customer interactions include not just the direct caregivers but a variety of other employees associated with the health care organization, such as receptionists, workers in the cafeteria, housekeeping employees, and billing clerks.

To measure interpersonal aspects of quality, patient satisfaction surveys have been widely used by various types of health care organizations. Ratings by consumers provide the most appropriate method for evaluating interpersonal quality (McGlynn and Brook 1996). Satisfaction surveys have been used to give physicians feedback on important dimensions of interpersonal communication and service quality. Evidence suggests that such feedback has achieved widespread acceptance by physicians, with more than three-fourths of the physicians affected by such surveys reacting positively to their use (Reed et al. 2003).

Quality of Life

The concept of quality of life has received a great deal of attention in recent years because patients with chronic and/or debilitating diseases are living longer but in a declining state of health. Chronic problems often impose serious limitations on patients' functional status (including physical, social, and mental functioning), access to community resources and opportunities, and sense of well-being (Lehman 1995). In a composite sense, during or subsequent to disease, a person's own perception of health, ability to function, role limitations stemming from physical or emotional problems, and personal happiness are referred to as health-related quality of life (**HRQL**).

An even narrower definition of quality of life has been proposed. Although a few basic measurements might be applicable to everyone in every situation (general HRQL), many more are relevant only to a particular patient or to patients suffering from a specific disease (disease-specific HRQL). General HRQL refers to the essential or common components of overall well-being. Disease-specific HRQL is associated with the potential quality of life impacts of a specific disorder and its treatment. Disease-specific HRQL focuses entirely on impairments that are caused by a specific disorder and the effects and side effects of treatments for that disorder. For example, arthritis quality of life is concerned with joint pain and mobility and the side effects of antiinflammatory agents; depression quality of life deals with the symptoms of depression (such as suicidal thoughts) and such medication side effects as blurred vision, dry mouth, constipation, and impotence (Bergner 1989); and cancer-specific HRQL may include anxiety about cancer recurrence (Ganz and Litwin 1996) and pain management.

Institution-related quality of life is also an important attribute of quality in addition to the clinical and interpersonal aspects. It refers to a patient's quality of life while confined in an institution as an inpatient. Factors contributing to institutional quality of life can be classified into three main groups: environmental comfort, self-governance, and caregiver attitudes. Cleanliness, safety, noise levels, odors, air circulation, environmental temperature, and furnishings are some of the key comfort factors that are particularly relevant to the physical aspects of institutional living. Factors associated with self-governance and staff attitudes, in particular, influence the emotional well-being of institutionalized patients. Self-governance means autonomy to make decisions, freedom to air grievances without fear of reprisal, and reasonable accommodation of personal likes and dislikes. Factors associated with caregiver attitudes are privacy and confidentiality, treatment from staff in a manner that maintains respect and dignity, and freedom from physical and/or emotional abuse.

The Macroview

The macroview encompasses systemwide efficiencies and outcomes, which include cost, access, and population health. Some of the other indicators of macro level quality are life expectancy, mortality rates, cause-specific mortality, low birth weight deliveries, and incidence and prevalence of specific diseases or chronic conditions. Access to health care has considerable influence on population health. The prospects of universal access in the United States are contingent on drastic reductions in health care expenditures. Without significant improvements in access, the US health care delivery system will continue to be rated behind most others in the developed world. From a systems standpoint, this predicament requires national policy initiatives, but it does not diminish the need to pursue quality improvements at the micro level over which practitioners, ancillary workers, and health care managers have more control.

Quality Assurance

The terms "quality assessment" and "quality assurance" are often encountered in literature on health care quality. Yet, these terms are not always well defined or differentiated. *Quality assessment* refers to the measurement of quality against an established standard. It includes the process of defining how quality is to be determined, identification of specific variables or indicators to be measured, collection of appropriate data to make the measurement possible, statistical analysis, and interpretation of the results of the assessment (Williams and Brook 1978). *Quality assurance* is synonymous with quality improvement. It is the process of institutionalizing quality through ongoing assessment and using the results of assessment for continuous quality improvement (CQI) (Williams and Torrens 1993). Quality assurance, then, is a step beyond quality assessment. It is a systemwide or organizationwide commitment to engage in the improvement of quality on an ongoing basis. Although the two activities— quality assessment and quality assurance— are related, quality assurance cannot occur without quality assessment. Quality assessment becomes an integral part of the process of quality assurance. On the other hand, it is possible to conduct quality assessment without engaging in quality assurance.

In the past, quality assurance focused on observing deviations from established standards by means of inspection techniques and was used in conjunction with punitive actions for noncompliance. The nursing home industry presents a typical case. Standards of patient care in nursing homes and the system for evaluating performance were developed mainly in conjunction with the certification of facilities for Medicare and/or Medicaid. Federal regulations developed by HCFA (now Centers for Medicare and Medicaid Services) are viewed as minimum standards or baseline criteria for defining quality of resident care in certified facilities. Compliance with the standards is monitored through annual inspections of the facilities (Singh 1997, 33–34), and serious noncompliance is punishable by monetary fines and threats of expulsion from Medicare and Medicaid. Although such external monitoring of quality is necessary (Lohr 1997), it is not quality assurance in the true sense. Rather, it is a rudimentary form of quality assessment that would be more appropriately referred to as "periodic monitoring of quality."

Quality assurance is based on the principles of total quality management (TQM), also referred to as CQI. The philosophy of TQM was developed and used in other industries before it was adapted for health care delivery. *TQM* is an integrative management concept of continuously improving the quality of delivered goods and services through the participation of all levels and functions of the organization (Evans 1993) to meet the needs and expectations of the customer. TQM encompasses five main elements: (1) Quality is an integrative concept. It must permeate everything that a health care organization does. In other words, it is not simply confined to the delivery of health services to patients, but applies equally to activities that support clinical care. Examples of supportive services include business office, housekeeping, and building and equipment maintenance functions. TQM must also have the support and commitment of the top management and managers at all levels. (2) The organization is committed to ongoing improvement. This means that the standards against which quality is assessed do not remain static. As soon as the current standards of performance are achieved, higher standards are set. The ultimate goal is to achieve a zero error rate or a 100% success rate. Even though such a state of perfection may never be attained, goals must nevertheless be set toward its achievement. (3) Everyone working in the organization plays a part in the production of quality goods and services. (4) TQM emphasizes the value of striving to exceed prevailing standards. This suggests an imperative to study the processes throughout the organization by which health care is produced and provided (Laffel and Blumenthal 1993). (5) TQM needs to be customer driven. The efforts of TQM are directed toward customer satisfaction. In a general sense, customers are the recipients (not necessarily the purchasers) of a service or product. From the organizational perspective, there are both internal and external customers. The organization's internal customers are the users of products or services that ultimately influence the quality of patient care. For example, nursing units are customers of the pharmacy, which must furnish the right medications as ordered by the physicians. The pharmacy is the customer of the physicians, who must prescribe legibly and correctly. Patients and communities are the external customers who ultimately benefit from the results of TQM. The adoption of TQM by many hospitals and health systems has streamlined administration, reduced lengths

of stay, improved clinical outcomes, and produced higher levels of patient satisfaction (HCIA Inc. and Deloitte & Touche 1997).

Quality Assessment

Quality assessment is particularly difficult because it requires the measurement of phenomena that are often subjective or qualitative. They must be quantified to be measured and compared. Measurement scales are developed to assess quality defined by qualitative concepts. Before these scales are used, their validity and reliability must be established. The *validity* of a scale is the extent to which it actually assesses what it purports to measure. If a measure is supposed to reflect the quality of care, one would expect improvements in quality to affect the measure positively. In other words, the measurement scale would show a higher score for improved quality and vice versa. *Reliability* reflects the extent to which the same results occur from repeated applications of a measure. The following sections survey some of the main criteria and mechanisms used to evaluate quality.

The Donabedian Model

In his well-known model to help define and measure quality in health care organizations, Donabedian proposed three domains in which health care quality should be examined: structure, process, and outcomes. Donabedian noted that all three domains are equally important. He also emphasized that these three approaches are complementary and should be used collectively to monitor care quality (Al-Assaf 1993b).

Structure, process, and outcomes are closely linked (Figure 2–10). The three

Figure 2–10 The Donabedian Model.

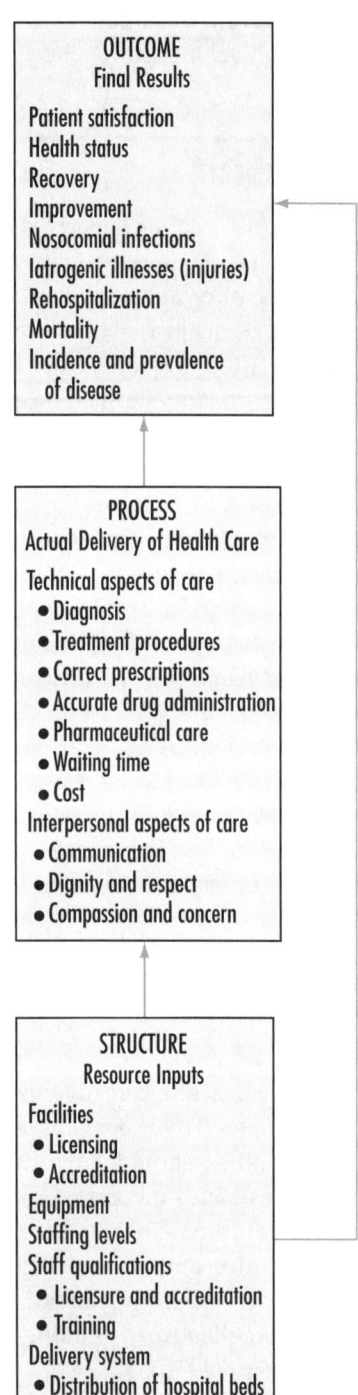

domains are also hierarchical. Structure is the foundation of the quality of health care. Good processes require a good structure. In other words, deficiencies in structure generally have a negative effect on the processes of health care delivery. Structure and processes together influence quality outcomes. Structure primarily influences process and has only a secondary direct influence on outcome. The model views quality strictly from the delivery system's perspective. It does not account for social and individual lifestyle and behavior factors that also have a significant influence on health status.

Structure

Structure has been defined as "the relatively stable characteristics of the providers of care, of the tools and resources they have at their disposal, and of the physical and organizational settings in which they work" (Donabedian 1980, 81). Structural criteria refer to the resource inputs, such as facilities, equipment, staffing levels, staff qualifications, programs, and the administrative organization (Guralnik et al. 1991; McElroy and Herbelin 1989). Structural measures indicate the extent to which health care organizations have the capability to provide adequate levels of care (Williams and Torrens 1993). Hence, structure provides an indirect measure of quality, under the assumption that a good structure enables health delivery professionals to employ good processes that would lead to good outcomes.

In the past, it was common to rely mostly on the evaluation of structural measures for quality assessment. As such, they were designed to ensure that certain minimum standards were met. Examples are licensing of facilities, accreditation of facilities by the Joint Commission on Accreditation of Healthcare Organizations (Joint Commission), and licensing and certification of health care professionals to ensure that they meet certain minimum qualifications. Training of personnel is designed to improve the structural elements of quality. From a system-wide macroperspective, structural elements include the number of physicians and hospital beds available per 1,000 population; the geographic distribution of physicians, hospitals, and nursing home beds; and the mix between primary care and specialist physicians.

Process

Process refers to the specific way in which care is provided. Examples of process are correct diagnostic tests, correct prescriptions, accurate drug administration, pharmaceutical care, waiting time to see a physician, and interpersonal aspects of care delivery. Peer review, discussed earlier in this chapter, was designed to serve a dual purpose: control costs and ensure that quality does not suffer. The activities of PROs rely mainly on process indicators in evaluating the quality of care provided to Medicare patients (Al-Assaf 1993a).

Like structure, process relates to patient care outcomes. In other words, structures and processes should be employed to achieve better outcomes. Some significant initiatives toward process improvement have been undertaken. Some main developments are clinical practice guidelines, cost-efficiency, critical pathways, and risk management.

Clinical Practice Guidelines

As discussed earlier, small area variations bring into question the appropriateness of care. In response, various professional groups, MCOs, and the government have embarked on the development of standardized practice guidelines. ***Clinical practice guidelines*** (also called medical practice guidelines) are explicit descriptions representing preferred clinical processes for specified conditions. A clinical practice guideline constitutes a plan to manage a clinical problem based on evidence whenever possible, and on consensus in the absence of evidence (Larsen 1996). Hence, clinical practice guidelines are designed to provide scientifically-based protocols to guide physicians' clinical decisions. Proponents believe that these guidelines simultaneously promote lower costs and better outcomes. Critics view guidelines as an administrative mechanism to reduce utilization. By the mid-1990s, 75 national organizations had developed approximately 1,800 sets of guidelines, and individual hospitals, MCOs, private researchers, and pharmaceutical manufacturers developed thousands of others (Firshein 1996).

The US Congress established the Agency for Health Care Policy and Research in 1989. This agency was reauthorized under the Healthcare Research and Quality Act of 1999, and was renamed Agency for Healthcare Research and Quality (AHRQ). Although the agency has a broad research agenda, one of its primary mandates is to build the scientific base of which health care practices work and which do not. In this role, the agency develops the information, tools, and strategies that decision-makers can use to make good clinical choices necessary to provide high-quality health care based on evidence. These activities have been mandated in the belief that they will eliminate inappropriate medical interventions and reduce health care costs (IOM 1990). AHRQ has established a National Guideline Clearinghouse (NGC) in partnership with the American Medical Association and the American

Association of Health Plans. The NGC is a comprehensive database of evidence-based clinical practice guidelines and related documents. It facilitates access to information produced by different organizations by making it all available at one site.

After some initial reluctance by physicians, current evidence suggests that clinical practice guidelines are being viewed positively. According to one report, among physicians affected by this care management tool, 66% expressed a positive view (only 8% were negative) on its overall effect on quality and efficiency of medical practice (Reed et al. 2003).

Cost-Efficiency

Also referred to as cost-effectiveness, ***cost-efficiency*** is an important concept in quality assessment. A service is cost-efficient when the benefit received is greater than the cost incurred to provide the service. Cost-efficiency uses the health production function to evaluate the relationship between increasing medical expenditures (or health risks) and improvements in health levels. As medical interventions and expenditures are increased, there is a curvilinear, rather than a constant, effect on improved health (Feldstein 1994, 26). At the start of medical treatment, each unit is likely to deliver benefits exceeding its costs, or benefits exceeding the potential risks. The marginal (i.e., additional) health benefits become smaller and risks become bigger, as more care is delivered and greater costs are incurred. An optimum point is reached when additional health benefits approximately equal the additional costs (or risks). Beyond this point, additional interventions result in fewer benefits in relation to the additional costs, or the risks are greater than the benefits. In economic terms, addi-

tional services beyond the optimum point produce diminishing marginal returns. This point also represents optimal quality, which serves as a point of demarcation between underutilization and overutilization.

Underutilization (underuse) occurs when the benefits of an intervention outweigh its risks or costs, and yet it is not used (Chassin 1991). Potential adverse health outcomes related to underutilization include hospitalizations that could be avoided by providing better medical access and timely care, low birth weight due to lack of prenatal care, infant mortality due to lack of early pediatric care, and low cancer survival rates due to lack of early detection and treatment. On the other hand, ***overutilization*** (overuse) occurs when the costs or risks of treatment outweigh its benefits, and yet additional care is delivered. When health care is overused, precious resources are wasted. Hence, inefficiency can be regarded as unethical because it deprives someone else of the potential benefits of health care. The principles of cost-efficiency indicate that health care costs can be reduced without lowering quality of care. Conversely, quality can be improved without increasing costs. A trade-off does not have to occur between cost and quality. Introduction of the prospective payment system (PPS) by Medicare is an example. The resulting discharge of patients "quicker and sicker" triggered by PPS initially raised some alarm concerning decreased quality, but it was found that processes of care in hospitals actually improved and mortality rates were unchanged or lower (Rogers et al. 1990). Other potential negative health outcomes that can be avoided by curtailing overuse include life-threatening drug interactions, nosocomial infections, and iatrogenic illnesses.

Critical Pathways

Critical pathways are outcome-based and patient-centered case management tools that are interdisciplinary, facilitating coordination of care among multiple clinical departments and caregivers. In the last few years, critical pathways have been used across multiple delivery settings. A critical pathway is a timeline that identifies planned medical interventions along with expected patient outcomes for a specific diagnosis or class of cases, often defined by a DRG. The outcomes and interventions included in the critical pathway are broadly defined. In addition to technical outcomes, pathways may measure such factors as patient satisfaction, self-reported health status, mental health, and activities of daily living (ADL). Interventions include treatments, medications, diagnostic tests, diet, activity regimens, consultations, discharge planning, and patient education. The critical pathway serves as a plan of action for all disciplines caring for the patient and incorporates a system for documenting and evaluating variances from the critical path plan. Critical pathways are unique to the institutions that develop them because they are based on the particular practices of that facility and its caregivers. A pathway also is customized to the patient population being served and the available patient care resources. Finally, critical pathways are meant to promote interdisciplinary collaboration within the environment of the hospital and its market. The latter occurs by making patients and families active participants in the process. For these reasons, critical pathways are difficult to replicate from one organization to another. Use of critical pathways reduces costs and improves quality by reducing errors, improving coordination among interdisciplinary players, streamlining case management functions, providing systematic data to assess care, and reducing variation in practice patterns (Giffin and Giffin 1994).

Risk Management

Risk management consists of proactive efforts to prevent adverse events related to clinical care and facilities operations and is especially focused on avoiding medical malpractice (Orlikoff 1988). Malpractice lawsuits are a deterrent to poor technical quality of care and provide redress for patients experiencing such care (Williams and Torrens 1993). In response to the threat of lawsuits, initiatives undertaken by a health care organization to review clinical processes and establish protocols for the specific purpose of reducing malpractice litigation can actually enhance quality. Because malpractice concerns also result in defensive medicine, risk management approaches should employ the principles of cost-efficiency along with standardized practice guidelines and critical pathways.

Threat of malpractice litigation also has a downside. Fear of litigation actually leads to a reluctance by hospitals and physicians to disclose preventable harm and actual medical errors. In this respect, it is believed that fear of litigation may actually conceal problems that may compromise patient safety (Lamb et al. 2003).

Outcomes

Outcomes refer to the effects or results obtained from utilizing the structure and processes of health care delivery. Outcomes are viewed by many as the bottom-line measure of the effectiveness of the health care delivery system (McGlynn and Brook 1996).

Positive outcomes suggest recovery from disease and improvement in health. They also suggest an overall improvement in health status through health promotion and disease prevention and adequate access to health care services. Outcomes are often gauged through a comparative assessment—between two time intervals—of the measures of morbidity, mortality, and health status. Other outcome measures include postoperative infection rates, nosocomial infections, iatrogenic illnesses, and rates of rehospitalization. Malpractice litigation is sometimes used as an outcome indicator because litigation seeks damages for negative outcomes. Another indicator of positive outcome is patient satisfaction (discussed earlier), which is assessed through questionnaires completed by patients and/or surrogates.

Quality outcomes are also evaluated using interview techniques and self-administered questionnaires to report on functional status, neuropsychiatric function, social function, and emotional and spiritual health. Determination of HRQL is an example. Typically, HRQL data are collected with self-report questionnaires, called "instruments," using survey research techniques. These instruments contain questions or items organized into scales. Each scale measures a different aspect or domain of HRQL. Some scales comprise dozens of items, whereas others may include only one or two items (Ganz and Litwin 1996). HRQL domains can be general, disease-specific, or institution-related.

None of the outcome measures provides a perfect assessment. Each measure focuses on a particular aspect of quality. Hence, using a combination of measures is likely to produce more objective results, but there is a cost and benefit trade-off. The greater the number of measures used for evaluating quality, the more costly the assessment process.

Quality Report Cards

The growing predominance of managed care raised concerns that efforts to control costs may jeopardize quality. The move to develop quality report cards for health plans responded to these concerns. The report cards can be used by employers and their employees to make health plan choices. Health Plan Employer Data and Information Set *(HEDIS)* has become the standard for reporting quality information on managed care health plans. This quality tool is a product of a partnership established in 1989 among health plans, employers, and the National Committee for Quality Assurance (NCQA), which now manages the HEDIS program. The latest edition is HEDIS 2007. Originally designed for private employers' needs as purchasers of health insurance, HEDIS has been adapted for use by the public, public insurers, and regulators. HEDIS 2007 contains over 70 measures across eight domains of care: effectiveness of care, access and availability of care, satisfaction with care, health plan stability, use of services, cost of care, informed health care choices, and health plan descriptive information (NCQA 2007). The HEDIS program has been criticized because disclosure is voluntary. In the absence of a national requirement, the voluntary aspect of reporting affords health plans the ability to restrict public disclosure and allows poorly performing health plans to escape public scrutiny (Thompson et al. 2003). Such selective nondisclosure undermines both informed consumer decision-making and public accountability (McCormick et al. 2002). However, MCOs seeking accreditation from NCQA are required to provide HEDIS results, which are audited by an NCQA certified auditor (NCQA 2003).

Summary

Increasing costs, lack of access, and concerns about quality pose the greatest challenges to health care delivery in the United States. To some extent, the three issues are interrelated. Increasing costs limit the system's ability to expand access, and without universal coverage for all Americans, they may never match the health status of populations in other developed countries. Despite spending the most resources on health care, the United States continues to rank in the bottom quartile among developed countries on outcome indicators, such as life expectancy and infant mortality. In fact, its relative ranking has been declining since 1960 (Anderson 1997).

Nations that have national health insurance can control systemwide costs through top-down controls, mainly in the form of global budgets. This approach is not possible in the United States because it has a multi-payer system. In the United States, regulatory approaches have been used to try to constrain the supply-side, but the major emphasis has been on constricting reimbursement to providers. Several competitive approaches have been used, mainly through the expansion of managed care. A move toward prospective payments and the growth of managed care can be largely credited with the brakes put on rising health care spending during the 1990s. However, the best current forecasts are for accelerated spending growth in the future, which means that a growing share of economic resources will be devoted to the delivery of health care.

Access to medical care is one of the key determinants of health status, along with environment, lifestyle, and heredity factors. Access is also regarded as a significant benchmark in assessing the effectiveness of the medical care delivery system. Access is explained in terms of enabling and predisposing factors, as well as factors related to health policy and health care delivery. Access has five dimensions: availability, accessibility, accommodation, affordability, and acceptability. Measures of access can relate to individuals, health care plans, and the health care delivery system.

Quality in health care has been difficult to define and measure, although it is receiving increasing emphasis. At the micro level, health care quality encompasses the clinical aspects of care delivery, the interpersonal aspects of care delivery, and quality of life. Indicators of quality at the macro level are commonly associated with life expectancy, mortality, and morbidity. Quality assessment is the measurement of quality against an established standard. Quality assurance emphasizes improvement of quality using the principles of CQI. Donabedian proposed that quality should be assessed along three dimensions: structure, process, and outcomes. These three approaches are complementary and should be used collectively to monitor quality of care. Reliability and validity are important concepts in the measurement of quality.

Test Your Understanding

Terminology

access	health planning	quality assessment
administrative costs	HEDIS	quality assurance
all-payer system	HRQL	reliability
certificate-of-need	institution-related quality	risk management
clinical practice guidelines	of life	small area variations
competition	outcomes	top-down control
cost-efficiency	overutilization	TQM
cost shifting	peer review	underutilization
critical pathways	PRO	validity
defensive medicine	QIO	
fraud	quality	

Review Questions

1. What is meant by the term "health care costs"? Describe the three different meanings of the term "cost."

2. Why should the United States control the rising costs of health care?

3. How do findings of the Rand Health Insurance Experiment reinforce the relationship between growth in third-party reimbursement and increase in health care costs? Explain.

4. Explain how, under imperfect market conditions, both prices and quantity of health care are higher than they would be in a highly competitive market.

5. What are some of the reasons for increased health care costs that are attributed to the providers of medical care?

6. What are some of the main differences between broad cost-containment approaches used in the United States and those used in countries with national health insurance?

7. Discuss the effectiveness of CON regulation in controlling health care expenditures.

8. Discuss price controls and their effectiveness in controlling health care expenditures.

9. Discuss the role of PROs (QIOs) in cost containment.

10. What are the four competition-based cost-containment strategies?

11. What are the implications of access for health and health care delivery?

12. What is the role of enabling and predisposing factors in access to care?

13. Briefly describe the five dimensions of access.

14. What are the four main types of access described by Anderson?

15. Describe the measurement of access at the individual, health plan, and delivery system levels.

16. What are some of the implications of the definition of quality proposed by the Institute of Medicine? In what way is the definition incomplete?

17. Discuss the dimensions of quality from the micro and macro perspectives.

18. Discuss the two types of health-related quality of life.

19. Distinguish between quality assessment and quality assurance.

20. What are the basic principles of TQM (or CQI)?

21. Give a brief description of the Donabedian model of quality.

22. Discuss the main developments in process improvement that have occurred in recent years.

REFERENCES

Aday, L.A. 1993. Indicators and predictors of health services utilization. In *Introduction to health services*. 4th ed., eds. S.J. Williams and P.R. Torrens, 46–70. Albany, NY: Delmar Publishers.

Aday, L.A., and R. Andersen. 1975. *Development of indices of access to medical care*. Ann Arbor, MI: Health Administration Press.

Aday, L.A. et al. 1980. *Health care in the US: Equitable for whom?* Newbury Park, CA: Sage.

Aday, L.A. et al. 1984. *Access to medical care in the US: Who has it, who doesn't?* Research Series No. 32. Chicago, IL: Center for Health Administration Studies, University of Chicago, Pluribus Press Inc.

Aday, L.A. et al. 1993. *Evaluating the medical care system: Effectiveness, efficiency, and equity*. Ann Arbor, MI: Health Administration Press.

Al-Assaf, A.F. 1993a. Introduction and historical background. In *The textbook of total quality management*, eds. A.F. Al-Assaf and J.A. Schmele, 3–12. Delray Beach, FL: St. Lucie Press.

Al-Assaf, A.F. 1993b. Outcome management and TQ. In *The textbook of total quality management*, eds. A.F. Al-Assaf and J.A. Schmele, 221–37. Delray Beach, FL: St. Lucie Press.

Altman, S.H., and J. Eichenholz. 1976. Inflation in the health industry: Causes and cures. In *Health: A victim or cause of inflation?* ed. M. Zubkoff, 1–32. New York: Milbank Memorial Fund.

Altman, S.H., and S.S. Wallack. 1996. Health care spending: Can the United States control it? In *Strategic choices for a changing health care system*, eds. S.H. Altman and U.E. Reinhardt. Chicago: Health Administration Press.

Andersen, R. 1968. *A behavioral model of families' use of health services*. Research Series No. 25. Chicago, IL: Center for Health Administration Studies, University of Chicago.

Andersen, R. 1997. Too big, too small, too flat, too tall: Search for "just right" measures of access in the age of managed care. Paper presented at the Association for Health Services Research Annual Meeting. Chicago, IL.

Anderson, G.F. 1997. In search of value: An international comparison of cost, access, and outcomes. *Health Affairs* 16, no. 6: 163–71.

Arnould, R.J. et al. 1993. Competitive reforms: Context and scope. In *Competitive approaches to health care reform*, eds. R.J. Arnould, R.F. Rich, and W.D. White, 3–18. Washington, DC: The Urban Institute Press.

Baucus, M., and E.J. Fowler. 2002. Geographic variation in Medicare spending and the real focus of Medicare reform. *Health Affairs Web Exclusives* 2002: W115–W117.

Bergner, M. 1989. Quality of life, health status, and clinical research. *Medical Care* 27, no. 3 (Supplement): S148–S156.

Borger, C., et al. 2006. Health spending projections through 2015: Changes on the horizon. *Health Affairs* 25, no.2: w61–w73.

Brown, K. 1992. Death and access: Ethics in cross-cultural health care. In *Choices and conflict: Explorations in health care ethics*, ed. E. Friedman. Chicago: American Hospital Publishing.

Catlin, A., et al. National health spending in 2005: The slowdown continues. *Health Affairs* (Millwood) 26, no.1:142–53.

Centers for Disease Control and Prevention (CDC). 2005. Annual Smoking-Attributable Mortality, Years of Potential Life Lost, and Productivity Losses—United States, 1997–2001. *MMWR* 54, no.25:625–8. Available at: *http://www.cdc.gov/mmwr/preview/mmwrhtml/mm5425a1.htm*.

Centers for Medicare & Medicaid Services. 2007. Pay for performance. *http://www.cms.hhs.gov/MedicaidSCHIPQualPrac/04_P4P.asp*.

Chassin, M.R. 1991. Quality of care—Time to act. *Journal of the American Medical Association* 266, no. 24: 3472–3.

Cordes, S.M. 1989. The changing rural environment and the relationship between health services and rural development. *Health Services Research* 23, no. 6: 757–84.

Coté, C.J. 2000. Adverse sedation events in pediatrics: A critical incident analysis of contributing factors. *Pediatrics* 105, no. 4: 805–14.

DeFriese, G.H., and T.C. Ricketts. 1989. Primary health care in rural areas: An agenda for research. *Health Services Research* 23, no. 6: 931–74.

Department of Health and Human Services (DHHS). 1996. *Health, United States, 1995*. Hyattsville, Maryland: National Center for Health Statistics.

Department of Health and Human Services (DHHS). 2002. *Health, United States, 2002*. Hyattsville, Maryland: National Center for Health Statistics.

Docteur, E.R. et al. 1996. Shifting the paradigm: Monitoring access in Medicare managed care. *Health Care Financing Review* 17, no. 4: 5–21.

Donabedian, A. 1980. *Explorations in quality assessment and monitoring: The definition of quality and approaches to its assessment.* Vol. 1. Ann Arbor, MI: Health Administration Press.

Donabedian, A. 1985. *Explorations in quality assessment and monitoring: The methods and findings of quality assessment and monitoring.* Vol. 3. Ann Arbor, MI: Health Administration Press.

Dranove, D. 1993. The case for competitive reform in health care. In *Competitive approaches to health care reform*, eds. R.J. Arnould, R.F. Rich, and W.D. White, 67–82. Washington, DC: The Urban Institute Press.

Easterbrook, G. 1987. The revolution. *Newsweek*, 26 January, 40–74.

Eddy, D.M. 1994. Clinical decision making: From theory to practice. In *The nation's health*. 4th ed., eds. P.R. Lee and C.L. Estes, 315–21. Boston: Jones & Bartlett Publishers.

Evans, J.R. 1993. *Applied production and operations management*. 4th ed. Minneapolis/St. Paul, MN: West Publishing Co.

Feldstein, P.J. 1993. *Health care economics*. 4th ed. Albany, NY: Delmar Publishers.

Feldstein, P. 1994. *Health policy issues: An economic perspective on health reform*. Ann Arbor, MI: AUPHA Press/Health Administration Press.

Finkelstein, E.A. et al. 2003. National medical spending attributable to overweight and obesity: How much, and who's paying? Health Affairs Web Exclusive, May 14. *http://www.healthaffairs.org/WebExclusives/Finkelstein_Web_Excl_051403.htm*.

Firshein, J. 1996. Measuring progress toward practice guidelines. *Business and Health* 14, no. 5: 38–42.

Fisher, E.S. et al. 2003a. The implications of regional variations in Medicare spending. Part 1: The content, quality, and accessibility of care. *Annals of Internal Medicine* 138, no. 4: 273–87.

Fisher, E.S. et al. 2003b. The implications of regional variations in Medicare spending. Part 2: Health outcomes and satisfaction with care. *Annals of Internal Medicine* 138, no. 4: 288–98.

Freeman, H.E. et al. 1982. Community health centers: An initiative of enduring utility. *Milbank Memorial Fund Quarterly/Health and Society* 60, no. 2: 245–67.

Gabel, J., and T. Rice. 1985. Reducing public expenditures for physician services: The price of paying less. *Journal of Health Politics, Policy and Law* 9, no. 4: 595–609.

Ganz, P.A., and M.S. Litwin. 1996. Measuring outcomes and health-related quality of life. In *Changing the US health care system: Key issues in health services, policy, and management*, eds. R.M. Anderson et al. San Francisco: Jossey-Bass Publishers.

Giffin, M., and R.B. Giffin. 1994. Market memo: Critical pathways produce tangible results. *Health Care Strategic Management* 12, no. 7: 1–6.

Gittelsohn, A., and N.R. Powe. 1995. Small area variation in health care delivery in Maryland. *Health Services Research* 30, no. 2: 295–317.

Gottlieb, S.R. 1974. A brief history of health planning in the United States. In *Regulating health facilities construction*, ed. C.C. Havighurst. Washington, DC: American Enterprise Institute for Public Policy Research.

Guralnik, J.M. et al. 1991. Morbidity and disability in older persons in the years prior to death. *American Journal of Public Health* 81, no. 4: 443–7.

HCIA Inc. and Deloitte & Touche. 1997. *The comparative performance of US hospitals: The sourcebook*. Baltimore, MD: HCIA Inc.

Health Care Financing Administration (HCFA). 1996. Overview of the Medicare program. *Health Care Financing Review: Medicare and Medicaid Statistical Supplement* 5.

Heffler, S. et al. 2002. Health spending projections for 2001–2011: The latest outlook. *Health Affairs* 21, no. 2: 207–18.

Hellander, I. et al. 1994. Health care paper chase, 1993: The cost to the nation, the states, and the District of Columbia. *International Journal of Health Services* 24, no. 1: 1–9.

Institute of Medicine (IOM). 1990. *Clinical practice guidelines: Directions for a new program*. Washington, DC: National Academy Press.

Institute of Medicine (IOM). 1993. *Access to health care in America*, ed. M. Millman. Washington, DC: National Academy Press.

Institute of Medicine (IOM). 2000. *To err is human: Building a safer health system*, eds. L.T. Kohn, J.M. Corrigan, and M.S. Donaldson. Washington, DC: National Academy Press.

Institute of Medicine (IOM). 2004. *Rewarding provider performance: Aligning incentives in Medicare*. Washington, DC: National Academy Press.

Laffel, G., and D. Blumenthal. 1993. The case for using industrial quality management science in health care organizations. In *The textbook of total quality management*, ed. A.F. Al-Assaf and J.A. Schmele, 40–50. Delray Beach, FL: St. Lucie Press.

Lapetina, E.M., and E.M. Armstrong. 2002. Preventing errors in the outpatient setting: A tale of three states. *Health Affairs* 21, no. 4: 26–39.

Lamb, R.M. et al. 2003. Hospital disclosure practices: Results of a national survey. *Health Affairs* 22, no. 2: 73–83.

Larsen, R.R. 1996. Narrowing the gray zone: How clinical practice guidelines can improve the decision-making process. *Postgraduate Medicine* 100, no. 2: 17–24.

Lehman, A.F. 1995. Measuring quality of life in a reformed health system. *Health Affairs* 14, no. 3: 90–101.

Levit, K. et al. 2003. Trends in US health care spending, 2001. *Health Affairs* 22, no. 1: 154–64.

Levy, D.E. 2006. Employer-sponsored insurance coverage of smoking cessation treatments. *American Journal of Managed Care* 12, no.9: 553–62.

Lohr, K.N. 1997. How do we measure quality? *Health Affairs* 16, no. 3: 22–5.

Loubeau, P.R., and V.F. Maher. 1996. Any-willing-provider laws: Point and counter point. *Medical Law* 15, no. 2: 219–26.

Lovitky, J.A. 1997. Health care fraud: A growing problem. *Nursing Management* 28, no. 11: 42, 44–5.

May, J. 1974. The planning and licensing agencies. In *Regulating health facilities constructions*, ed. C.C. Havighurst. Washington, DC: American Enterprise Institute for Public Policy Research.

McCormick, D. et al. 2002. Relationship between low quality-of-care scores and HMOs' subsequent public disclosure of quality-of-care scores. *Journal of the American Medical Association* 288, no. 12: 1484–90.

McElroy, D., and K. Herbelin. 1989. Assuring quality of care in long-term care facilities. *Journal of Gerontological Nursing* 15, no. 7: 8–10.

McGlynn, E.A. 1997. Six challenges in measuring the quality of health care. *Health Affairs* 16, no. 3: 7–21.

McGlynn, E.A., and R.H. Brook. 1996. Ensuring quality of care. In *Changing the US health care system: Key issues in health services, policy, and management*, eds. R.M. Andersen, T.H. Rice, and G.F. Kominski, San Francisco: Jossey-Bass Publishers.

Minino, A.M., and B.L. Smith. 2001. Deaths: Preliminary data for 2000. *National Vital Statistics Reports* 49, no. 12. National Center for Health Statistics.

Mitchell, J. et al. 1988. *Impact of the Medicare fee freeze on physician expenditures and volume: Final report*. Baltimore, MD: Health Care Financing Administration.

National Center for Health Statistics. 2002. *National Vital Statistics Reports* 49, no. 12. Centers for Disease Control and Prevention.

National Center for Health Statistics. 2006. Health, United States, 2006. Hyattsville, MD: US Department of Health and Human Services.

National Committee for Quality Assurance (NCQA). 2007. HEDIS 2007 Summary Table of Measures and Product Lines. *http://www.ncqa.org/programs/hedis/2007/MeasuresList.pdf.*

National Committee for Quality Assurance (NCQA). 2003. Managed care organization accreditation. *http://web.ncqa.org/tabid/67/Default.aspx.*

Norton, C.H., and M.A. McManus. 1989. Background tables on demographic characteristics. *Health Services Research* 23, no. 6: 807–48.

Orlikoff, J.E. 1988. *Malpractice prevention and liability control for hospitals.* 2nd ed. Chicago: American Hospital Publishing.

Penchansky, R., and J.W. Thomas. 1981. The concept of access: Definition and relationship to consumer satisfaction. *Medical Care* 19: 127–40.

Public Health Service. 1997. *Smoking cessation: A systems approach.* Rockville, MD: Department of Health and Human Services (AHCPR Publication No. 97–0698), April.

Reed, M. et al. 2003. Physicians and care management: more acceptance than you think. *Issue brief* [Center for the Study of Health System Change], January (60): 1–4.

Reinhardt, U.E. 1994. Providing access to health care and controlling costs: The universal dilemma. In *The nation's health.* 4th ed., eds. P.R. Lee and C.L. Estes, 263–78. Boston: Jones & Bartlett Publishers.

Reinhardt, U.E. et al. 2002. Cross-national comparisons of health systems using OECD data, 1999. *Health Affairs* 21, no. 3: 169–81.

Rogers, W.H. et al. 1990. Quality of care before and after implementation of the DRG-based prospective payment system: A summary of effects. *Journal of the American Medical Association* 264, no. 15: 1989–94.

Ross, J.S., et al. 2007. Certificate of need regulation and cardiac catheterization appropriateness after acute myocardial infarction. *Circulation* 115, no. 8:1012–19.

Rowland, D., and B. Lyons. 1989. Triple jeopardy: Rural, poor, and uninsured. *Health Services Research* 23, no. 6: 975–1004.

Sardell, A. 1988. *The US experiment in social medicine, the Community Health Center Program, 1965–1986.* Pittsburgh, PA: University of Pittsburgh Press.

Sheils, J., and Haught, R. 2004. The cost of tax-exempt benefits in 2004. *Health Affairs* (Millwood) W4: 106–12.

Shekelle, P.G., and D.L. Schriger. 1996. Evaluating the use of the appropriateness method in the Agency for Health Care Policy and Research clinical practice guideline development process. *Health Services Research* 31, no. 4: 453–68.

Sherman, A. 1991. *Falling by the wayside: Children in rural America.* Washington, DC: Children's Defense Fund.

Singh, D.A. 1997. *Nursing home administrators: Their influence on quality of care.* New York: Garland Publishing.

Svarstad, B.L. 1986. Patient-practitioner relationships and compliance with prescribed medical regimens. In *Applications of social sciences to clinical medicine and health policy*, eds. L.H. Aiken and D. Mechanic. New Brunswick, NJ: Rutgers University Press.

TECH Research Network. 2001. Technology change around the world: Evidence from heart attack care. *Health Affairs* 20, no. 3: 25–42.

Thompson, J.W. et al. 2003. Health plan quality-of-care information is undermined by voluntary reporting. *American Journal of Preventive Medicine* 24, no. 1: 62–70.

Tucker, J. 1997. Obey says future Medicare cuts inevitable. *PT Bulletin*, 27 June, 10.

Van de Water, P.N., Lavery, J. 2006. Medicare finances: Findings of the 2006 trustees report. *Medicare Brief* 13: 1–8.

Weisbrod, B. 1991. The health care quadrilemma: An essay on technological change, insurance, quality of care, and cost containment. *Journal of Economic Literature* 29 (June): 523–52.

Wendling, W., and J. Werner. 1980. Nonprofit firms and the economic theory of regulation. *Quarterly Review of Economics and Business* 20, no. 3: 6–18.

Wennberg, J.E. 2002.Unwarranted variations in healthcare delivery: Implications for academic medical centres. *British Medical Journal* 325, no. 7370: 961–4.

Wennberg, J.E. et al. 1987. Are hospital services rationed in New Haven or over-utilized in Boston? *Lancet* 1, no. 8543: 1185–9.

Wennberg, J.E., and A. Gittelsohn. 1973. Small area variations in health care delivery. *Science* 183: 1102–8.

Williams, S.J. 1995. *Essentials of health services*. Albany, NY: Delmar Publishers.

Williams, K.N., and R.H. Brook. 1978. Quality measurement and assurance. *Health Medical Care Services Review* 1: 3–15.

Williams, S.J., and P.R. Torrens. 1993. Influencing, regulating, and monitoring the health care system. In *Introduction to health services*. 4th ed., eds. S.J. Williams and P.R. Torrens, 377–396. Albany, NY: Delmar Publishers.

Wilson, F.A., and D. Neuhauser. 1985. *Health services in the United States*. 2nd ed. Cambridge, MA: Ballinger Publishing Co.

Wong, M.D. et al. 2001. Effects of cost sharing on care seeking and health status: Results from the medical outcomes study. *American Journal of Public Health* 91, no. 11: 1889–94.

Chapter 3

Leiyu Shi, DrPH, MBA, MPA, and Douglas A. Singh, PhD, MBA

Health Policy

Learning Objectives

- To understand the definition, scope, and role of health policy in the United States
- To recognize the principal features of US health policy
- To comprehend the process of legislative health policy
- To become familiar with some of the critical health policy issues in the United States

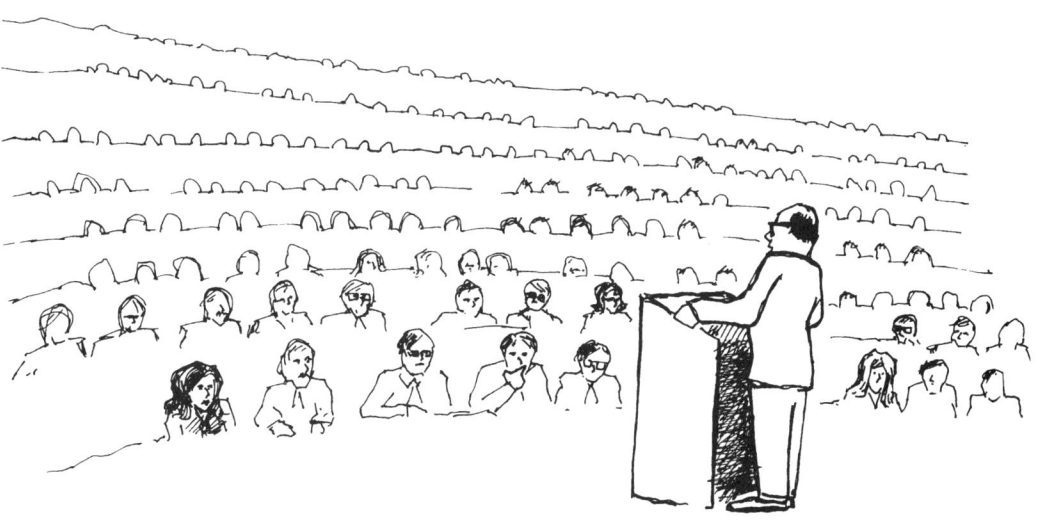

"Ladies and Gentlemen, to come up with a uniform health policy, we will now break up into 31 different groups."

95

Introduction

Even though the United States does not have a centrally controlled system of health care delivery, it does have a history of federal, state, and local government involvement in health care and health policy. Americans possess an incredible desire to be healthy. They contend that their individual health contributes to the overall health of the nation and, consequently, to the economy. It is, therefore, not surprising that the government is so keenly interested in health policy. This chapter first defines what health policy is and explores the principal features of health policy in the United States. Next, it describes the development of legislative policy and gives examples of critical health policy issues. Finally, it provides an outlook for the future of health policy in the United States.

What Is Health Policy?

Public policies are authoritative decisions made in the legislative, executive, or judicial branches of government intended to direct or influence the actions, behaviors, or decisions of others (Longest 1994). When public policies pertain to or influence the pursuit of health, they become health policies. Therefore, *health policy* can be defined as "the aggregate of principles, stated or unstated, that . . . characterize the distribution of resources, services, and political influences that impact on the health of the population . . ." (Miller 1987, 15).

Public policies are supposed to serve the interests of the public; however, the term "public" has been interpreted differently in the political landscape. At the most general level, the term "public" refers to all Americans. "Public" also can refer to voters or likely voters; that is, the subset of Americans who directly determine the outcomes of political elections. Finally, the term can refer to only those who are politically active. The latter group consists of those Americans who communicate directly with their representatives by either writing or calling, contribute money to politicians or political groups, attend protests or other forums on behalf of a particular interest or candidate, or in other ways make their voices and policy preferences heard. Legislators and policymakers are most responsive to the views or wishes of these active Americans, particularly when they are constituents from within their legislative districts. People who are older, have more years of education, and have strong party identification are more likely to be politically active.

Different Forms of Health Policies

Health policies often come as a by-product of public social policies enacted by the government. For example, important changes in the US health care system came about after World War II due to policies that excluded fringe benefits from income or Social Security taxes and a Supreme Court ruling that employee benefits, including health insurance, could be legitimately included in the collective bargaining process. As a result, employer-provided health insurance benefits grew rapidly in the mid-20th century (Health Insurance Association of America 1992). In 1965, adoption of the Medicare and Medicaid legislation expanded the health sector by providing publicly subsidized health insurance to the elderly and the indigent. In 1997, Congress approved the State Children's Health Insurance Program (SCHIP), which extends health coverage to children whose families have incomes above the eligibility level for Medicaid, but who cannot afford private coverage. All of these developments in public policy have shaped the way health services are delivered in this country.

The American health care system has been developed under extraordinarily favorable public policies. For example, the nation has a long history of support for the development of medical technology through policies that directly support biomedical research and encourage private investments in such research. The National Institutes of Health (NIH) had a budget of about $10 million when the agency was established in the early 1930s. Today, following exponential growth, the proposed FY 2008 NIH budget is nearly $29 billion (NIH 2007). Encouraged by policies that permit firms to recoup their investments in research and development, private industry also spends a significant amount on biomedical research and development.

Health policies pertain to health care at all levels, including policies affecting the production, provision, and financing of health care services. Health policies affect groups or classes of individuals, such as physicians, the poor, the elderly, or children. They can also affect types of organizations, such as medical schools, health maintenance organizations (HMOs), nursing homes, medical technology producers, or employers. In the United States, each branch and level of government can influence health policy. For example, both the executive and legislative branches at the federal, state, and local levels can establish health policies, and the judicial branch can uphold, strike down, or modify existing laws affecting health and health care at federal, state, or local levels.

Health policies can be made through the private sector or the public policymaking process. An example of private-sector health policies is the decisions made by insurance companies regarding their product lines, pricing, and marketing. Their focus is to restrict the public policymaking process and the public-sector health policies that result from this process. Examples of public health policies include (1) major reforms in medical education, as suggested in the 1910 Flexner report, which encouraged a university/hospital-based model for education; (2) the 1965 legislation that established the Medicare and Medicaid programs; (3) an executive order regarding operation of federally funded family planning clinics; (4) a court's decision that the merger of two hospitals violates federal antitrust laws; (5) a state government's decision about its procedures for licensing physicians; (6) a county health department's decision about its procedures for monitoring sanitation standards in restaurants; (7) and a city government's enactment of an ordinance banning smoking in public places within the city. Thus, health policies can take several different forms.

Statutes or laws, such as the statutory language contained in the 1983 Amendments to the Social Security Act that authorized the prospective payment system (PPS) for reimbursing hospitals for Medicare beneficiaries, are also considered policies. Another example is the certificate-of-need (CON) programs through which many states seek to regulate capital expansion in their health care systems.

The scope of health policy is limited by the political and economic system of a country. In the United States, where pro-individual and pro-market sentiments dominate, public policies are likely to be fragmented, incremental, and noncomprehensive. National policies and programs are typically based on the notion that local communities are in the best position to identify strategies that will address their unique needs. However, the type of change that can be enacted at the community level is clearly limited.

Regulatory Tools

Health policies may be used as *regulatory tools* (Longest 1994). They call on government to prescribe and control the behavior of a particular target group by monitoring the group and imposing sanctions if it fails to comply. Examples of regulatory policies are abundant in the health care system. Federally funded quality improvement organizations (QIOs, formerly peer review organizations), for instance, develop and enforce standards concerning appropriate care under the Medicare program. State insurance departments across the country regulate health insurance companies in an effort to protect customers from default on coverage in case of financial failure of an insurance company, excessive premiums, and mendacious practices.

Some health policies are "self-regulatory." For example, physicians set standards of medical practice, hospitals accredit one another as meeting the standards that the Joint Commission on Accreditation of Healthcare Organizations has set, and schools of public health decide which courses should be part of their graduate programs in public health (Weissert and Weissert 1996).

Allocative Tools

Health policies may also be used as *allocative tools* (Longest 1994). They involve the direct provision of income, services, or goods to certain groups of in-

dividuals or institutions. Allocative tools in the health care arena are distributive or redistributive. *Distributive policies* spread benefits throughout society. Typical distributive policies include funding of medical research through the NIH, the development of medical personnel (e.g., medical education through the National Health Service Corps), the construction of facilities (e.g., hospitals under the Hill-Burton program during the 1950s and 1960s), and the initiation of new institutions (e.g., HMOs). *Redistributive policies*, on the other hand, take money or power from one group and give it to another. This system often creates visible beneficiaries and payers. For this reason, health policy is often most visible and politically charged when it performs redistributive functions. Redistributive policies include Medicaid, which takes tax revenue from the more affluent and spends it on the poor in the form of free health insurance. Other redistributive policies include the State Children's Health Insurance Program (SCHIP), welfare, and public housing programs. Redistributive policies, in particular, are believed to be essential for addressing the fundamental causes of health disparities.

The Principal Features of US Health Policy

Several features characterize US health policy, including government as subsidiary to the private sector; fragmented, incremental, and piecemeal reform; pluralistic (interest group) politics; the decentralized role of the states; and the impact of presidential leadership. These features often act or interact to influence the development and evolution of health policies.

Government as Subsidiary to the Private Sector

In much of the developed world, national health care programs are built on a consensus that health care is a right of citizenship and that government should play a leading role in the provision of health care. In the United States, however, health care is not seen as a right of citizenship or as a primary responsibility of government. Instead, the private sector plays a dominant role. Similar to many other public policy issues, Americans generally prefer market solutions as opposed to government intervention in health care financing and delivery. For this reason, a strong preference prevails to minimize the government's role in the delivery of health care.

Americans have typically harbored a general mistrust of government. The Declaration of Independence defined the new nation in a great protest over government intrusion on personal liberty. The United States is a capitalist nation where the presumption is that private markets best determine the production and consumption of goods and services, including health care services. One result is that Americans have developed social insurance programs far more reluctantly than most industrialized democracies. In addition, American public opinion often presumes these programs are overly generous.

Generally speaking, the government's role in US health care has grown incrementally, mainly to address perceived problems and negative consequences. Some of the most-cited problems associated with government involvement include escalating costs, bureaucratic inflexibility, excessive regulation, red tape, irrational paperwork, arbitrary and sometimes conflicting public directives, inconsistent enforcement of rules and regulations, and fraud and abuse. Other problems include inadequate reimbursement schedules, arbitrary denial of claims, insensitivity to local needs, consumer and provider dissatisfaction, and charges that government programs tend to promote welfare dependence rather than a desire to seek employment (Longest 1994).

The most credible argument for policy intervention in the nation's domestic activities begins with the identification of situations in which markets fail or do not function efficiently. Health care in the United States is a big industry, but certain specific characteristics and conditions of the health care market distinguish it from other businesses. The market for health care services in the United States violates the conditions of a competitive market in several ways. The complexity of health care services almost eliminates the consumer's ability to make informed decisions without guidance from the sellers (providers). Sellers' entry into the health care market is heavily regulated. Widespread insurance coverage also affects the decisions of buyers and sellers regarding cost and utilization. These and other factors determine that the markets for health care services do not operate competitively, thus inviting policy intervention.

Government spending for health care has been largely confined to filling the gaps in the private sector. This intervention includes environmental protection, preventive services, communicable disease control, care of special groups, institutional care of the mentally and chronically ill, provision of medical care to the indigent, and support for research and training. With health coverage considered a privilege or even a luxury for those who are offered insurance through their employer, the government is left in a gap-filling role for the most vulnerable of the uninsured population.

Another important example of the subsidiary role of government was the enactment of the Hospital Survey and Construction Act in 1946 (also known as the Hill-Burton Act). This legislation expanded the availability of health services and improved hospital facilities after the unregulated markets had failed to provide adequate access to inpatient hospital care. The program, intended to provide funds for hospital construction, marked the beginning of extensive federal developmental subsidies to increase the availability of health services.

Fragmented, Incremental, and Piecemeal Reform

Public power in the United States is enormously fragmented. This system follows the design of the founding fathers, who developed a structure of "checks and balances" to limit government's power. Federal, state, and local governments pursue their own policies with little coordination of purpose or programs. The subsidiary role of the government and the attendant mixture of private and public approaches to the provision of health care also resulted in a complex and fragmented pattern of health care financing, in which: (1) The employed are predominantly covered by voluntary insurance provided through contributions that they and their employers make. (2) The aged are insured through a combination of coverage financed out of Social Security tax revenues (Medicare Part A) and government-subsidized voluntary insurance for physician, supplementary, and prescription drug coverage (Medicare Part B and Part D). (3) The poor are covered through Medicaid via federal, state, and local revenues. (4) Special population groups—for example,

veterans, American Indians, members of the armed forces, Congress, and the executive branch—have coverage that the federal government provides directly.

US health policies have been incremental and piecemeal, resulting from compromises involving the resolution of a variety of competing interests. An example is the broadening of the Medicaid program since its start in 1965. Congress has enacted policies to expand Medicaid eligibility to enroll more children into the program. In 1984, the first steps were taken to mandate coverage of pregnant women and children in two-parent families who met income requirements and to mandate coverage for all children five years old or younger who met financial requirements. When the federal government mandates Medicaid eligibility or benefits, it is telling the states that they must expand their programs accordingly to continue receiving federal matching dollars.

In 1986, states were given the option of covering pregnant women and children up to five years of age in families with incomes below 100% of federal poverty income guidelines, regardless of their participation in the Aid to Families with Dependent Children (AFDC) program. In 1988, that option was increased to cover families at 185% of federal poverty income. In 1988, Congress required that Medicaid coverage for families leaving the AFDC program be continued for six months, and they gave states the option of adding another six months. In addition, as part of the Medicaid Catastrophic Act, which remains in effect today, Congress mandated coverage for pregnant women and infants in families with incomes below 100% of federal poverty guidelines. In 1989, it was expanded to 133% of the poverty income, and the age of covered children was raised to six. In the early 1990s, states began experimenting with waivers allowing for expansion of Medicaid managed care programs. In 1996, the Personal Responsibility and Work Opportunity Act (PRWORA) ended the formal link between AFDC benefits and Medicaid benefits. In 1997, the Balanced Budget Act created SCHIP, which allows states to use Medicaid expansion to extend insurance coverage to uninsured children who otherwise are not qualified for existing Medicaid programs. This illustrates how a program is reformed and/or expanded through successive legislative action. In typical American fashion, the Medicaid program has been reformed through incremental change, but without ensuring access to medical care for all of the nation's uninsured. Among the uninsured are millions of Americans who are not categorically eligible for services. These uninsured consist mostly of adults younger than 65 years of age with no dependent children. Congress has demonstrated the desire and political will to address the needs of a small number of the uninsured perceived to be the most vulnerable (e.g., pregnant women and children) but has not developed a consensus on more dramatic steps to move beyond incremental adjustments to existing programs.

Institutional fragmentation is vividly clear in the process of legislative development of health policy. Thirty-one congressional committees and subcommittees try to claim some fragment of jurisdiction over health legislation. The conglomeration of reform proposals that emerges from these committees faces a daunting political challenge—separate consideration and passage in each chamber, negotiations in a joint conference committee to reconcile the bills passed by the two houses, and then return to each chamber for approval. In the Senate, 41 of the 100 members can thwart the whole process at any point.

Once a bill has passed in Congress, however, it is not a fait accompli. Multiple levels of federal and state bureaucracy must interpret and implement the legislation. Rules and regulations must be written. During this process, politicians, interest groups, or project beneficiaries may influence the program's ultimate design. Sometimes, the result can differ significantly from its sponsors' intent. This complex and seemingly anarchic process of policy formulation and implementation makes fundamental, comprehensive policy reform extremely difficult. Ideology and government organization reinforce the tendency toward a standstill. It usually takes a great political event—a landmark election, a popular upheaval, a war, or a domestic crisis—to overcome the tilt toward inaction.

Pluralistic and Interest Group Politics

Perhaps the most common explanation for US health policy outcomes takes into full account the demands of interest groups and the incremental policies resulting from compromises struck to satisfy those demands. Traditionally, the policy community has included (1) the legislative committees with jurisdiction in a policy domain, (2) the executive branch agencies implementing policies, and (3) private interest groups. The first two supply the policies demanded by the third.

Established groups resist innovative, nonincremental policies because these measures undermine the bargaining practices that reduce threats to existing interests. The system's stability is ensured because most groups are satisfied with the benefits they receive; however, the result for any single group is less than optimal. Interest groups' pluralism affects health policy just as it does any other policy debate in American politics.

Powerful interest groups involved in health care politics adamantly resist any major change (Alford 1975). Each group fights hard to protect its own best interests.

Well-organized interest groups are the most effective "demanders" of policies. By combining and concentrating their members' resources, organized interest groups can dramatically change the ratio between the costs and benefits of participation in the political markets for policy change. These interest groups represent a variety of individuals and entities, such as physicians in the American Medical Association; senior citizens allied with AARP (formerly called the American Association of Retired Persons); institutional providers such as hospitals belonging to the American Hospital Association; nursing homes belonging to the American Health Care Association; and the companies making up the Pharmaceutical Research and Manufacturers of America.

Physicians have often found it hard to lobby for their interests with a single voice because they include so many specialty groups. For example, the American Academy of Pediatrics is involved in advocacy for children's health issues. Other groups include Physicians for a National Health Program, the American Society of Anesthesiologists, and the Society of Thoracic Surgeons. Though driven by their specific interests, they can come together on issues that threaten the entire group, such as the 1992 decision by the Office of Management and Budget to reduce total Medicare payments when implementing a reimbursement system based on resource-based relative values.

Not only do the traditional members of the health policy community find themselves split over questions of optimal health policy, but the community has also grown considerably as new interest groups have formed and joined. Business is the major new member, although it too is split, mainly along the lines of large and small employers. Other, newer members of the health policy community represent consumer interests, but consumer interests are not uniform, nor are the policy preferences of their interest groups. Consumers often lack financial means to organize and advocate for their interests.

To overcome pluralistic interests and maximize policy outcomes, diverse interest groups form alliances among themselves and with legislators to protect and enhance the interests of those receiving benefits from government programs. Each alliance member receives benefits from current programs. Legislators can show their constituencies the economic benefits of government spending in their districts, agencies can expand their programs, and interest groups benefit directly from government programs.

The policy agendas of interest groups typically reflect their interests. For example, the AARP advocates programs to expand financing for long-term care for the elderly and was a major advocate for prescription drug coverage for Medicare beneficiaries, which went into effect on January 1, 2006. Organized labor has been among the staunchest supporters of national health insurance. The primary concerns of educational and research institutions and accrediting bodies are embedded in policies that would generate higher funding to support their educational and research activities. Other policy concerns of these groups include licensure and practice guidelines, and anything that may influence future demand for their graduates and affiliates. The Food and Drug Administration's job is to ensure that new pharmaceuticals meet safety and efficacy standards. Quality Improvement Organizations (QIOs) ensure that Medicare beneficiaries receive only needed and appropriate procedures.

Pharmaceutical and medical technology organizations are concerned with detecting changes in health policy and influencing the formulation of policies concerning approval and monitoring of drugs and devices. Three main factors drive health policy concerns about medical technology: (1) medical technology is an important contributor to rising health costs, (2) medical technology often provides health benefits, and (3) the utilization of medical technology also provides economic benefits. These factors are likely to remain important determinants of US policies on medical technology. Another factor driving US technology policy is the policymakers' desire to develop cost-saving technology and to expand access to it. The government is spending more and more money on outcome studies to identify the value of alternative technologies that promise to provide better care at lower cost.

American employers' health policy concerns are shaped mostly by the degree to which they provide health insurance benefits to their employees and their dependents, and to their retirees. Many small business owners adamantly oppose health policies requiring them to cover employees because they believe they cannot afford it. Employees also pay attention to health policies that affect worker health or the labor-management relations experienced by employers. For example, employers have to comply with federal and state regulations on employee health and well-being, and on the prevention of job-related illnesses and injuries. Employers are often inspected by regulatory agencies to ensure that they adhere to workplace health and safety policies.

The health policy concerns of consumers and the groups that represent them reflect the rich diversity of the American people. African Americans and, more recently, the rapidly growing numbers of Hispanic Americans face special health problems. Both groups are underserved by many health care services and underrepresented in all of the health professions in the United States. Their health policy interests include getting their unique health problems (e.g., higher infant mortality, higher exposure to violence among adolescents, higher levels of substance abuse among adults, and earlier deaths from cardiovascular disease and various other causes) adequately addressed. Exhibit 3–1 summarizes the major concerns of dominant interest groups.

Decentralized Role of the States

In the United States, individual states play a significant role in the development and implementation of health policies. The role of individual states has taken several forms: financial support for the care and treatment of the poor and chronically disabled, which includes the primary responsibility for the administration of the federal/state Medicaid and SCHIP programs; quality assurance and oversight of health care practitioners and facilities (e.g., state licensure and regulation); regulation of health care costs and insurance carriers; health personnel training (states pay most of the costs to train health care professionals); and authorization of local government health services.

Most of the incremental policy actions of recent years originated in state governments. One action, taken by 24 states, was to create a special program called an "insurance risk pool." These programs help people acquire private insurance otherwise unavailable

Exhibit 3–1 Interest Group Preferences

Federal and state governments
- Cost containment
- Access to care
- Quality of care

Employers
- Cost containment
- Workplace health and safety
- Minimum regulation

Consumers
- Access to care
- Quality of care
- Lower out-of-pocket costs

Insurers
- Administrative simplication
- Elimination of cost shifting

Practitioners
- Income maintenance
- Professional autonomy
- Malpractice reform

Provider organizations
- Profitability
- Administrative simplification
- Bad debt reduction

Technology producers
- Tax treatment
- Regulatory environment
- Research funding

to them because of the medical risks they pose to insurance companies. Most of these programs are financed by a combination of individual premiums and taxes on insurance carriers.

Other state-initiated programs have addressed additional vulnerable populations. New Jersey developed a program to ensure access to care for all pregnant women. Florida began a program, called Healthy Kids Corporation, which linked health insurance to schools. Washington developed a special program for the working poor that uses HMOs and preferred provider organizations to provide care within the state's counties. Maine established a program, MaineCare, to offer HMO-based coverage at moderate prices to small businesses with 15 or fewer employees. The state subsidized premiums on a sliding-fee scale based on the employer's ability to contribute (Lemov 1990). Minnesota created a program, Children's Health Plan, designed to provide benefits to children up to age nine who lived in families with incomes below 185% of the poverty level, but who do not qualify for Medicaid. Colorado and New York have also enacted similar legislation. Several states, including Massachusetts, Hawaii, and Oregon, have experimented with more comprehensive programs designed to provide universal access to care within their jurisdictions. Most notably, Massachusetts recently passed legislation requiring about 515,000 people (most of the state's uninsured) to obtain health insurance by July 1, 2007, or face penalties including the potential loss of a personal income tax deduction. To bring the plan to fruition, Massachusetts expanded Medicaid eligibility, reconfigured its $1 billion free care pool, and established rules to help insurance companies create more affordable health plans (Belluck 2007). Exhibit 3–2 lists the arguments often cited in favor of decentralizing health programs at the state level.

Arguments have also been made against too much state control over health policy de-

Exhibit 3–2 Arguments for Enhancing States' Role

- Americans distrust centralized government in general and lack faith in the federal government as an administrator in particular.
- The federal government has grown too large, intrusive, and paternalistic.
- The federal government is too impersonal, distant, and unresponsive.
- State and local governments are closer to the people and more familiar with local needs; therefore, they are more accessible and accountable to the public and better able to develop responsive programs than federal agencies.
- National standards reduce flexibility and seriously constrain the ability of states to experiment and innovate.
- States are equipped to take on such functions (i.e., more full-time legislators, more professional staffs and bureaucrats).
- States are more likely to implement and enforce programs of their own making.
- States have served as important laboratories for testing different structures, approaches, and programs and for providing insight into the political and technical barriers encountered in enactment and implementation.
- States respond to crises faster.
- It is easier to change a state law than a federal one.
- States are more willing to take risks.

cisions. The greater control states have, the more difficult it becomes to develop a coordinated national strategy. For example, it is difficult to plan a national disease-control program if all states do not participate, or if they do not collect and report data in the same way. Moreover, some argue that disparities among states may lead to inequalities in access to health services. This might, in turn, lead to migration from states with poor health benefits to those with more generous programs. Finally, states may interpret federal incentives in ways that jeopardize the policy's original intent. For example, many states took advantage of federal matching grants for Medicaid programs by including a number of formerly state-funded services under an "expanded" Medicaid program. This allowed states to gain increased federal funding while providing exactly the same level of services they had provided before. This phenomenon, called Medicaid maximization, although pursued by only a few states, had an impact outside of those states and may have contributed nationally to rising health care costs in the early 1990s (Coughlin et al. 1999).

Impact of Presidential Leadership

Americans often look to strong presidential leadership in the search for possible sources of major change in health policies. President Lyndon Johnson's role in the passage of Medicare and Medicaid is often cited as a prime example. Presidents have important opportunities to influence congressional outcomes through their efforts to develop compromises that get bills passed with at least some of their preferred agendas.

Some important health policies have been passed since President Harry Truman's administration. The major piece of health legislation passed under Truman was the Hill-Burton Hospital Construction Act. In 1965, Johnson achieved the passage of Medicare and Medicaid because of an unusually favorable level of political opportunity and his leadership skills. Two major pieces of health legislation were passed during Nixon's presidency: (1) the actions leading to federal support of HMOs in 1973 and (2) the enactment of the National Health Planning and Resources Development Act of 1974 (CON legislation). This act represented an additional effort to restrain rapidly rising health care costs and included a fairly elaborate system of required approvals for new equipment and new hospital construction. Under Reagan, new Medicare cost-control approaches for hospitals and physicians were created, and additional Medicare coverage for the elderly was established. Even though Clinton's comprehensive reform efforts failed, his incremental initiatives have succeeded. Examples include the Health Insurance Portability and Accountability Act of 1996 and SCHIP.

Many political lessons can be learned from the failure of Clinton's health care reform initiative (Litman and Robins 1997). Presidents can achieve landmark changes in health policies only when political opportunity, political skill, and commitment converge. Opportunities were uniquely abundant for Johnson in 1965, and he effectively handled his legislative role. Presidents Truman, Kennedy, and Carter might have promoted their proposals with greater skill but were fundamentally thwarted by the lack of a true window of opportunity. Clinton enjoyed a uniquely high level of public interest in health care reform but failed in part because of other weaknesses in his level of opportunity, especially his failure to act within the "window of opportunity" (the first 100 days after his election). The complexity of the ever-changing details of his proposal was another major flaw and ultimately proved too hard for the public to grasp and too easy for adversaries to distort.

The health policy agenda of President George W. Bush has focused less on broad, sweeping reform, and more on market-based, individualistic, incremental policies, such as health savings accounts and implementation of health information technology.

The Development of Legislative Health Policy

The making of US health policy is a complex process that involves private and public sectors (including multiple levels of government) and reflects (1) the relationship of the government to the private sector, (2) the distribution of authority and responsibility within a federal system of government, (3) the relationship between policy formulation and implementation, (4) a pluralistic ideology as the basis of politics, and (5) incrementalism as the strategy for reform.

The Policy Cycle

The formation and implementation of health policy occurs in a policy cycle comprising five components: (1) issue raising, (2) policy design, (3) public support building, (4) legislative decision-making and policy support building, and (5) legislative decision-making and policy implementation. These activities are likely to be shared with Congress and interest groups in varying degrees.

Issue raising is clearly essential in the policy formation cycle. The enactment of a new policy is generally preceded by a variety of actions that first create a widespread sense that a problem exists and needs to be addressed. The president may form policy concepts from a variety of sources, including campaign information; recommendations from advisers, cabinet members, and agency chiefs; personal interests; expert opinions; and public opinion polls.

The second component of policymaking is the design of specific policy proposals. Presidents have substantial resources to develop new policy proposals. They may call on segments of the executive branch of government, such as the Centers for Medicare and Medicaid Services and policy staffs within the Department of Health and Human Services (DHHS). The alternative preferred by both Kennedy and Johnson was the use of outside task forces.

In building public support, presidents can choose from a variety of strategies, including major addresses to the nation and efforts to mobilize their administration to make public appeals and organized attempts to increase support among interest groups.

To facilitate legislative decision-making and policy support building, presidents, key staff, and department officials interact closely with Congress. Presidents generally meet with legislative leaders several mornings each month to shape the coming legislative agenda and to identify possible problems as bills move through various committees.

Suppliers of Policy

All three branches of government—legislative, executive, and judicial—are suppliers of policy. Of these, the legislative branch is the most active in policymaking, which is particularly evident from policies that take the form of statutes or laws. Legislators play central roles in providing policies demanded by their various constituencies.

Members of the executive branch also act as suppliers of policies. Presidents, governors, and other high-level public officials propose policies in the form of proposed legislation and push legislators to enact their preferred policies. Top executives, as well as executives and managers in charge of departments and agencies of government, make policies in the form of rules and regulations used to implement statutes and programs. In this manner, they interpret congressional interest and thereby become intermediary suppliers of policies.

The judicial branch of government also is a policy supplier. Whenever a court interprets an ambiguous statute, establishes judicial precedent, or interprets the US Constitution, it makes policy. These activities are not conceptually different from legislators enacting statutes or members of the executive branch establishing rules and regulations for the implementation of the statutes. All three activities concur with the definition of policy in that they are authoritative decisions made within government to influence or direct the actions, behaviors, and decisions of others.

Legislative Committees and Subcommittees

The legislative branch creates health policies and allocates the resources necessary to implement them. Congress has three important powers that make it extremely influential in the health policy process. First, the Constitution grants Congress the power to "make all laws which shall be necessary and proper for carrying into execution." The doctrine of implied powers states that Congress may use any reasonable means not directly prohibited by the Constitution to carry out the will of the people. This mandate gives it great power to enact laws influencing all manner of health policy. Second, Congress possesses the power to tax, which allows it to influence and regulate the health behavior of individuals, organizations, and states. Taxes on cigarettes, for example, are intended to reduce individual cigarette consumption, whereas tax relief for employer benefits is designed to promote increased insurance coverage for working people. Third, Congress possesses the power to spend. This ability allows for direct expenditures on the public's health through federal programs, such as Medicare and the NIH, but the power to allocate resources also gives Congress the ability to induce state conformance with federal policy objectives. Congress may prescribe the terms with which it dispenses funds to the states, such as mandating the basic required elements of the federal/state-funded Medicaid program.

At least 14 committees and subcommittees in the House of Representatives, 24 in the Senate, and more than 60 other such legislative panels directly influence legislation (Falcone and Hartwig 1991). Of these, five committees—three in the House and two in the Senate—control most of the legislative activity in Congress (Longest 1994) and are discussed below.

House Committees

The US Constitution provides that all bills involving taxation must originate in the US House of Representatives. The organization of the House gives this authority to the Ways and Means Committee. Hence, the Ways and Means Committee is the most influential by distinction of its power to tax. This committee was the launching pad for much of the health financing legislation passed in the 1960s and early 1970s under the chairmanship of Representative Wilbur Mills (D-AR). Ways and Means has sole jurisdiction over Medicare Part A, Social Security, unemployment compensation, public welfare, and health care reform. It also shares jurisdiction over

Medicare Part B with the House Commerce Committee. This committee, formerly Energy and Commerce, has jurisdiction over Medicaid, Medicare Part B, matters of public health, mental health, health personnel, HMOs, foods and drugs, air pollution, consumer products safety, health planning, biomedical research, and health protection.

The Committee on Appropriations is responsible for funding substantive legislative provisions. Its subcommittee on Labor, Health and Human Services, Education, and Related Agencies is responsible for health appropriations. Essentially, this committee holds the power of the purse. The committee and the subcommittee are responsible for allocating and distributing federal funds for individual health programs (except for Medicare and Social Security, which are funded through the Social Security Trust Fund).

Senate Committees

The Committee on Labor and Human Resources has jurisdiction over most health bills, including the Public Health Service Act, the Federal Drug and Cosmetic Act, HMOs, health personnel, and mental health legislation (e.g., Community Mental Health Centers Act). This committee formerly included a subcommittee on Health and Scientific Research, which was used by its then chairman Senator Edward Kennedy (D-MA) as a forum for debate on whether the United States should have a national health care program. When the full committee came under Republican control in the 1980s, the subcommittee was abolished.

The Committee on Finance and its Subcommittee on Health, similar to the Ways and Means Committee in the House, has jurisdiction over taxes and revenues, including matters related to Social Security, Medicare,

Medicaid, and Maternal and Child Health (Title V of the Social Security Act). It is responsible for many of the Medicare and Medicaid amendments, such as professional standards review organizations, PPS, and amendments controlling hospital and nursing home costs.

The Legislative Process

When a bill is introduced in the House of Representatives, the Speaker assigns it to an appropriate committee. The committee chair forwards the bill to the appropriate subcommittee. The subcommittee forwards proposed legislation to agencies that will be affected by the legislation, holds hearings ("markup") and testimonies, and may add amendments. The subcommittee and committee may recommend, not recommend, or recommend tabling the bill. Diverse interest groups, individuals, experts in the field, and business, labor, and professional associations often exert influence on the bill through campaign contributions and intense lobbying. The full House then hears the bill and may add amendments. The bill can be approved with or without amendments. The approved bill is sent to the Senate.

In the Senate, the bill is sent to an appropriate committee and next forwarded to an appropriate subcommittee. The subcommittee may send the bill to agencies that will be affected. It also holds hearings and testimonies from all interested parties (e.g., private citizens, business, labor, agencies, experts). The subcommittee votes on and forwards the proposed legislation with appropriate recommendations. Amendments may or may not be added. The full Senate hears the bill and may add amendments. If the bill and House amendments are accepted, the bill

goes to the president. If the Senate adds amendments that have not been voted on by the House, the bill must go back to the House floor for a vote.

If the amendments are minor and noncontroversial, the House may vote to pass the bill. If the amendments are significant and controversial, the House may call for a Conference Committee to review the amendments. The Conference Committee consists of members from equivalent committees of the House and Senate. If the recommendations of the Conference Committee are not accepted, another Conference Committee is called.

After the bill has passed both the House and Senate in identical form, it is forwarded to the president for signature. If the president signs the legislation, it becomes law. If the president does not sign the legislation, at the end of 21 days it becomes law unless the president vetoes the legislation. If less than 21 days are left in the congressional session, presidential inaction results in a veto. This is called a "pocket veto." The veto can be overturned by a two-thirds majority of the Congress; otherwise the bill is dead.

Once legislation has been signed into law, it is forwarded to the appropriate agency for implementation. The agency publishes proposed regulations in the Federal Register and holds hearings on how the law is to be implemented. A bureaucracy only loosely controlled by either the president or Congress writes (publishes, gathers comments about, and rewrites) regulations. Then the program goes on to the 50 states for enabling legislation, if appropriate. There, organized interests hire local lawyers and lobbyists and a completely new political cycle begins. Finally, all parties may adjourn to the courts, where long rounds of litigation shape the final outcome.

Critical Policy Issues

Government health policies have been enacted to resolve or prevent perceived deficiencies in health care delivery. Over the last four decades, most health policy initiatives have focused on access to care, cost of care, and quality of care (Falcone and Hartwig 1991). Some Americans contend that they have the right (access) to the best care (quality) at the least expense (cost), despite their level of income or social class. Legislative efforts have been specific to issues in access (expanding insurance coverage, outreach programs in rural areas), cost containment (PPS, relative-value scales), and quality (creating the Agency for Health Care Policy and Research [now Agency for Health Care Research and Quality] and calling for clinical practice guidelines, see Chapter 2).

With the publication of Healthy People 2010, elimination of health disparities across sociodemographic subpopulations has emerged as a bold policy objective. Since health disparities are caused primarily by nonmedical factors, the advancement of this goal signals a new policy direction that integrates health policy with broader public policy. Although it is highly unlikely this goal will be fulfilled within the first decade of the 21st century, the promotion of this policy objective reflects a significant government commitment. In the remainder of this section, critical policy issues related to access to care, cost of care, and quality of care, the three areas of greatest health policy concerns, are highlighted.

Access to Care

Underlying support for government policies enhancing access to care is the social justice principle that access to health care is a right that should be guaranteed to all American citizens. There are two variations on this argument: (1) All citizens have a right to the same level of care, and (2) all citizens have a right to some minimum level of care. The latter is more prevalent in the United States. However, significant debate exists over which health care services ought to be included in a basic tier. However, the conclusion that all citizens are entitled to a minimum level of services remains intact. Policies on access are aimed primarily at providers and financing mechanisms to expand care to the most needy and underserved populations, including the elderly, children, minorities, rural residents, those of low-income, and persons with acquired immune deficiency syndrome (AIDS).

Providers

Several groups of providers deliver health care. Policy issues include ensuring a sufficient number and desirable geographic distribution of each. The debate over the supply of physicians is an important public policy issue because policy decisions influence the number of persons entering the medical profession, and that number, in turn, has implications for other policies. The number of new entrants into the profession is influenced by programs of government assistance for individual students and by government grants made directly to educational institutions. An increased supply of physicians, particularly specialists, may result in increased health care expenditures because of increased demand for care induced by the physicians. An increased supply of physicians, particularly primary care physicians, may help alleviate shortages in certain regions of the country. Programs enacted to expand delivery of care, particularly to the underserved, have included the National Health Service Corps, legislation supporting rural health clinics to expand geographic access, student assistance programs to expand the pool of health care workers, legislation to expand a system of emergency medical services, and the establishment of community health centers in inner cities and rural areas.

Public Financing

Although a national health care program is seen by many people as the best way to ensure access, the United States focuses instead on the needs of particular groups. As early as the Truman administration, and certainly by 1958, congressional attention turned to the health care needs of the elderly (Marmor 1973). In 1960, Congress enacted the Kerr-Mills program (P.L. 86–778), which provided federal grants to state government programs assisting the elderly. Medicare, and its companion program Medicaid (care for the poor was added to Medicare in part to compromise with a physician-drafted proposal), established the precedent that government should facilitate access to health care among those unable to secure it for themselves. Over the years, policies have been enacted to provide access to health care for specific groups otherwise unable to pay for and receive care. These groups include the elderly (Medicare), poor children (Medicaid and SCHIP), poor adults (Medicaid and local or state general assistance), the disabled (Medicaid and Medicare), veterans (Department of Veterans Affairs), Native Americans (Indian Health Service), and patients with end-stage renal disease (Social Security benefits for kidney dialysis and transplants).

Access continues to be a problem in many communities, partly because health policies enacted since 1983 have focused on narrowly defined elements of the delivery system. The United States has not had a unified strategy of reforming the system based on a policy of integrated services. Since the diminution of health planning in the early 1980s, the United States has approached the access problem on a piecemeal basis—one group, one type of geographic location, and one type of service at a time. The fact that many Americans remain uninsured is reason to expect ongoing debate toward a public policy on this issue.

Access and the Elderly

Two main concerns dominate the debate about Medicare policy. First, spending should be restrained to keep the program viable. Current emphasis is on using market-based mechanisms to deliver services more efficiently. Second, the program needs to be made truly comprehensive by adding services not currently covered (e.g., comprehensive nursing home coverage). Both concerns originate from the assumption that the elderly need public assistance to finance their health care.

Access and Minorities

Minorities are more likely than Whites to face access problems and to warrant special attention. Hispanics, African Americans, Asian Americans, and Native Americans, to name the most prevalent minorities, all face barriers accessing the health care delivery system. In some instances, the combination of low-income and minority status creates difficulties; in others, the interaction of special cultural habits and minority status causes problems. With the exception of Native Americans, no other minority population has programs specifically designed to serve its needs. Resolving the problems confronting minority groups would require policies designed to target the special needs of minorities, to encourage professional education programs sensitive to their special needs, and to develop programs to expand the delivery of services to areas populated by minorities. Many of these areas are known to be short of health care professionals.

Access in Rural Areas

Delivery of health care services in rural communities has always raised the question of how to bring advanced medical care to residents of sparsely settled areas. Financing high-tech equipment for a few people is not cost efficient, and finding physicians who want to live in rural areas is difficult. The medical model of health services delivery evident in large teaching institutions makes specialists and expensive diagnostic equipment readily available. This is not the case in rural medical practices, making those practices less desirable to many medical school graduates. Reimbursement systems based on average costs make it difficult for rural hospitals with few patients to survive financially.

In the Omnibus Budget Reconciliation Act (OBRA) of 1986, Congress began to address the particular problems of rural hospitals with three important provisions. The act separated the urban and rural pools of funds used to pay for outliers, those cases in which excessive expenditures above the PPS allotment are incurred. This ended the practice of using revenues otherwise intended for rural hospitals to reimburse expensive cases in urban hospitals. It provided early payments to hospitals with fewer than 100 beds. It also changed the criteria for rural referral centers to allow more hospitals to qualify for funds.

The OBRA of 1987 included provisions that (1) provided a greater increase in reimbursement to rural hospitals than to urban hospitals, (2) allowed rural hospitals located adjacent to metropolitan statistical areas to be defined as urban hospitals, (3) authorized a rural health care transition program to provide assistance to hospitals and others wishing to adopt new service delivery strategies, (4) required a report on the appropriateness of separate urban and rural rates, (5) and authorized small rural hospitals to serve as residency training sites for physicians (Patton 1988).

Shortages of personnel translate into access problems for rural residents. The federal government designates certain areas as health professions shortage areas, based on having a population-to-primary care physician ratio of at least 3,500:1 and being an area adjacent to others in which primary medical care personnel are overused.

Providing funding for the National Health Service Corps is another major step toward redressing the problem of personnel shortages in rural areas. The Corps affects only the percentage of graduating physicians practicing in shortage areas, and then only for a limited period for each student. Additional programs increase the total supply of physicians and create incentives for permanent practice in rural areas as needed.

Access and Low Income

Low-income mothers and their children have problems accessing the health care system, because they lack insurance and because they generally live in medically underserved areas. Limited access among children creates problems of untreated chronic health conditions that lead to increased medical expenditures and loss of productivity to society.

Low-income mothers face the same problems as their children in accessing medical services. Pregnant women in low-income families are far less likely to receive prenatal care than are women in higher income categories. The SCHIP program, signed into law August 5, 1997, gave states some flexibility in how to spend federal funds allocated for children's health coverage over five years (States Face a Welcome Dilemma 1997). After a period of enthusiastic outreach efforts and program expansion, a severe economic downturn, beginning in 2002, forced states to implement enrollment barriers for SCHIP (and Medicaid). As of January 2007, approximately 9 million children remain uninsured, despite the fact that a majority of them are eligible for Medicaid or SCHIP (Kaiser Family Foundation 2007a). As SCHIP undergoes federal reauthorization in 2007, funding decisions will critically affect whether this number of uninsured children can be reduced.

Access and Persons with AIDS

Persons with AIDS, who have progressed from infection by human immunodeficiency virus to actually having the disease and therefore needing more expensive treatment, also have problems obtaining health care. People with AIDS have difficulty obtaining insurance coverage, and their illness leads to catastrophic health care expenditures. Financial access can be a barrier, particularly for persons without adequate health insurance benefits. The AIDS epidemic presents a special challenge to policymakers committed to universal access to health care services. The services required are expensive, and the population in need is relatively small. Further, the care is directed toward patients who are terminally ill. In 2003, President

Bush pledged $15 billion over five years to combat HIV/AIDS in the developing countries, with a particular focus on Africa. As of September 2006, the President's Emergency Plan for AIDS Relief (PEPFAR) supported prevention of mother-to-child transmission of HIV in over 6 million pregnancies and antiretroviral treatment for 822,000 people (US President's Emergency Plan for AIDS Relief 2007). On the other hand, funding to help AIDS victims at home remains inadequate by many accounts. According to The Foundation for AIDS Research (amfAR), Congress has provided significant increases for HIV/AIDS research, care, treatment, and prevention in the United States; however, domestic agencies still lack adequate resources to effectively combat the HIV/AIDS epidemic (Foundation for AIDS Research 2007).

Cost of Care

The strengths of the US health care delivery system also contribute substantially to its weaknesses. The United States has the latest developments in medical technology and well-trained specialists, but these advances amount to the most expensive means possible to provide care to patients, making the US health care system the most costly in the world. No other aspect of health care policy has received more attention during the past 20-plus years than efforts to contain increases in health care costs. Cost containment has become a major policy priority because of the government's increasing role in financing of health care services. Government programs, especially Medicare, Medicaid, Veterans Affairs, armed services, and federal employee benefit programs, are under constant pressure from Congress to keep costs down.

The National Health Planning and Resources Development Act of 1974 (P.L. 93–641) became law in 1975. This act marked the transition from improvement of access to cost containment as the principal theme in federal health policy. Advocates for both objectives supported health planning; however, the purpose rapidly became defined solely in terms of containing health care expenditures by the 1970s and health service researchers showed that the increased supply of health care facilities also increased expenditures. When Congress was considering expanding programs such as the Hill-Burton construction grants for health facilities through comprehensive health planning, policy analysts concluded that unneeded health care facilities were causing increases in health expenditures. In health care, unneeded supply generates demand. Therefore, it seemed logical to enact a policy that would allow construction of only those facilities that were actually needed. Need for facilities could be determined through a planning process, and final decisions would include some input from the citizens of the community.

Health planning, through CON review, was used as a policy tool to contain hospital costs; however, hospital charges continued to increase throughout the 1970s. The 1980 election signaled formal changes in the policy environment. One major change in the health policy environment was a new system of paying hospitals for Medicare clients, the PPS, enacted in 1983 (Mueller 1988). By 1982, members of Congress and the administration were convinced that voluntary efforts to contain hospital expenditures were failing. Congress used the Tax Equity and Fiscal Responsibility Act of 1982 as the legislative vehicle to reduce reimbursement for hospitals by $5 billion over three years. Congress commissioned the DHHS to develop a

new system for reimbursement that would pay hospitals on a prospective basis rather than a retrospective basis. In lieu of tight regulation of charges established by individual hospitals, the PPS serves as a general fee schedule and establishes a prospective payment for general categories of treatment (based on diagnosis-related groups) that applies to all short-stay hospitals. PPS has proved to be the most successful tool for controlling hospital expenditures. As cost containment continued to be the dominant theme in the 1980s, health planning was no longer viewed as a national policy priority.

The election of Ronald Reagan in 1980 marked a general shift in policy that was geared to a reduction of federal government activity in domestic policy issues and toward an acceleration of deregulation throughout the domestic economy. The CON program, the cornerstone of cost containment through health planning, was retained by 38 states after Congress repealed the national law requiring such a program. The targets of CON laws may not always be hospitals, which were the subject of debates and legislation in the 1970s. Instead, the concerns of the 1990s became nursing homes, psychiatric facilities, and long-term hospitals. The owners of these facilities are less powerful than hospitals in influencing fiscal policy.

States use health planning in ways other than the review of petitions to add capital expenditures. More than 35 states have established state offices of rural health. Many of these programs use methods of health planning (i.e., needs assessment and consideration of alternative strategies for delivering services) to assist medical care providers and rural communities. A few states have used a direct regulatory approach to determine how much hospitals and nursing homes would be reimbursed. A variety of methods have been used, including limiting payments to a fixed percentage of the institution's charges, reimbursing only what the state determines is a reasonable amount for a given service, and determining in advance the total expenditures to be paid to hospitals and nursing homes for the coming year.

The policy focus on cost containment is also influenced by the private sector. Major corporations have awakened from the habit of passively paying medical bills. They are now aggressively pursuing ways to restrain the escalation of medical costs. These large purchasers are buying medical services in volume, at wholesale prices, and even dictating the terms of service. This method is a radical change from the long-held custom of individuals or their insurers paying for health care retail on a case-by-case basis. Institutional buyers want to know what they are getting for their money. The answers require detailed data, close scrutiny, and, ultimately, outside judgment of whether the services are worth their cost.

Expenditures are a function of the price of services times the quantity of services delivered. Most policies enacted to date have focused on the price of services. Policymakers are reluctant to consider restricting the quantity of services, fearful of interpretations that they are sacrificing quality of care for cost containment. These concerns are warranted as the media fuel the frenzy over denial of services by managed care organizations.

Increased debate over the right to die and the value of life-extending services provides an opportunity to discuss limiting reimbursable services. So far, the federal government has been reluctant to adopt an explicit rationing strategy to contain expenditures, but state governments can be expected to experiment with various means of

cost containment. Interest in Oregon's rationing policies of the 1990s indicates that the issue may be addressed by state legislatures seeking to contain rising medical expenditures.

The fragmented multi-payer system in the United States does not lend itself to a centralized policy of cost containment. This is one main reason why health care expenditures in the United States will remain above per capita expenditures in other countries.

Quality of Care

Along with access and cost, quality of care is the third main concern of health care policy. Funding to evaluate new treatment methods and diagnostic tools is increasing dramatically. Funding for research to measure the outcome of medical interventions has also increased. This research is focused on the question of appropriateness of medical procedures.

The federal government began its actions to relieve the malpractice crisis and devoted greater attention to policing the quality of medical care with the Health Care Quality Act of 1986. This legislation mandated the creation of a national database within the DHHS to provide data on legal actions against health care providers. This information helps people recruiting physicians in one state to know of actions against those physicians in other states. Additional national legislation has been suggested to reform legal proceedings to lower the cost of malpractice claims and, therefore, reduce the premiums charged to providers.

In 1989, the federal government embarked on a major effort to sponsor research to establish guidelines for medical practice. In the OBRA of 1989, Congress created a new agency, the AHCPR, formerly called the

National Center for Health Services Research, and more recently called the Agency for Healthcare Research and Quality (AHRQ), and mandated it to conduct and support research with respect to the outcomes, effectiveness, and appropriateness of health care services and procedures (House of Representatives 1989). In the late 1980s, AHCPR (now AHRQ) established funding for patient outcomes research teams (PORTs) that focus on particular medical conditions. The PORTs are part of a broader effort, the medical treatment effectiveness program, which "consists of four elements: medical treatment effectiveness research, development of databases for such research, development of clinical guidelines, and the dissemination of research findings and clinical guidelines" (Salive et al. 1990). Today, the PORTs continue to produce valuable and applicable research findings on quality of care for various diseases and conditions, such as schizophrenia, diabetes, and stroke prevention. In March 2001, the Institute of Medicine (IOM) issued a comprehensive report, Crossing the Quality Chasm. Building on the extensive evidence collected by the IOM committee, the report identified six areas for quality improvement: (1) Safety. Patients ought to be as safe in health care facilities as they are in their homes. (2) Effectiveness. The health care system should avoid overuse of ineffective care and underuse of effective care. (3) Patient-centeredness. Respect for the patient's choices, culture, social context, and special needs must be incorporated into the delivery of services. (4) Timeliness. Waiting times and delays should be continually reduced for both patients and caregivers. (5) Efficiency. Health care should engage in a never-ending pursuit to reduce total costs by curtailing waste, such as waste of supplies, equipment, space, capital, and the innovative

human spirit. (6) Equity. The system should seek to close racial and ethnic gaps in health status (Berwick 2002).

Policies designed to increase activities that promote good health are targeting individual behavior. Smoking cessation programs are designed to eliminate a specific behavior known to be related to the onset of several critical illnesses, including cancer, heart problems, and chronic obstructive lung disease. Data on the nation's health behavior indicators are published regularly by the US Office of Disease Prevention and Health Promotion. The US Environmental Protection Agency continues to monitor the quality of the air and water, and reports on cities and states not complying with federal standards.

Research and Policy Development

The research community can influence health policymaking through documentation, analysis, and prescription (Longest 1994). The first role of research in policymaking is documentation; that is, the gathering, cataloging, and correlating of facts that depict the state of the world that policymakers face. This process may help define a given public policy problem or raise its political profile. A second way in which research informs, and thus influences, policymaking is through analysis of what does and does not work. Examples include program evaluation and outcomes research. Often taking the form of demonstration projects intended to provide a basis for determining the feasibility, efficacy, or practicality of a possible policy intervention, analysis can help define solutions to health policy problems. The third way in which research influences policymaking is through prescription. Research that demonstrates that a course of action being contemplated by policymakers may (or may not) lead to undesirable or unexpected consequences can contribute significantly to policymaking.

The Future of Health Policy

Many of the problems confronted in US health care policy exist because policymakers have not adopted a comprehensive approach. Instead, single issues have been approached individually, and not all dimensions of any one issue have been considered when developing specific policies. Given the political system, the future of health policy is likely to continue in a piecemeal, fragmented, disjointed, and largely state-based manner aimed at enhancing access, containing cost, and improving quality. The recent policy goal of elimination of health disparities could not be realized without concerted efforts and coordinated strategies across health and non-health sectors.

Health Insurance Reform

The US health care system is criticized for many reasons. One common criticism is that the United States is the only industrialized nation that fails to assure universal access to basic health care. Over 44 million people— mostly adults and children in wage-earning families—lack health insurance. Nor does holding onto a job guarantee coverage. Seven out of every 10 Americans depend on their employers for their insurance, but in today's tight economy employers are chipping away at benefits, compelling employees to pay more of the cost and even eliminating coverage entirely. Being without health insurance often means being without medical care, especially for many of the adult poor

and minorities (Freeman et al. 1990). One critical future policy concern is to ensure that most, if not all, Americans have adequate health insurance. If and when the time comes for a comprehensive reform of the current health care system, policy debate is likely to include several different proposals. These proposals are addressed in Chapter 4.

States as Leaders

From the 1930s through the 1950s, states' involvement in health care was limited to basic public health functions, such as control of communicable diseases, direct delivery of certain services, such as care for the chronically mentally ill, and administration of federal grants-in-aid. With the start of the health insurance industry in the 1940s and 1950s, states also began to regulate both Blue Cross and Blue Shield plans and commercial policies.

The states' role in health care diminished considerably in the 1970s as Medicare and Medicaid grew well beyond most of their creators' predictions and as other federal programs, such as support for community health centers, expanded in scope.

During the 1980s, President Reagan ushered in a new era characterized by an effort to return greater control and discretion over the financing, delivery, and regulation of health care to the states. *Block grants*, which consolidate funds from many different categorical programs into one lump sum that is distributed to the states on a formula basis, became a key vehicle to achieve all three goals.

By the mid-1990s, states faced the prospect of gaining even greater control and flexibility for the administration and financing of health and human service programs. In 1995, Congress seriously considered a proposal to turn the entire Medicaid program over to state governments by giving them a block grant with few federal strings attached.

States are vested with broad legal authority to regulate almost every facet of the health care system. They license and regulate health care facilities and health professionals; restrict the content, marketing, and price of health insurance (including professional liability or malpractice insurance); set and enforce environmental quality standards; and enact a variety of controls on health care costs.

All states bear a large responsibility for financing health services for the poor, primarily through the Medicaid program, for which financing is shared with the federal government. States also pay the costs of providing health coverage to state employees and retirees, and sometimes for other publicly employed workers, such as teachers and police. In addition, most states also help subsidize some costs of delivering health services to those without any coverage at all. An example is Oregon, which, in 1989, embarked on a controversial experiment that expands Medicaid coverage to more than 100,000 additional people by reducing the Medicaid benefit package (Bodenheimer 1997).

By far, however, the states' most significant effort to contain costs was to increase enrollment of Medicaid beneficiaries into HMOs and other managed care arrangements, starting in the 1990s. By 2001, over half of Medicaid beneficiaries received services via managed care (Kaiser Family Foundation 2001). A review of studies on the effects of Medicaid managed care programs confirmed cost savings of 10% to 15% below those of the regular fee-for-service system; however, this cost savings may now be in jeopardy because many states, as part of their Medicaid maximization strategies, have crafted their programs to include safety net providers and mental health benefits. As the

federal government closes the loopholes that allow for Medicaid maximization, this strategy may lead to higher costs for states, which could ultimately undermine the purpose of moving Medicaid beneficiaries to managed care: to increase access and quality of care (Coughlin et al. 1999).

Medicaid's inability to cover all the poor is one reason that approximately 44.6 million Americans lack health coverage (Kaiser Family Foundation 2007b). Often, it falls on the state governments, along with city and county governments, to help subsidize the costs of caring for those who lack health insurance coverage. Although many of these individuals are served by public health agencies or public hospitals that provide direct care to those without health insurance, many states also administer programs to provide coverage to these people.

One of the oldest and most fundamental state roles has been protecting the public's health. Originally, this meant controlling the spread of communicable diseases. The roles have expanded exponentially over the past several decades to include protecting the environment, workplace, housing, food, and water; preventing injuries and promoting health behaviors; responding to disasters and assisting communities in recovery efforts; ensuring the quality, accessibility, and accountability of medical care and providing basic health services when otherwise unavailable; monitoring population health status and changes in the health care system; and developing policies and plans that support individual and community health improvement. The Institute of Medicine (1988), in its study of the future of public health, condensed these various activities into three basic functions: assessment of health status and systems; policy development; and assurance of personal, educational, and environmental health services.

The biggest challenge facing state public health agencies today is strengthening their capacity to protect and promote the public's health while ensuring that basic health services are still available to those who cannot pay. Personal health services funded or provided by states, often in cooperation with local governments, range from public health nursing and communicable disease control to family planning and prenatal care, to nutritional counseling and home health services.

The challenge before state public health agencies is to seek partnerships with the private sector or with local governments. The goal is not merely to decrease their role in direct care but rather to engage private-sector and local government partners in efforts that will improve overall health status. One of the benefits of a managed care approach in the private health care market is managed care's emphasis on population-based services.

As discussed previously in this chapter, states are already undertaking their own comprehensive reforms. They have made important strides in expanding coverage to low-income uninsured groups through SCHIP, subsidy programs, Medicaid expansions, and insurance reforms. Many states have implemented effective cost-containment programs, such as hospital rate setting and setting limits on insurance premium increases.

Growth Initiative for Health Centers

One of the few goals that Republicans and Democrats seem to agree upon is preserving Community Health Centers as a safety-net health care provider for the uninsured. Acting on the recommendation of President Bush, Congress passed a significant increase in health center funding in the Omnibus Appropriations Act of 2003. The federal Health Centers program received $1.5 billion, $161

million more than the previous year. The President, who has pledged to double the size of the health center program, has continued to support increased funding for the health center program each year since then. In 2006, federal health center program allocations totaled $1.78 billion (NACHC 2006).

In addition to the President's request for 1,200 new and expanded sites, the increased health center funding will stabilize present health centers financially; they had been deteriorating in the light of state and local funding reductions, the rising number of uninsured, and the full impact of mandated Medicaid managed care in a more competitive health care marketplace. Significant progress toward the President's goals has been accomplished: as of 2004, the President's initiative had resulted in more than 600 new or expanded health center sites (Shi 2007).

Medical Malpractice

President Bush has asked Congress to set a $250,000 cap on noneconomic or so-called pain-and-suffering damages. Doctors in some parts of the country are facing double-digit increases in their malpractice insurance premiums and blaming the problem on runaway jury verdicts in malpractice suits. According to DHHS, the malpractice litigation "crisis" threatens access to health care. Many states have already limited damage awards in malpractice cases. But trial lawyers and consumer groups say malpractice suits are not out of control. They claim that insurance companies are raising premiums because of poor underwriting decisions and low investment returns. They also warn that limiting lawsuits hurts victims of egregious medical mistakes and reduces incentives to protect patient safety. Doctors contend that high liability expenses drive up health care costs, thus reducing access to treatment.

Mental Health Benefits

More than 30 million Americans suffer from schizophrenia, severe depression, and other mental disorders. Historically, employers' insurance has paid much lower treatment benefits for mental problems than for medical illness. The 1996 Mental Health Parity Act (MHPA) requires that annual or lifetime dollar limits on mental health benefits be no lower than any such dollar limits for medical and surgical benefits offered by a group health plan or health insurance issuer offering coverage in connection with a group health plan (US Dept of Labor 2007). Congress has considered broadening the MHPA, but conservative lawmakers and business lobbies claim the cost of parity is too high.

Steps to a Healthy United States

To advance President Bush's goal of helping Americans live longer, better, and healthier lives, the DHHS has launched the Steps to a Healthy US initiative. The initiative unites all relevant programs of the Health and Human Services agencies, including the Centers for Disease Control and Prevention, the Centers for Medicare and Medicaid Services, the Food and Drug Administration, and the National Institutes of Health. The initiative will also highlight health promotion programs to motivate and support responsible health choices, community initiatives to promote and enable healthy choices, health care and insurance systems that put prevention first by reducing risk factors and complications of chronic disease, state and federal policies that invest in the prevention for all Americans, and cooperation among policymakers, local health agencies, and the public to invest in disease prevention. Although the initiative's goals are lofty and worthy, concrete, workable strategies are yet to be developed and implemented.

Summary

Health policies are developed to serve the public's interests; however, public interests are diverse. The public often holds conflicting views. A 2007 New York Times/CBS News poll found a majority of Americans support access to health insurance for all. Sixty percent of respondents said they would be willing to pay more in taxes to support such a policy (NY Times 2007). However, while the public supports the goal of national health insurance, it also rejects the idea of the federal government running the health care delivery system. Similarly, while the public wants the government to control health care costs, it also believes that the federal government already controls too much of Americans' daily lives.

In the future, policymakers' challenge will be to find a balance between governmental provisions and control and the private health care market to improve coverage and affordability of care. Successful health policies are more likely to be couched in terms of cost containment (a market justice, economic, business, and middle-class concern) than improved or expanded access, and reducing or eliminating health disparities (a social justice, liberal, labor, low-income issue). However, cost-related policies are unlikely to significantly affect the quality of care or reduce health disparities.

Test Your Understanding

Terminology

allocative tools   *health policy*   *regulatory tools*
block grants   *public policies*
distributive policies   *redistributive policies*

Review Questions

1. What is health policy? How can health policies be used as regulatory or allocative tools?

2. What are the principal features of US health policy? Why do these features characterize US health policy?

3. Identify health care interest groups and their concerns.

4. What is the process of legislative health policy in the United States? How is this process related to the principal features of US health policy?

5. Describe the critical policy issues related to access to care, cost of care, and quality of care.

6. What do you think the future of health policy will look like in the United States?

REFERENCES

Alford, R.R. 1975. *Health care politics: Ideology and interest group barriers to reform.* Chicago: University of Chicago Press.

Belluck P. Jan. 9, 2007. Massachusetts could serve as a guide in California's health insurance bid. New York: *The New York Times.*

Berwick, D.M. 2002. A user's manual for the IOM's "Quality Chasm" report. *Health Affairs* 21, no. 3: 80–90.

Bodenheimer, T. 1997. The Oregon health plan—Lessons for the nation. *New England Journal of Medicine* 337, no. 9: 651–655.

Coughlin, T. et al. 1999. A conflict of strategies: Medicaid managed care and Medicaid maximization. *Health Services Research* 34, no. 1: 281–293.

Falcone, D., and L.C. Hartwig. 1991. Congressional process and health policy: Reform and retrenchment. In *Health policies and policy.* 2nd ed., eds. T. Litman and L. Robins, 126–144. New York: John Wiley & Sons.

Foundation for AIDS Research (amFAR). 2007. Public Policy. *http://www.amfar.org/cgi-bin/iowa/ programs/publicp/record.html?record=9.*

Freeman, H.E. et al. 1990. Uninsured working-age adults: Characteristics and consequences. *Health Services Research* 24 (February): 811–823.

Health Insurance Association of America. 1992. *Source book of health insurance data.* Washington, DC.

House of Representatives. 1989. Omnibus Budget Reconciliation Act of 1989: Conference report to accompany H.R. 3299. Washington, DC: Government Printing Office, 21 November.

Institute of Medicine, Committee for the Study of the Future of Public Health. 1988. *The future of public health.* Washington, DC: National Academy Press.

Kaiser Family Foundation, Commission on Medicaid and the Uninsured. 2007a. State Children's Health Insurance Program at a Glance. *http://www.kff.org/medicaid/upload/7610.pdf.*

Kaiser Family Foundation, Commission on Medicaid and the Uninsured. 2007b. Characteristics of the uninsured. *http://www.kff.org/uninsured/upload/7613.pdf.*

Kaiser Family Foundation, Commission on Medicaid and the Uninsured. 2001. Medicaid and managed care fact sheet. *http://kff.org/medicaid/loader.cfm?url=/commonspot/security/getfile.cfm&PageID=13724.*

Lemov, P. 1990. Health insurance for all: A possible dream? *Governing* (November): 56–62.

Litman, T., and L. Robins. 1997. The relationship of government and politics to health and health care—A sociopolitical overview. In *Health politics and policy.* 3rd ed., eds. T. Litman and L. Robins, 3–45. New York: John Wiley & Sons.

Longest, B.B. 1994. *Health policymaking in the United States.* Ann Arbor, MI: Health Administration Press.

Marmor, T. 1973. *The politics of Medicare.* Chicago: Aldine Publishing Co.

Miller, C.A. 1987. Child health. In *Epidemiology and Health Policy*, eds. S. Levine and A. Lillienfeld. New York: Tavistock Publications.

Mueller, K.J. 1988. Federal programs do expire: The case of health planning. *Public Administration Review* 48 (May/June): 719–735.

National Association of Community Health Centers (NACHC). 2006. A sketch of community health centers: Chart book 2006. *http://www.nachc.com/research/Files/Chart%20Book%202006.pdf.*

National Institutes of Health. 1991. *NIH data book.* Washington, DC.

National Institutes of Health. 2007. Summary of the FY 2008 President's Budget. *http://officeofbudget.od.nih.gov/PDF/Press%20info-2008.pdf.*

Patton, L.T. 1988. *The rural health care challenge.* Staff Report to the Special Committee on Aging, US Senate. Washington, DC: Government Printing Office, October.

Salive, M.E. et al. 1990. Patient outcomes research teams and the Agency for Health Care Policy and Research. *Health Services Research* 25 (December): 697–708.

Shi, L., P.B. Collins, and K.F. Aaron. 2007. Health center financial performance: National trends and state variation, 1998–2004. *J Public Health Management and Practice* 13(2):133–50.

States face a welcome dilemma: How to best spend $24 billion to cover nation's uninsured children. 1997. *State Health Watch* 4, no. 8: 1, 4.

US Department of Labor. 2007. Mental Health Parity Fact Sheet. *http://www.dol.gov/ebsa/newsroom/fsmhparity.html.*

US President's Emergency Plan for AIDS Relief. 2007. *http://www.pepfar.gov/.*

Weissert, C., and W. Weissert. 1996. *Governing health: The politics of health policy.* Baltimore: Johns Hopkins University Press.

Chapter 4

Leiyu Shi, DrPH, MBA, MPA, and Douglas A. Singh, PhD, MBA

The Future of Health Services Delivery

Learning Objectives

- To assess the trends in private and public health insurance
- To evaluate the challenges faced by managed care
- To discuss future financing and insurance options in the current system
- To discuss various options for a universal health insurance system
- To understand future challenges in wellness and prevention, chronic care, and long-term care
- To identify trends in the spread of infectious diseases attributed to globalization
- To foresee the evolving role of public health under new threats
- To explore the future outlook of US hospitals
- To address issues pertaining to the future needs for a well-prepared health care workforce.
- To understand the value of collaborative teamwork and cross-training in the delivery of health care
- To appreciate the emphasis on customer service and potential barriers
- To get an overview of new frontiers in clinical technology
- To survey the unfolding era of evidence-based health care

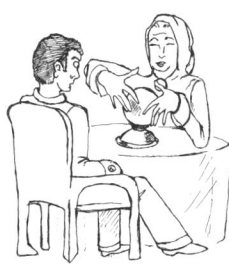

"Will the U.S. have universal health insurance?"

Introduction

Predicting the future direction of health care delivery in the United States is predicated upon major current developments and the course they might take in the foreseeable future. Future change also relies on historical precedents and a society's fundamental values. These elements come into play particularly when any kind of a sweeping transformation is proposed. For instance, in 1993, President Clinton proposed his national health care initiative in an economic, social, and political environment in which health care expenditures were getting out of hand and a significant number of Americans were without health insurance. However, the majority of Americans did not think that nationalized health insurance was the right way to address these issues. Most Americans were opposed to uninvited government intervention. The insured Americans were particularly fearful of losing their existing coverage with which they were reasonably satisfied. Middle-class Americans have also held a widespread belief that they pay more than their reasonable share of taxes to support Medicare and Medicaid programs to help the underprivileged. Besides the American middle class, the Clinton Plan was also opposed by most providers, particularly by physicians in private practice.

Rejection of the Clinton plan based on ingrained American values provided the impetus for a widespread shift toward managed care, which at that time had already started to emerge as a growing force. Managed care became the natural choice for injecting competition into the financing, insurance, delivery, and payment functions of health care.

At this point, the foundational values of American society remain intact. Hence, no sweeping changes are expected. However, medical cost escalation and cost of health insurance premiums continue to outpace both general inflation and general economic growth. For example, premiums for family coverage have risen by 87% since 2000 (Claxton et al. 2006). Faced with such a cost burden, fewer employers are offering health insurance coverage to their workers. The percentage of firms offering health insurance has fallen from 69% in 2000 to 61% in 2006 (Claxton et al. 2006). Also, since the mid-1990s, there has been steady erosion in retiree health benefits. Buchmueller and colleagues (2006) estimated that in 2003 only about 25% of private-sector employees worked at establishments that offered retiree health benefits, down from 32% in 1997. At the same time, Americans' appetite for new medical breakthroughs remains unabated. Amid these transitions, any major health care reform on a national scale has remained a nonissue. But, in April 2006, Massachusetts restructured its own health insurance markets, imposed assessments on employers who did not provide health insurance to their workers, and pooled private and public resources to cover many of the uninsured. If successful, this model may open the way for other states to initiate health insurance reforms.

At the time of this writing, the United States has also undergone a major political change with the Democrats gaining majority in both houses of Congress and control of the powerful Ways and Means Committee in Fall 2006. The presidential election of 2008 will be of significant interest because of major uncertainties on several fronts.

Any attempts to project the future of health care provoke more questions than answers. Even though precise forecasts cannot be made, certain fundamental features of health care delivery in the United States are assured at least for the foreseeable future. The stable features of US health care essentially recapitulate some of the points made in earlier chapters. In addition, this chapter provides some insights into current directions that might impact the future financing and delivery of health care. Other discussions revolve around what might be achievable, given the right configuration of broader socioeconomic, cultural, and technological forces, particularly in view of some of the major issues that must be addressed.

Trends in Private and Public Health Insurance

Trends in Employment-Based Insurance

During the era marked by the rapid growth of managed care, the proportion of nonelderly who had employment-based health insurance increased from 64.4% in 1994 to 66.8% in 2000. This was also a period of economic expansion and shortage of skilled workers that created stiff competition for labor. Since then, employment-based coverage has been eroding. It went down to 62.4% in 2004, which is below the level in 1994 (Gold 2006). Between 2000 and 2004, declines in employment-based coverage were the steepest for younger and low-income people (Holahan and Cook 2005). In addition, as the US workforce continues to age, the composition of enrollees in employment-based insurance will shift toward older adults, which portends an acceleration in the rate of premium growth. Well before we see the effects of baby boomers' enrollment in Medicare, rising premiums in private health plans could place more pressure on an already strained employment-based health insurance system (Keenan et al. 2006).

Public sector employers, particularly state and local governments, also face challenges similar to those in the private sector. As are major private employers, the public sector is experimenting with numerous cost-containment strategies, including disease and case management, aggressive management of pharmacy benefits, and contracting with managed care (McKethan et al. 2006).

Given the existing conditions, at least some commentators regard employers as ineffective and unenthusiastic managers of the health benefits they sponsor (Galvin et al. 2005). It is suggested that, if possible, employers would like to get out of the business of offering health benefits altogether, but it is unlikely to happen (Galvin and Delbanco 2006). Research suggests that employers, both large and small, hold a positive view of the value of health benefits in attracting and retaining workers, improving morale, and increasing workers' productivity. The same employers also believe that all employers should share in the cost of health insurance (Whitmore et al. 2006). It appears that employers are sensitive to having to carry the cost burden of those employed elsewhere, such as spouses of employees.

High-Deductible Health Plans

Faced with escalating health insurance premiums, employers appear to be embracing increased responsibility and higher cost sharing by the employees as strategies for reducing their health care costs (Claxton et al. 2005a). One emerging health plan type, the high-deductible health plan (HDHP), seems to be gaining some initial momentum. For example, in 2006, among firms that offered employment-based health insurance, 7% offered a HDHP. It was estimated that out of 155 million Americans covered under employment-based health insurance, as many as 2.7 million may be covered under a HDHP (Claxton et al. 2006). However, these plans may become more popular in the future because they carry the lowest premium compared to HMO, PPO, and POS plans, they offer tax advantages to workers and give the insured control over how the money is spent. Hence, these plans are also loosely referred to as consumer-directed health plans.

There are two basic types of HDHPs. The first type, called health reimbursement arrangements (HRAs), grew out of federal regulations made by the Internal Revenue Service in 2002. The second type, health savings accounts (HSAs), were authorized in the Medicare Prescription Drug, Improvement, and Modernization Act (MMA) of 2003.

An **HRA** is a medical care reimbursement plan sponsored by an employer. HRAs are typically offered in conjunction with a health plan that carries a high deductible. Generally, health plans that carry at least $1,000 deductible for a single plan and $2,000 for a family plan are considered **high-deductible health plans**. In this arrangement, employers typically commit a predetermined amount of funds that the employee (and eligible dependents) can use to pay for medical expenses and for premium costs for the HDHP. Once the allocated funds are exhausted, the HDHP health insurance kicks in, in which the employee must first meet the deductible requirements out of pocket. Once the deductible is met, the plan becomes similar to a traditional health plan (Claxton et al. 2005b).

An **HSA** is a savings account created by an individual to pay for health care. To be eligible to create an HSA, a person must be covered by a "qualified health plan," which is a HDHP but also meets other legal requirements. Employers can offer qualified

health plans, and both employers and employees can contribute to an HSA, but employer contributions are optional. An HSA offers certain tax advantages to the employee. Any contributions made by the employer are nontaxable. Employee contributions are on a pre-income tax basis. Funds in the HSA are invested and the earnings from investments are tax free. Withdrawals from the account to pay for health care are nontaxable; only withdrawals for nonmedical purposes are taxable. The savings account can build up over time, it belongs to the employee, and is portable (Claxton et al. 2005b). HSAs are an improvement over medical savings accounts (MSAs) that were authorized under the Health Insurance Portability and Accountability Act of 1996, but were available only to small businesses, the self-employed, and the uninsured.

The major problem with HDHPs as a reform effort is that they do not achieve universal coverage, and no one knows their impact on the control of health care cost growth. Poor families and individuals with limited tax liability are unlikely to benefit from HSAs' tax incentives. Also, people may skimp on care and delay seeking medical treatment for fear of depleting their accounts, thus jeopardizing their health.

Insurance Restructuring in Massachusetts

In April 2006, Massachusetts became the first state to break the gridlock between Democrats and Republicans, and passed a bipartisan plan that would achieve nearly universal coverage in the state. The plan was implemented in July 2007. The "individual mandate" part of the legislation requires all state residents to have health insurance or face legal penalties. The "employer mandate" part of the legislation requires all employers with more than 10 workers to offer at a minimum a Section 125 cafeteria plan that permits workers to purchase health insurance with pre-tax dollars (The Henry J. Kaiser Family Foundation 2006a). Large government subsidies would enable low-income individuals to buy insurance. People whose incomes are less than the federal poverty level will have their premiums paid by the state. Those earning up to 300% of the federal poverty level will pay a subsidized premium.

At the core of the plan is the reorganization of a large part of the state's private insurance system into a "single market" structure with uniform rules and a central clearinghouse or "Connector" to facilitate the purchase and administration of private health insurance coverage. The Connector relieves employers of the burden of obtaining and administering health insurance coverage. Only plans approved by the state's insurance department may be sold through the Connector (Haislmaier and Owcharenko 2006).

The plan is expected to cost $1.2 billion over three years. This funding will be derived from redistribution of existing funding that includes federal Medicaid payments that were previously paid to safety net providers under a federal waiver. Actually, the potential loss of this federal funding is what prompted the state to reform its health care system. Also noteworthy is the fact that Massachusetts had enacted a play-or-pay (see explanation of this option later in this chapter) mandate in 1988, but it was never implemented.

Unknown at this point are some key questions regarding the availability of private plans that the state would consider "affordable," whether employers would continue to offer current health insurance or switch to

the Section 125 plan, which would be cheaper, and whether the plan can be financed over the long term.

The key features of what the program offers are quite appealing. If successful, the plan is likely to be emulated by other states. The plan has three main desirable features, as described by Haislmaier and Owcharenko 2006: (1) Insurance through the Connector is available to all residents of the state. (2) Coverage can become portable among employers within the state, and the coverage can be retained during periods of unemployment, part-time employment, or self-employment. (3) The program will provide a choice of plans. Once a year, participants will be allowed to switch coverage on a guaranteed-issue basis at standard prices. However, the plan faces many challenges and unknowns, and its full effects will not become known for several months.

Trends in Medicare and Medicaid

The Medicare Part D prescription drug benefit requires beneficiaries to receive drug coverage through private plans. The MMA of 2003 also provides new incentives, including sizable payment increases, to expand the role of private managed care plans to provide all Medicare covered services under the Medicare Advantage option (Biles et al. 2004). The policy is intended to attract more beneficiaries into managed care from the traditional fee-for-service option. Although only 14% of Medicare beneficiaries have chosen to enroll in Medicare Advantage, the Centers for Medicare and Medicaid Services estimates that by 2013 the proportion of beneficiaries in Medicare Advantage will rise to 30%. This estimate is perhaps based on the current levels of increased payments to private plans, but there is no certainty that Congress will maintain the payment increases when faced with future budget constraints. The program will very likely face budget constraints as, by 2015, annual Medicare expenditures are projected to reach $792 billion, which is more than double the amount of spending in 2005, and represents an average annual increase of 9%. In comparison, national health expenditures are expected to grow at an average rate of 7.2% between 2005 and 2015 (Borger et al. 2006).

The MMA has also attached a means-test feature to Medicare for both Part B and Part D premiums. In Part B, for example, single beneficiaries earning less than $80,000 per year ($160,000 per couple) will pay the standard premium, whereas those earning more will pay a higher income-based premium. As originally crafted, Medicare was not to be a means-tested program. Means-tested premiums may have opened the way for future reforms in which the wealthy would be asked to share a greater cost burden for financing the program.

Total enrollment in Medicaid has increased from 33.5 million in 2000 to 44.5 million in 2005 (Sanofi-Aventis US 2006), and expenditures have jumped from $118 billion to $179 billion (Catlin et al. 2007), or from $3,522 to $4,022 on a per capita basis, during the same period. Between 2005 and 2015, Medicaid spending is projected to grow at an average annual rate of 7.8%. Spending is projected to reach $384.4 billion in 2015 (Borger et al. 2006), which is more than double the amount spent in 2005. In 2005, 10 states had at least 90% of their Medicaid recipients enrolled in managed care. Nationwide, 62.2% of Medicaid recipients were in managed care, up from 58.4% in 2003 (Sanofi-Aventis US

2006). There is some evidence that Medicaid recipients enrolled in HMOs incur less overall expenditures (Kirby et al. 2003). Hence, it is expected that more states will mandate HMO enrollment in the future.

Future Options in Financing and Insurance

National health expenditures are projected to reach $4 trillion by 2015, approximately double the total spending in 2005, despite the fact that health care expenditures are expected to grow at a moderate rate of 7.2% annually. The amount of spending is projected to consume 20% of the gross domestic product (GDP) in 2015 (Borger et al. 2006), up from 16% in 2005. Although 88% of insured Americans rate their own health insurance coverage as excellent or good, approximately 20% are dissatisfied with the costs. Also, among the insured, 60% are at least somewhat worried about being able to afford the cost of their health insurance over the next few years, mainly if they lost their jobs. People's inability to pay for care when needed is on the rise; one in four Americans indicated they had a problem paying for care sometime during the previous year (The Henry J. Kaiser Foundation 2006b).

Some innovative approaches in health care financing and insurance have already started to emerge. This section also includes proposals that might reduce the number of uninsured through innovative financing policies. Given that one out of every five dollars would be consumed by health care, Americans will have to forego some other goods and services. This will likely lower, at least to some degree, the overall standard of living that Americans have become accustomed to. Erosion in the standard of living is perhaps best reflected in the growing number of poor in the United States. This is simply another social ill effect that unrestrained growth in health care will bring.

Defined Contribution Plans

Currently, the majority of employers offer what is referred to as a ***defined benefit plan***. The employer selects a health insurance plan and commits to providing the health benefits package, generally on a cost sharing basis. Large employers generally offer a choice of plans that vary in cost. Employees can choose from more expensive and less expensive plans. In the defined benefit health insurance arrangement, consumers have no financial incentives to be prudent purchasers, and patients are almost totally removed from the cost of care. But, the consumer of health insurance and health care is likely to bear more responsibility in the future. The defined contribution approach holds this promise. Defined contribution health insurance products that make use of Internet technologies are also getting some attention. Under a ***defined contribution plan***, employers commit to a fixed dollar amount for health benefits rather than to a predetermined package of health benefits.

The model for a defined contribution approach has, for some time, been used for retirement benefits. A shift occurred in the 1980s on the retirement benefits front when employers began moving away from defined benefit (or pension) plans toward defined contribution (or savings) plans (White 2001). Many employers see adoption of the defined contribution approach for health care benefits as compatible with the need to give employees a greater role in purchasing health insurance as well as health care services (Christianson et al. 2002). Actually, both

HRAs and HSAs, discussed earlier, use certain features of defined contribution arrangements. In the future, other variations of defined contribution arrangements are likely to emerge.

A defined contribution plan could take one of two basic forms. On the more conservative side, employees would simply use the defined contribution to choose among several health plans selected by their employer. On the more radical side, employees could take their defined contribution dollars and purchase their own health insurance. In either case, the employer's share of premium costs is capped at a predetermined fixed dollar amount. One way to ensure that the money is actually applied to health care is to directly deposit the employer's contribution into employees' HSAs, which the employees are responsible for managing (White 2001).

In the future, the Internet is likely to play a major role in the purchase of health insurance and in the management of HSAs. Internet-based ***e-health plans*** will enable consumers to tailor plans according to individual needs, obtain instant quotes, and make online purchases. Managed care organizations are likely to play a major role by adapting their existing structures to meet the new demand. On the other hand, many of the emerging e-health plans have secured partners, such as Merrill Lynch, Chase Capital Partners, Hewitt Associates, Pricewaterhouse Coopers, and even the Mayo Clinic. These developments may indicate the emergence of the next wave of health care financing (White 2001). In any event, "consumer choice," "affordability," "cost effectiveness," and "better value" are going to be tomorrow's buzzwords.

Defined contribution plans also have implications for the health insurance market.

With consumers in the driver's seat, aided by the ability to shop on the Web, insurers will have to come up with differentiated plans that would serve a variety of needs and fit different budgets.

Public Entitlement Programs

Care for the future elderly, particularly as the first wave of baby boomers turns 65 in 2011, has serious implications for the Medicare program. Today's elderly account for 13% of the US population, yet they get more than 60% of all federal social spending (Lamm and Blank 2005). By 2020, the elderly will constitute 16% of the population, which will put unprecedented financial strains on the younger generations.

The RAND Corporation, in collaboration with Stanford University and the VA system of Greater Los Angeles, explored how changes in medical technology, disease, and disability would affect health care spending for the elderly population. Their key finding: Medical innovations will result in better health and longer life, but they will likely increase, not decrease, Medicare spending. Even though the health of the population over age 65 has been improving since the early 1980s, cumulative Medicare spending is relatively unaffected by the health status of new beneficiaries because healthier people live longer and have more years in which to accumulate costs. As in the past, new technologies will increase health care expenditures even though such technologies may improve health. The reason is that the reduction in spending resulting from better health will be outweighed by the costs of technologies themselves and by health expenditures during the additional years of life that the technologies may make possible. In short, there are no silver bullets for Medi-

care's fiscal crisis on the foreseeable horizon (RAND 2005). Given the grim prospects, Medicare will require a major reform effort and political will to carry out the needed reforms. Means testing has already been addressed earlier. Other reforms will most likely be coordinated along with reforms for the Social Security system which will also face severe financial shortfalls. Since there is no single magic bullet to cure these programs, the main options will likely include a combination of raising eligibility age, increasing premiums and other mechanisms to shift costs from the program to the beneficiaries, reducing reimbursement to providers, and curtailing benefits. Given the expansion of benefits in recent years, the latter option will be the most controversial, but will likely become necessary.

Given the cost projections presented earlier, the Medicaid program will also have to choose various options to curtail spending, similar to the ones just discussed, but for a couple of exceptions. Age limitation does not apply because eligibility is means tested, and there is perhaps little room, if any, to raise income-based eligibility thresholds. Secondly, shifting costs to the beneficiaries will be impractical because the program serves the indigent. Experiences of some states during the 2001–2003 recession might provide some lessons for the future. A study by Coughlin and Zuckerman (2005) concluded that states relied on a range of short-term solutions instead of reassessing their basic tax structures and policies. By resorting to short-term approaches, some states have created structural deficits that will profoundly influence state policymaking for many years to come (Coughlin and Zuckerman 2005). The implication here is that Medicaid reform will require tax hikes at both the federal and state levels.

Tax Credits and Vouchers

McClellan and Baicker (2002) argued that President Bush's proposal to introduce tax credits for the purchase of health insurance would enable millions of Americans to purchase private health insurance. It would also improve the functioning of private markets, empower patients to make informed decisions, and increase the use of high-value health care while reducing inappropriate use. To this effect, Congress passed the Trade Adjustment Assistance Act of 2002, which includes health insurance tax credits for displaced workers and retirees who have lost their employer coverage. The work of Patel (2002) suggests that affordable individual health insurance is available for most Americans, but one main barrier is the lack of consumer awareness. A variation of this approach is to issue the tax credits in advance in the form of vouchers that enable people, particularly the poor, to purchase insurance.

High-Risk Pools

Tax credits would still leave some people uninsured, particularly those who are considered high risk due to severe illnesses or chronic conditions. *High-risk pools* target groups that cannot purchase health insurance on their own because of poor health. Over 30 states currently have set up high-risk pools that enable hard-to-insure people to purchase subsidized coverage. In almost all cases, premium rates are capped at 125% to 150% of the average market rate. Deductibles are generally $1,000 or less, and an 80–20 coinsurance is common. Proposals that the federal government should help states establish these pools are based on the premise that the federal government already is the insurer of last resort in case of major

natural catastrophes, and in the housing mortgage market through loan guarantees (Swartz 2002). Under the Trade Adjustment Assistance Reform Act of 2002, the Centers for Medicare and Medicaid Services (CMS) awarded the entire $80 million dollars that the bill had appropriated. The Deficit Reduction Act of 2005 reauthorized federal funds through fiscal year 2010. Federal grants provide seed money to create new high-risk pools and to cover operational losses.

Future Challenges for Managed Care

The role of managed care, as we know it, is assured in American health care at least for the foreseeable future. For now, status quo has been maintained in employer-sponsored health insurance as employers have been able to pass increased insurance costs to the employees through higher cost sharing in insurance premiums and higher deductibles and co-payments. However, pressures to control health care costs are beginning to mount. Once again, managed care will have to adapt and change to remain competitive.

Management of Risk

The greatest challenge in insurance is maintaining a balance between healthy and sick enrollees. However, 30% of persons 21 to 24 years of age are uninsured compared to 13.7% of people 55 to 64 years of age (Serota 2002). With the shifting demographics of the health insurance pool, managed care in the future will have to focus on managing the risk of an increasing number of people with potentially debilitating chronic illnesses, and also the sickest people in society. As discussed earlier, a growing number of Medicaid and Medicare beneficiaries, most of whom are high risk, are receiving care through managed care plans. Reforms in Medicaid, Medicare, and managed care will be necessary for MCOs to do a better job of managing health risk and for keeping costs under control. Future trends point to managed care as a risk-driven health care payment system. Instead of diagnosis and treatment as its principal business, the health care system will have to predict health risk and try to manage that risk before it turns into illness and cost (Institute of Medicine 1996, 54). Managing risk will involve population-based efforts to improve overall health status and an increased emphasis on prevention.

Accountability

MCOs in the future will have to be more accountable to both employers and enrollees. Although the choice of health plans by employers is driven primarily by the cost of premiums, accountability measures will be useful for enrollees in making informed decisions about which plan to choose. Such measures would be necessary if e-health programs catch on with the implementation of

defined contribution benefits. Clinical practice guidelines to assess and improve the quality of care in MCOs will also become more common.

Comprehensive Reform: If and When It Occurs

At some point, debate over comprehensive reforms leading to universal coverage is likely to arise again. In a system driven by incremental reforms, experimentation with additional ad hoc arrangements is eventually likely to run out of viable options. Comprehensive reform may come up for debate, particularly if employer-based health coverage continues to erode, or if powerful politicians believe Americans are ready for comprehensive reform. The last situation occurred in 1992 when Clinton became president. Past proposals likely to be considered again have included a single-payer system, managed competition, and employer-based play-or-pay (see Exhibit 4–1 for summaries of major approaches to finance health care).

Exhibit 4–1 General Approaches for Health Care Financing Reorganization

---

Option 1: A laissez-faire, free-market approach ("piecemeal")

Pros:
- Builds on the current system rather than replacing it.
- Promotes managed care concepts (HMOs, PPOs) that incorporate mechanisms to control costs.
- Gives people an incentive to price-shop for insurance and medical care, improving individual choice and reducing personal costs.
- Maintains private market-based approach.
- Significantly restricts government involvement and regulation compared with the other approaches.

Cons:
- Does not mandate coverage for everyone.
- Requires consumers to have a sophisticated knowledge of insurance plans.

Exhibit 4–1 continued

- Relies primarily on questionable cost-control strategies already in place.
- Does not address administrative waste.
- Continues a two-tier medical system in which those who can afford it have greater coverage, while low income people receive minimum coverage.
- Lacks coverage for long-term care services.

Option 2: Government-financed public health care system ("single-payer" or "national health insurance")

Pros:
- Guarantees access to care for all individuals.
- Ensures coverage regardless of health status, economic status, job loss, or job change.
- Reduces or eliminates many out of pocket costs.
- Controls costs by setting payment rates and global limits on total health care spending.
- Removes employers' responsibility to provide health insurance, though they continue to pay for coverage through taxes.
- Greatly reduces multiple payers, thus lowering administrative costs.
- Spreads risk and cost across entire population.

Cons:
- Requires a substantial increase in taxes.
- Puts government in charge of whole system, which could lead to budgetary constraints affecting choice, quality, and use of new technologies.
- May result in waiting lists and shortages due to supply-side rationing.
- Significantly curbs need for private insurance coverage, resulting in thousands of lost jobs throughout the insurance industry.
- Could allow political and ideological biases to influence scientific decisions.

Option 3: Employer-based regulatory approach ("play-or-pay")

Pros:
- Provides coverage for everyone.
- Builds on the current system rather than replacing it.
- Eliminates exclusions for preexisting conditions.
- Reduces out of pocket costs substantially for many groups of people.
- Maintains competition among private-market insurance companies.
- Spreads risk and cost across entire population.

Cons:
- May offer no real incentive for some employers to "play" because tax route may be cheaper, which could shift millions of employed people into government pool.
- Mandates small businesses to pay, through either health insurance ("play") or higher taxes ("pay").
- Enables many insurance companies to continue to operate, which means some of the administrative costs (e.g., advertising) also continue.
- Increases taxes, although less than for government-based approaches.

Assuming that a major reform of the US health care system does occur in the future, the single-payer proposal is the least likely to be adopted because this will be the most drastic of the three approaches. Employer mandates enacted in Hawaii in 1974 are also discussed in this section, but are unlikely to be an option today because they will be highly resisted by employers.

Although a universal health insurance program will cover all citizens, access will be restricted to essential care. People wanting access to services beyond what is determined to be essential will have to pay for them (Ginzberg 1999). Besides, those who currently have good coverage will have to settle for a system that imposes supply-side rationing, and the delivery system will quickly become overburdened with an unanticipated surge in demand for services. Cost-effectiveness criteria will become the gold standard for rationing medicine. There are three major problems with proposals for universal health insurance. (1) To financially sustain such a system Americans will have to "give up a cherished dream: the dream of total, universal care for any ailment freely available on demand" (Lamm and Blank 2005). (2) Proposed options (discussed below) only deal with insurance financing. They do not address the potential problem with access—how an overburdened system will meet increased demand for services. (3) Americans will have to be willing to pay increased taxes to sustain such a system.

Single-Payer

A *single-payer health plan* would place the responsibility for financing health care with a central agency (most likely the federal government). One major advantage of this system is that all Americans and lawful residents would be entitled to benefits regardless of individual or family income. Private insurance plans and government entitlement programs (Medicaid, Medicare, TriCare, and the Federal Employee Health Benefits Program) would no longer be necessary under a single-payer system, although the market for some private insurance will remain for those desiring coverage beyond what a basic government plan might offer.

According to one proposal, financing would come from an employer excise tax (8.7%) on annual revenues and a payroll tax levied on employees' salaries (2.2%), similar to federal or state income tax (LAPSR 1996). Additionally, the unemployed, disabled, and elderly would be subsidized through federal and state funds based on their ability to pay (LAPSR 1996, 1). Health care providers would be reimbursed on a fee-for-service scale. Hospitals, nursing homes, and other institutional facilities would be given an annual prospective budget to provide all required care.

A single-payer system could accomplish two major goals of health care reform: (1) provide universal coverage and (2) contain costs. By eliminating private health insurance, the single-payer system can lower administrative costs. But, the bulk of savings will come from supply-side rationing, which is the hallmark of all national health insurance programs.

A single-payer system has other drawbacks. Financing this type of plan primarily with an employer tax would place a financial burden on small businesses. Very likely, an increase in general taxes will also become necessary to support a burgeoning system. In addition, a single-payer system will likely create bureaucratic problems associated with the centralized administrative process. These problems include lack of flexibility and enhanced power and control over providers and businesses. Open rationing of health services will be highly resisted by the American public.

Managed Competition

President Clinton's proposed Health Security Act of 1993 was based largely on the principles of ***managed competition***. The plan proposed to guarantee every citizen the right to receive a comprehensive package of health care benefits. Under the proposal, regional alliances would be established to ensure that every citizen was enrolled in a plan. The alliances would function very much like the Connector in the Massachusetts health plan discussed earlier, that is, act as the fiscal intermediary between the plans and enrollees. Financing for the proposed program was based on cost sharing between employers (80%) and employees (20%).

The advantage of adopting a managed competition arrangement is that the medical infrastructure is already in place, and the private insurance industry, the would-be administrator of care, is well established in the United States. This could facilitate a smooth transition, whereas the single-payer system would require redesigning the entire health care delivery system. Also, compared to a single-payer system, managed competition calls for a smaller government bureaucracy.

Unfortunately, managed competition cannot guarantee that everyone would have equal access to care. Inner cities and rural areas in particular would have difficulty attracting enough health plans. A fundamental problem with managed competition is that unless several plans are competing against each other in a given geographic area, the system cannot drive down the cost of health care.

Play-or-Pay

Employer-based ***play-or-pay*** was introduced as a Senate bill in 1989 to achieve universal coverage. Under this system, employers must either provide their employees health insurance (play) or pay into a public health insurance program. The plan requires private or public insurance entities to provide identical benefits to working Americans and their dependents. Medicaid and Medicare would remain to provide care to the elderly, disabled, and poor.

If the employer chooses to pay, financing is through a payroll tax paid by the employer and the employee. The employee is still responsible for co-payments, premiums, and deductibles. Employees could also purchase supplemental health care benefits privately or through their employers.

Because an employer-based system is already in place, this type of plan is less disruptive than a single-payer system. Since many Americans who are uninsured are actually employed, this program could considerably reduce the number of uninsured.

Much like a single-payer system, play-or-pay would place an undue economic burden on small businesses because of mandatory employer financing. However, given the choice of "not to play, but pay" many employers, including those who currently provide health insurance to their workers, will choose to pay because, as the recent experience in Massachusetts indicates, it will be cheaper to pay than to play. Consequently, a greater cost burden would fall on the public who will have to pay higher taxes. This was precisely the reason why Massachusetts did not implement its 1988 enactment of a play-or-pay mandate. California is another state that passed a play-or-pay mandate in 2003, but the law was repealed through a ballot referendum. Another drawback of a play-or-pay system is that it focuses only on the financing of care, and does not address other areas of concern, such as access to care, utilization of services, and quality of care.

Employer Mandates

Employer mandates require employers to help pay for their employees' coverage. Despite the seeming appeal of an employer mandate, only Hawaii has implemented this type of reform. States' ability to adopt employer mandates has been thwarted by the federal Employee Retirement Income Security Act (ERISA), which exempts self-insured businesses from state insurance regulations and taxes. Hawaii is the only state that received a Congressional exemption from ERISA for its employer mandate. In spite of employer mandates, almost 10% of the population in Hawaii is uninsured (DHHS 2006, 420).

Most employers not offering health insurance to their workers would actually like to offer it, but they find it too costly. Other employers do not offer health insurance because most of their employees already have coverage (often from a spouse's employer) or because health insurance is not regarded as necessary to attract or retain the types of employees needed (Friedland 1996). This is often the case in low-skill jobs.

National and Global Challenges

To restrain the mounting burden of health care spending, wellness and disease prevention will have to be incorporated into health care delivery. On the other hand, the demands of chronic care and new and resurgent infectious diseases must also be incorporated into medical practice. New health care roles are required to coordinate the needs of people with chronic illnesses. Health care institutions and private practitioners must coordinate their efforts with public health agencies to identify emergent diseases and contain the spread of infection.

Future of Wellness, Prevention, and Health Promotion

Because of the changing causes of death, disease patterns, and the economic burden of disease, future health care emphasis will shift from acute to preventive care. To keep health benefit costs under control, employers are likely to promote employee health. Coile (2002) proposed that employers might have to take a long-term view instead of depending on short-term solutions. Employers would have to proactively identify employees and dependents with health risk factors, and support health promotion strategies to reduce health risks through smoking cessation, weight reduction, and stress management programs (Coile 2002, 14). Hospitals and managed care plans must continue as the leaders in integrating wellness and health promotion into medical care delivery. The goals and objectives laid out in Healthy People 2010 are also consistent with this kind of shift in emphasis. However, the epidemic of overweight and obesity threatens to undo much of the progress that has been made in controlling cardiovascular disease, diabetes, and cancer (Satcher 2006).

The former US Surgeon General, David Satcher, laid out a three-point plan to increase investment in prevention: (1) At the first level, labeled "downstream," the focus is on the individual and his or her lifestyle and behaviors. For example, regular physical activity, good nutrition, and scheduled immunizations are emphasized here, as well as the importance of avoiding toxins such as tobacco, alcohol, and harmful drugs. (2) At the second level, labeled "midstream," the focus is on the community. For example, investments are needed in public infrastructures that support walking, biking, and physical recreation. Schools should provide physical education. (3) At the third level, labeled "upstream," the focus is on health policy that supports prevention. An example is legislation that promotes physical activity and good nutrition programs in schools (Satcher 2006). Although putting such a plan into practice will be a challenge, it will require public-private partnership.

Challenges of Chronic Illness Care

In one century, the United States and most other nations have made significant gains in health status and life expectancy—mainly by conquering communicable diseases and developing more affluent lifestyles. However, with a higher life expectancy, such chronic disorders as heart disease and cancer have become the major causes of death. Future trends project an increase in affluence-related diseases, including cardiovascular, oncotic, and degenerative diseases. The more successful health care is at vanquishing disease symptoms and prolonging life, the more people will have to face the inevitable physical deterioration of the aging process.

Changing patterns of diseases are occurring in the shift to more chronic and multifaceted illnesses—a shift that will affect the demand for services and the type of services required. The future health care delivery system will have to be configured to meet these impending challenges. At a fundamental level, the shift will be from a reactive approach that responds to illness and its accompanying complications to a proactive approach that focuses on managing the underlying medical conditions.

Approximately one-third of Americans with chronic illnesses report that they are in fair to poor health, and too many chronically ill patients are not equipped to deal with their medical problems. According to one report, only 30% of patients with chronic illnesses felt very confident about their ability to decide something as basic as when it is appropriate to see a physician, 20% were not very confident about taking their medications in an appropriate manner, almost 50% had low levels of confidence about eating right, and about 50% could count on a high level of social support. On the other hand, people who suffer from chronic illnesses continue to engage in risky behaviors at rates comparable to the general population, despite the higher risks to their health. The chronically ill also face barriers because of affordability and physical access even though the vast majority has private or public insurance. The frequently expressed need for home care and special transportation services remains unmet for the vast majority of patients (Foundation for Accountability 2001). On the other hand, expenditures for long-term care are projected to increase at 2.6% annually above inflation to $154 billion in 2010, $195 billion in 2020, and a staggering $270 billion in 2030 (Congressional Budget Office-CBO-1999). Clearly, the future's health care delivery system will need to improve drastically to meet the growing demand for effective chronic care. The system needs to shift decisively from the current acute care model to a chronic care model.

Some of the main initiatives to improve the quality of care and reduce costs of care for the chronically ill have occurred through Medicare policy. For example, Section 721 of the MMA establishes the Chronic Care Improvement Program (CCIP). The CCIP, a new service that is predicated on disease management, is being introduced on a pilot basis with the fee-for-service option in Medicare. Other demonstration programs called for by previous legislative action such as the Medicare, Medicaid, and State Children's Health Insurance Program Benefits Improvement and Protection Act of 2000 are in various stages of planning and implementation. However, past demonstration projects have had a less than optimal record of achieving their intended objectives. Hence, more comprehensive, multifaceted innovations that simultaneously address provider practice, patient education, and patient self-management are necessary. Also, given the well-established influence of reimbursement on physician behavior, payment strategies should be restructured to facilitate transition of chronic care principles to the health care delivery system (Wolff and Boult 2005). Reimbursement systems must change in a way that also includes compensation for the services of nonphysician providers, such as nurse practitioners and community health nurses. In addition, health care professionals, including physicians, need to receive appropriate training in the management and coordination of the special needs of people suffering from chronic illnesses.

Challenges in Long-Term Care

The financing and delivery of long-term care will remain a major challenge. The good news is that long-term care is typical-ly needed later in life. Even though the first wave of baby boomers will start retiring in 2011, they are not likely to need professional long-term care services until 2025 or later. However, the system must be reformed before that time comes. In their report to the National Commission for Quality Long-Term Care, Miller and Mor (2006) identified six main areas of concern that must be addressed: financing, resources, infrastructure, workforce, regulation, and information technology.

Financing

Currently, most middle-class families are unprepared to meet long-term care expenses. Most people think that Medicare would pay for their long-term care needs. But, Medicare covers only short-term post-acute care. It is estimated that less than 10% of the elderly have private long-term care insurance (Burke et al. 2005). Unless policy initiatives are established to promote long-term care health insurance plans, the public sector will see its expenditures grow rapidly. Purchasing long-term care insurance is both expensive and confusing. The Congressional Budget Office (CBO 2004) recommended improving the way private markets for LTC insurance currently function. For instance, private insurance could be made more attractive to consumers by standardizing insurance policies to allow competing policies to be more easily compared. Currently, state insurance regulations do not require insurance carriers to offer policies that conform to particular design standards. Standardized policies could also stimulate price competition among insurers and help keep premiums lower than they would otherwise be. However, reform is also needed in a public financing system, particularly Medicaid, that pays for the bulk of long-term care costs. The Deficit Reduction Act (DRA) of 2005 tightened Medicaid eligibility rules. The law also extended the time period for asset transfers (called the look-back period) to qualify for Medicaid (Crowley 2006). In 2004, Medicaid and Medicare financed roughly 60% of all long-term care costs (CBO 2004). Without reform, these programs will put enormous financial pressure on the future working population.

Resources

Currently, financing for long-term care in the United States is tilted quite heavily in favor of institutional services rather than community-based services. Costs can be reduced if people who otherwise would be placed in nursing homes can have their needs met using community-based care. However, the Home and Community Based Waiver (HCBW) program has been too restrictive. Some provisions have been made in the DRA to extend community-based care to a larger number of people.

Infrastructure

The institutional long-term care sector has been going through a cultural change that has led to the creation of enriched living environments in nursing homes. New architectural designs, living arrangements, and worker and patient empowerment are improving the quality of life in nursing facilities that have adopted the innovative models such as Eden Alternative, Green House Project, and Wellspring. Over time, traditional living and care arrangements will be replaced by these and other innovative models.

Workforce

The aging of America will shrink the overall pool of workers. Experts think that this will have a particularly drastic effect on the health care sector, and long-term care in particular because of low pay and hard work. It is estimated that between 2000 and 2010 alone, when the baby boomers are about to reach retirement age, an additional 1.9 million direct care workers will be needed in long-term care settings (Department of Health and Human Services 2003). Another issue that must be addressed is a lack of training in geriatrics among the current workforce (discussed later).

Regulation

Currently, many experts see fundamental contradictions between the existing regulatory mechanisms that address quality issues in nursing facilities through periodic inspections and sanctioning, and regulations that require the same nursing facilities to implement quality improvement programs. Also, one of the most disconcerting aspects of government regulation of long-term care is its inconsistent application both within and across regions over time (Miller and Mor 2006). These issues need to be resolved.

Information Technology

Interoperable IT systems will enable providers to track patients' care across hospitals, nursing homes, home health agencies, and physicians' offices. Such systems are particularly critical in long-term care because the elderly frequently make transitions between long-term care and non-long-term care settings. Currently, such transitions rarely occur smoothly because of high rates of missing or inaccurate information (Miller and Mor 2006).

Infectious Diseases and Challenges of Globalization

The much-needed shift to chronic disease and disability does not mean that infectious disease prevention and control efforts will become unnecessary. In fact, intensified efforts will be required to combat emergent and resurgent infectious diseases. For instance, the sudden appearance in the early 1980s of a previously unknown disease we now call AIDS challenged the widely held belief that infectious diseases were under control. Since then, other deadly bacterial infections, such as Lyme disease, have appeared. Even though some of the newer infections have not created the panic that AIDS did, the scientific community is baffled by some ordinary bacterial infections that have turned lethal. Another cause of concern is that certain strains of bacteria have become antibiotic-resistant from the inadvertent overuse of antibiotics, which presents fresh challenges from infectious diseases, new and old. New forms of influenza virus have periodically raised alarms in the United States. Hantavirus, which is believed to have originated in Korea, has caused some lethal infections in the United States. National public health alerts made headlines in 2002 when encephalitis cases in New York were attributed to the West Nile Virus, which then traveled 3,000 miles west to California. This infection had never before been identified in the Western Hemisphere (Novick 2001), and its emergence in the United States has been attributed to global flow of goods, services, and people. Increase in air travel resulted in the spread of Severe Acute Respiratory Syndrome (SARS) from China to Canada in 2003, and of polio virus from India to northern Minnesota in 2005 (Milstein et al. 2006).

The above examples demonstrate that infectious diseases and health care must be viewed from a global perspective. The HIV/AIDS epidemic, for instance, has so far affected Africa the most. The African epidemic received little attention from the United States until very recently when it was recognized that the epidemic posed growing risks to US interests due to increasing globalization. Immigration of people from other countries to the United States, international travel to and from the United States, and shipments coming to the United States from other countries have made it increasingly possible for deadly infections to cross international borders. Data show that the US death rate from infectious diseases has doubled since 1980, and treatment of these diseases uses 15% of total US health spending (Kassalow 2001). HIV/AIDS, Hepatitis C, and other infectious diseases, some currently known and some as yet unknown, will pose growing threats to US interests, particularly as the AIDS crisis is expected to spread rapidly through India, Russia, China, and Latin America, which make up almost 40% of the world's population (Gow 2002).

The global aspect of infectious diseases emphasizes the need to link together the nation's foreign policy and public health policy. Globalization presents social and economic opportunities from which nations can benefit, but it also holds the potential for a global catastrophe. International cooperation, sharing of information, and technical and financial assistance will be necessary to avert any major health mishaps that could affect millions of people around the world.

Bioterrorism and the Transformation of Public Health

Public health has always been about protecting the population's health. More recently, emphasis on homeland security has lifted public health to a new level of respect and recognition as an instrument to protect the public against new threats to their health and well-being. Actually, the interest in public health in America has been like a seesaw, going up during times of danger to people's health and safety, and coming down when no present dangers loom. The importance of public health and deficiencies in the existing public health system received national attention during terrorism-related attempts to bring about an anthrax epidemic in October 2001, soon after the terrorist attacks and destruction of the World Trade Center in New York City on September 11, 2001. Since then, a heightened awareness of potential threats posed by chemical and biological weapons, and low-grade nuclear materials has prompted public officials nationwide to review and revamp the system. Most experts believe that the threat of terrorism on American soil will remain with us for the foreseeable future. The nation's central public health agency, the Centers for Disease Control and Prevention (CDC), will continue to play a vital role in recognizing emerging threats and in developing measures to contain any unexpected outbreaks. Public health agencies at local, state, and federal levels have been identifying infrastructure weaknesses and reevaluating plans to protect the American public (Baker and Koplan 2002). Public health must prepare for threats other than those posed by "imported" infectious diseases (discussed earlier); possible use of chemical, biological, and nuclear agents; and natural disasters such as Hurricanes Katrina and Rita in the Gulf Coast. Safeguarding the nation's food and water supplies is equally important.

The future effectiveness of public health will involve cooperation among public health agencies at the federal, state, and local levels; other departments of the government, such as the Department of Justice, and the Food and Drug Administration; private and public organizations, such as hospitals, clinics, and nursing homes; private practitioners, such as physicians and nurses; volunteer agencies, such as the American Red Cross and numerous other voluntary organizations; civil defense agencies, such as police and fire departments; businesses; and individuals and groups within communities.

To protect the health and safety of American communities, public health agencies will need to strengthen the 10 core public health functions enumerated by the National Association of County Health Officials (1994) in its *Blueprint for a Healthy Community: A Guide for Local Health Departments*:

1. ***Conduct a community diagnosis.*** Collect, manage, and analyze health-related data for information-based decision-making.

2. ***Prevent and control epidemics.*** Investigate and contain diseases and injuries.

3. ***Provide a safe and healthy environment.*** Maintain clean and safe air, water, food, and facilities.

4. ***Measure performance, effectiveness, and outcomes of health services.*** Monitor health care providers and the health care system.

5. **Promote healthy lifestyles.** Provide health education to individuals and communities.

6. **Provide laboratory testing.** Identify disease agents.

7. **Provide targeted outreach and form partnerships.** Assure access to services for all vulnerable populations and the development of culturally appropriate care.

8. **Provide personal health care services.** Treat illness, injury, disabling conditions, and dysfunction (ranging from primary and preventive care to specialty and tertiary treatment).

9. **Promote research and innovation.** Discover and apply improved health care delivery mechanisms and clinical interventions.

10. **Mobilize the community for action.** Provide leadership and initiate collaboration.

Effective public health responses will also require revamping the infrastructure and improving skills. Some priorities include workforce development; technical leadership skills for top-level public health professionals; modern information and communication systems; state-of-the-art disease surveillance systems, including early-warning systems; resources to maintain front-line public health response teams in a state of readiness; and rapid deployment of antidotes and vaccines when needed. In addition, periodic readiness assessment, ongoing research, and the upgrading of laboratory capabilities will be needed to ensure readiness for new and yet unknown challenges.

Local and state public health agencies will remain safety-net providers by continuing to deliver certain health care services to those in need. Increasingly, however, these governmental agencies will form partnerships with organized health care providers to ensure that population-based prevention is available to everyone. To increase efficiencies, consolidation will be effected by regionalizing public health jurisdictions. This would diminish the number of local public health jurisdictions from approximately 3,000 to somewhere between 500 and 1,000 (Mays et al. 2000). In some jurisdictions, the privatization of public health services using contractual arrangements with private providers will continue in ways that improve efficiency (Baker and Koplan 2002).

The Future Outlook for US Hospitals

It appears that a nationwide hospital construction boom is under way to expand capacity, replace aged facilities, or build new full-service or specialty hospitals. Many hospitals are replacing existing semi-private patient rooms with all private rooms. In many instances, hospitals are also increasing capacity in operating rooms, diagnostic radiology, telemetry observation beds, critical care for newborns and children, and outpatient services. For increasing capacity, the most notable market factor is population growth, particularly in areas where such populations are well insured. At this point, there is little evidence, however, as to how the benefits of increased capacity will balance with the increased costs (Bazzoli et al. 2006). Recent research shows that contrary to popular opinion, the aging of the baby boomers and increased longevity in general will have less of an impact on the future of hospital demand than local population trends and changing practice patterns attributable to advancing medical technology (Strunk et al. 2006).

Cost increases in the health care system have also been primarily attributed to hospitals. For example, it is estimated that hospitals were responsible for about 28% of the $528 billion increase in health care spending between 1998 and 2003 (D'Cruz and Welter 2005). Hence, hospitals will come under increased scrutiny to contain costs and improve efficiencies.

Hospitals will also be expected to continue to respond to other pressures from their external environments. They will increasingly develop a continuum of medical care services, and will continue to engage in providing one-stop shopping for all health care needs. Hospitals will also continue to reinvest capital in the development of integrated delivery networks, including joint ventures with other hospitals, physician practices, and managed care organizations.

The hospital of the future will be a health center, not just a medical center. Keeping people healthy will continue to receive a great deal of emphasis, and hospitals will increasingly engage in offering valuable resources to the community on matters of health and well-being, and will be held increasingly accountable for the community's health status. Hospitals will work not only to improve community health services but also to develop better programs to measure outcomes.

Other freestanding institutions of health care delivery will continue to exert competitive pressures on hospitals. On the other hand, concerns about Medicare's solvency and pick up in cost escalation will impose fiscal pressures. With the growing number of uninsured patients, the workloads of emergency departments are likely to increase, but without any additional reimbursement. Especially public hospitals and those located in urban centers will face increasing utilization and financial pressures because these hospitals end up sharing a larger burden of uncompensated care.

Cost pressures are likely to require hospitals to focus on greater labor productivity and reductions in overall staffing. This will require emphasis on multiskilled workers and labor-saving technology.

Future of the Health Care Workforce

Health care delivery influences, and is influenced by, the characteristics of the health care workforce. Some of the factors influencing the workforce include changes in the utilization of hospital-based and other health care services, an increasing elderly population, training and availability of skilled and semi-skilled workers, and more women and minorities entering the health care workforce. The future health care workforce will also be impacted by individual career choices and enrollments in training programs, and immigration of trained foreign workers in areas of high labor demand. Shortage of nurses is one of the dominant issues today. However, whether this shortage will continue is debated. Currently, pharmacists, technicians, and therapists are also in short supply (Coile 2002).

Supply and Demand for Physicians

The Council on Graduate Medical Education (COGME) assessed the likely future supply, demand, and need for physicians in the United States through 2020 for both generalist and specialist physicians. The report concluded that between 2000 and 2020, the number of practicing physicians would rise from approximately 781 thousand full-time equivalent (FTE) to 1.02 million FTEs under the most probable aggregate assumptions that take into account physician lifestyle factors such as working fewer hours, and increased productivity as a result of new technologies. These figures translate to 283 FTEs per 100,000 population in 2000, and 313 FTEs per 100,000 population in 2020 (Department of Health and Human Services 2005). On the surface, these figures may indicate a surplus of physicians. However, there are two main factors that suggest that the demand for physicians is likely to grow more rapidly than the supply (Department of Health and Human Services 2005): (1) A greater proportion of elderly in the population, and (2) the changing age-specific per capita physician utilization rates, with those age 45 and above using more services. When these assumptions are factored in, the demand for physicians in 2020 will be between 1.02 million and 1.24 million. Hence, there could actually be a shortage of physicians by 2020. Also, the problems of specialty maldistribution and geographic maldistribution are likely to continue. By 2010, the number of specialists is expected to reach 152 per 100,000 population (from 140 in 2000), and the number of generalists is expected to remain stable at 67 per 100,000 population (Institute for the Future 2000). These projections represent a generalist to specialist ratio of 31:69. The COGME forecasted a similar mix for 2020. A shortage of generalists will have serious consequences in a health care system that needs to focus more on addressing multiple chronic conditions. Two major forces will negatively affect the supply of generalist physicians in rural America—the number of residency graduates in primary care and the increasing feminization of the physician workforce. During the 1990s, growth of managed care had sparked a renewed interest among medical graduates in pursuing residencies in prima-

ry care because a shortage of generalists was widely forecast. Consequently, family practice residencies increased 54% between 1993 and 2000, a trend that would have had a sizable impact on the rural physician workforce (Colwill and Cultice 2003). However, the new century has seen a remarkable drop in student interest in primary care. The second factor, feminization of the physician workforce, is also believed to negatively affect the supply of rural practitioners because women have been less likely to select rural practice. The proportion of women in family medicine is expected to double to 40% by 2020 (Colwill and Cultice 2003).

Supply and Demand for Nurses

The recent shortage of RN-trained nurses in the United States has received much attention. Nurse shortages in the past have been cyclical. The current shortage began in 1998, and in 2006 entered its ninth year, making it the longest shortage in the past 50 years (Auerbach et al. 2007). In response, hospitals have used a mix of short-term and long-term strategies to deal with shortages. Among the long-term solutions are investments in training by expanding existing training capacity, opening new schools, and adding fringe benefits focused on education; and improvement of work environments through lengthening or redesigning of orientation programs for new nurses, increasing staffing levels, and work redesign (May et al. 2006). Only time will tell if these strategies will produce a lasting effect in alleviating the problem. Other factors, however, seem to suggest that the shortage of nurses will persist in the future. Unlike previous age cohorts of nursing students in the 1970s and 1980s, large numbers of people are entering the profession in their late 20s and early 30s. Based on revised projections taking into account this recent pattern of entry into nursing schools, the total RN workforce size is expected to be 2.45 million in 2012 and 2.47 million in 2020. The authors of these projections, Auerbach and colleagues (2007), used the demand data produced by the Health Resources and Services Administration, and estimated a shortfall of 340,000 nurses in 2020. The authors also comment that future changes in the economy, immigration, educational incentives, retirement trends among nurses, wages, delivery of health care, and societal values in general could affect future cohorts' propensities to enter nursing.

Deficits in Geriatric Training

Based on current trends, a shortage of health care professionals schooled in geriatrics is a critical challenge. It is estimated that only about 9,000 practicing physicians in the United States (2.5 geriatricians per 10,000 elderly) have formal training in geriatrics. This number is expected to drop down to 6,000 in the near future. Among nurses, less than 0.05% have advanced certification in geriatrics (CDC and Merck Institute of Aging and Health–CDC/Merck 2004).

The elderly use the majority of home health care services and nursing home care, about half of hospital inpatient days, and approximately a quarter of all ambulatory care visits. Growth of the elderly population will impose increased challenges on the health care delivery system, which has thus far ignored the need for specialized geriatrics training. Many elderly patients suffer from chronic conditions. Their care is complicated by the presence of comorbidities, use of multiple drug prescriptions, and an increased prevalence of mental conditions and dementia. Evidence shows that care of older adults

by health care professionals prepared in geriatrics yields better physical and mental outcomes without increasing costs (Cohen et al. 2002a). Current trends in the education and training of health care professionals shows the future demand will far outstrip the supply of physicians, nurses, therapists, social workers, and pharmacists with geriatrics training. This problem is compounded due to a shortage of faculty in colleges and universities who are trained in geriatrics. Only 600 medical school faculty out of 100,000 list geriatrics as their primary specialty. Due to this and perhaps other reasons, only 3% of medical students take any elective geriatric courses. In other disciplines, such as nursing, pharmacy, medicine, and dentistry, the majority of educational curricula do not require geriatric training. For example, 60% of nursing schools have no geriatric faculty (CDC/Merck 2004). A shortage of workforce members prepared in geriatrics affects all settings, but it especially affects nursing facilities that serve large numbers of frail elderly. Geriatrics training is also important in other types of health services, such as oncology, neurology, rehabilitation, and critical care (Kovner et al. 2002). Even though there are some encouraging signs that initiatives are being taken by educational institutions in recognition of a critical deficit in geriatric training, it is not clear how the nation will deal with the impending need.

Workforce Diversity

Women's continual entry into the workforce in large numbers is likely to affect health services delivery. Although further research and time will clarify this impact, health services managers should be prepared to improve the work environment to accommodate the needs of female workers. Examples include day care services and flexible work schedules. MCOs are likely to select women for their staff physicians, nurses, social workers, and case managers. Female physicians are expected to prefer managed care to private practice because MCOs are more likely to provide secure income and regular hours.

The increase in the proportion of non-Whites, particularly in the most populous cities and states, is another change. Already, the states of California, Texas, New York, New Jersey, and Florida have significant minority populations. And estimates say near the middle of this century, more than half of US citizens will be non-White (US Census Bureau 2001, 17). Consequently, the future health care workforce will be much more diverse ethnically and racially. Preparation of a culturally competent health care workforce is a growing challenge. The term *cultural competence* refers to knowledge, skills, attitudes, and behavior required of a practitioner to provide optimal health care services to persons from a wide range of cultural and ethnic backgrounds. Development of cultural competence is necessary because most future health care professionals will be called upon to deliver services to many patients with backgrounds far different from their own. To do so effectively, health care providers need to understand how and why different belief systems, cultural biases, ethnic origins, family structures, and many other culture-based factors influence the manner in which people experience illness, comply with medical advice, and respond to treatment. These variations have implications for outcomes of care (Cohen et al. 2002b).

Changes in the racial/ethnic and gender makeup of the workforce will continue to influence the management of health services organizations. Managers will have to consider cultural backgrounds and attitudes to-ward work as well as employees' potential language and educational disparities. Having more women in the workforce will require awareness of gender pay disparities and the need to address family issues, such as childcare and maternity leave.

Work Organization

In many health care settings, multidisciplinary team approach, collaboration, and cross-training will be used to improve quality and productivity. These approaches improve communication, enable practitioners to address complex clinical cases from different perspectives, and improve productivity by avoiding duplication.

Collaborative Team Approach

Consistent with the concept of total quality management is the use of multidisciplinary teams to provide patient services. The team approach concept is intended to provide comprehensive care and to eliminate duplication of services. For example, diabetes is not only a growing health concern in the United States, but it is also a complex chronic disease. Care for diabetes requires significant daily self-care that includes medication management, proper diet, and physical activity. Insulin dependency creates additional daily tasks such as monitoring of blood glucose levels, administrating proper dosages of insulin, and managing hypoglycemic episodes. Further, depression is a common comorbidity accompanying diabetes that can lower physical and mental functioning, which can lead to decreased ability to adhere to the self-care regimens. The result can likely be complications that can eventually lead to serious problems such as blindness, heart disease, and kidney failure. In diabetes management, a collaborative team approach provides numerous benefits to patients and practitioners. Also, a collaborative approach can provide medical students valuable cross-training (Robinson et al. 2004). A multidisciplinary team approach is also indispensable in ethical decision-making. Most medium- and large-sized hospitals have ethics committees that generally include multiple disciplines, such as physicians, nurses, social workers, administrators, ethicists, and clergy. Development of medical science and new technology create new challenges regarding clinical decisions that defy straightforward answers.

Health services providers and managers are more likely to involve key stakeholders, including patients and the population, in decision-making (Issel and Anderson 1996, 82). By involving the patient in decision-making, health care organizations hope to improve customer service and control costs. In a wellness-care system, it will become apparent that dictating a treatment regimen that customers do not like, and will not comply with, will not meet the goals of the organization or the customer (Issel and Anderson 1996, 82).

Cross-Training

Cross-training of health service workers can include teaching an employee to assume additional clinical or clerical roles or training an employee to work in several different areas (D'Aunno et al. 1996). The ultimate objectives are to improve staff flexibility, realize greater efficiency, and reduce costs. However, cross-training also benefits the employees by furnishing them with a larger set of skills than they would otherwise have. Although licensure issues can hamper worker cross-training in a number of areas, in other areas licensure conflicts do not arise. For example, one tertiary care setting used a cross-training program to evaluate the feasibility of floating a medical/surgical floor nurse to the medical intensive care unit, and both units have been jointly managed (Gilbert and Counsell 2000).

Training workers to become multiskilled health practitioners (MHPs) has several advantages. MHPs are an asset to small rural hospitals that may have difficulty obtaining or maintaining staff in certain specialties. Workers trained in multiple areas can respond to changing needs and demands in the health services industry. Continuity of care may also be enhanced by the use of MHPs because cross-trained nurses can attend to patients throughout their care rather than attending to them in a specific care level setting (D'Aunno et al. 1996).

Enhanced Focus on Customer Service

Market forces have increased competition among health care providers and networks of providers. Competition has brought with it more input from payers as well as consumers, increased scrutiny of services, and accountability for outcomes. In response, the health care industry is placing more emphasis on patient satisfaction. In a consumer-choice market, an institution's client satisfaction ratings may be the best predictor of future success (Coile 2002). Health care organizations will undoubtedly become more service oriented because those regulations and economic factors that made the industry substantially immune to competition are being dismantled (Eisenberg 1997).

Health services will not make the transition to service orientation without challenge. Eisenberg (1997) cited four barriers that must be overcome: (1) Health care environments are highly regulated on everything from waste disposal to records maintenance. To comply with the extensive regulations requires a great deal of time and resources, which can impede focusing on the consumer. (2) The health care industry has a traditional resistance to entrepreneurship. Incentives for efficiency and cost management are uncommon. This is partly because of the large number and various types of payers and the traditional view of health services as a noble and charitable enterprise (Eisenberg 1997, 22). (3) Health services are typically paternalistic. Because hospitalization generally occurs not by choice but because of necessity, consumers are often in a subordinate role without much decision-making power about what happens to them in the hospital. (4) The traditional medical model tends to depersonalize the patient. Patients are categorized by their condition. Training for health careers predominantly focuses on scientific and technical levels, ignoring customer relations.

To compete in a changing health care environment, health services will have to overcome these barriers and make a commitment to customer satisfaction and patient relations. This goal can be accomplished by adopting customer service principles as part of the overall mission and philosophy, empowering staff, improving both internal and external communications, creating feedback systems measuring patient satisfaction, and making service environments more user-friendly (Eisenberg 1997).

New Frontiers in Clinical Technology

Technological progress is behind much of the growth in the health services industry. The Institute for the Future (2000) predicted that eight types of medical technologies would especially affect future delivery of patient care—rational drug design, advances in imaging, minimally invasive surgery, genetic mapping and testing, gene therapy, vaccines, artificial blood, and xenotransplantation.

1. Rational drug design is a step beyond the painstaking and costly random search for new pharmaceuticals that is characterized by trial and error. Now, scientists can study the structure and composition of a receptor or enzyme, and actually design new chemicals or molecular entities that bind to the receptors or enzymes. Rational drug design will shorten the drug discovery process. The chief candidates for this process are drugs to treat neurological and mental disorders, and antiretroviral therapies for HIV/AIDS, encephalitis, measles, and influenza.

2. Imaging technologies present an enhanced visual display of tissues, organ systems, and their functions. Current research focuses on four areas: (a) Finding new energy sources and focusing an energy beam to avoid damage to adjacent tissue and to minimize residual damage. (b) Use of microelectronics in digital detectors and advances in the contrast media for a finer detection of abnormalities. (c) Faster and more accurate analysis of images using 3-D technology. (d) Improvements in display technology to produce higher resolution displays.

3. The latest advances in minimally invasive surgery include image-guided

brain surgery, minimal access cardiac procedures, and the endovascular placement of grafts for abdominal aneurysms. The overall impact of minimally invasive procedures on cost-efficiency and the patients' quality of life from early recovery assures the growth of this technology and the growth of ambulatory surgi-centers.

4. Genetic mapping has enabled the identification of a wide range of genes that can cause complex diseases, such as diabetes, cancer, heart disease, Huntington's disease, and Alzheimer's disease. The discovery of genetic susceptibility to certain diseases will improve preventive techniques. The term *genometrics* is used for the association of genes with specific disease traits.

5. Gene therapy is a therapeutic technique in which a functioning gene is inserted into targeted cells to correct an inborn defect or to provide the cell with a new function. The future challenge in this area is to develop methods that discriminately deliver enough genetic material to the right cells. Cancer treatment is receiving much attention as a prime candidate for gene therapy since current techniques (surgery, radiation, and chemotherapy) are effective in only half the cases.

6. Vaccines have traditionally been used prophylactically to prevent specific infectious diseases, such as diphtheria, smallpox, and whooping cough. However, the therapeutic use of vaccines in the treatment of noninfectious diseases, such as cancer, has opened new fronts in medicine. At the same time, development of new vaccines for emerging infectious diseases remains on the research agenda. Making today's vaccines safer for wide-scale preventive use against bioterrorism, in which such agents as smallpox and anthrax may be used, will also be an ongoing challenge.

7. Research will continue on the development of fluids that, in many instances, could be used as substitutes for real blood in transfusions, particularly in war and in natural disasters when supplies may fall short.

8. Transplantation of organs is one of the 20th century's great medical advances. It treats a life-threatening chronic disease by replacing the diseased organ. However, a critical shortage of transplantable tissues remains a major concern. *Xenotransplantation*, in which animal tissues are used for transplants in humans, is a growing research area. New knowledge and methods in molecular genetics, transplantation biology, and genetic engineering look promising.

The Era of Evidence-Based Health Care

Wide variations in clinical practice (see Small Area Variations in Chapter 2) have finally caught the attention of mainstream media in the United States, raising public awareness of the quality and cost implications of clinical variations (Schaeffer and McMurtry 2004). There is little evidence that high-spending providers deliver better outcomes. The goal of evidence-based medicine (EBM) is to increase the value of medicine. Even though consumers, as well as practitioners, often fear that reducing costs translates into lower quality, this is not necessarily true. Quality of care can be improved while reducing costs—thus increasing the value of medical care—by reducing misuse and overuse (Slawson and Shaughnessy 2001). The tools for the practice of evidence-based medicine have been developed for several years, mainly in the form of clinical practice guidelines. Evidence-based practice guidelines are intended to represent "best practices" and "proven therapies."

Several countries have undertaken some significant initiatives in the research and application of EBM. For example, in the United States, the Agency for Healthcare Research and Quality (http://www.ahrq.gov) leads national efforts in the use of evidence to guide health care decisions. The establishment of the National Institute for Health and Clinical Excellence (http://www.nice.org.uk) in England, the Scottish Intercollegiate Guidelines Network (http://www.sign.ac.uk), and the National Institute for Clinical Studies (http://www.nicsl.com.au) in Australia have similar responsibilities for developing evidence-based guidelines and for providing information on the clinical and cost-effectiveness of interventions (Gerrish et al. 2007).

There is at least some evidence that practitioners may have begun to incorporate EBM into their clinical decision-making. For example, Halm and colleagues (2007) reported a remarkable reduction in the proportion of patients undergoing carotid endarterectomy (a surgical procedure that removes the inner lining of the carotid artery if it has become thickened or damaged by plaque) for inappropriate reasons subsequent to the publication of several large international randomized controlled trials that rationalized the use of the procedure.

On the other hand, the use of guidelines is not widespread in the medical community. Even though the research community has known about clinical variations since the 1970s, and evidence has mounted since then, relatively little has been done to translate this research into actual practice. Many physicians think that guidelines and protocols are either too simple or too complicated, promote "cookbook care," lack creditable authors or evidence, are biased, decrease flexibility, reduce autonomy, and are not applicable to the practice population (Oeyen 2007).

Future strategies are needed to improve guidelines and protocols, and their adherence. At least six recommendations can be made for the future:

1. The issue of practice variations will require the attention of practitioners, payers, and policymakers.

2. Computer-based models will have to be developed to incorporate EBM into medical decision-making. Models that are easily usable and understandable are essential.

3. Ongoing clinical trials will be the backbone of EBM. Adherence to clinical guidelines is higher when the recommendations are supported by evidence from randomized controlled trials (Leape et al. 2003).

4. Guidelines and protocols must be revised and kept current to incorporate subsequent scientific evidence.

5. Future practice guidelines must incorporate economic analysis. Mounting health care expenditures will pressure society to make rational choices about when certain types of services become unwarranted. Treatments with cost-effectiveness ratios

greater than a widely agreed upon standard may have to be eliminated from recommended practice. Also, future technological change will be driven by assessments that show clear-cut clinical and economic advantages.

6. Financial incentives, including provider payments and patient cost sharing, must be restructured. Reimbursement methods should focus on paying for best achievable outcomes and the most effective care over the course of treatment instead of paying for units of service (Gauthier et al. 2006).

In the future, EBM will also transcend what physicians do. For example, the practice of nursing, pharmacology, and other disciplines allied with the practice of medicine will be governed by EBM. Eventually, EBM will become the standard that will govern the multidisciplinary process of health care delivery.

Summary

At the dawn of the 21st century, the only certainty facing health care is change. Future directions will be determined mainly by social, cultural, technological, and economic changes. Lack of access for the uninsured and cost inflation will continue to haunt the system. In the short run, greater cost shifting will move more expense from employers to employees. A defined contribution from employers is likely to replace the existing defined benefit program. To what extent this shift will occur and to what extent employers may actually abdicate their responsibility to be directly involved in purchasing health insurance will depend largely on the state of the economy and labor markets. Managed care's vast infrastructure will not be easily dismantled. Instead, it is more reasonable to assume that in a changing environment, managed care itself will have to evolve, since employers once again will be in a position to exert enough influence to bring about certain desired changes. Better management of risk and more accountability for cost and quality will be demanded. Given the right set of circumstances, universal health care could once again appear on the national policy agenda. If a national health care system becomes a reality, universal access will be restricted to essential care. Those wanting access to services beyond the essentials will have to pay for them.

Under growing cost pressures, wellness and public health will be more strongly emphasized. In a reformed health care system, a major challenge will be to forge partnerships between communities and all levels of government. Coordinating functions and developing needed infrastructures have become even more critical due to increased threats of bioterrorism and outbreaks of new infectious diseases.

A rapidly growing elderly population that requires care for chronic ailments and long-term care will pose increased challenges. Physicians will need training to function more effectively in a chronic care environment.

Composition of the health care workforce will undergo changes because of a decline in inpatient hospital care, an increasing elderly population, and more women and minorities entering the health care workforce. Despite recent efforts to bring about some parity, the problems associated with specialty maldistribution and geographic maldistribution will continue. Even though currently there is a surplus of physicians in the United States, by 2020, a shortage could exist. A shortage of nurses has also been projected, but factors such as economic conditions, immigration, and educational incentives could change the outlook.

As minority populations continue to increase and the workplace becomes increasingly diverse, health care managers face the challenge of preparing a culturally competent health care workforce. The health care workforce also needs to be schooled to give geriatric care. Additional workforce issues include cross-training and the team approach to addressing complex problems.

Health care is often seen as developing into a consumer-choice market. Client satisfaction and customer services will increasingly determine the success of health care organizations in a competitive market. However, industry regulations, lack of incentives, paternalism, and predominance of the medical model pose critical barriers to service orientation.

New frontiers will be opened in the application of clinical, informational, and telematics technology. Technologies such as new drugs, safer procedures, gene therapy, and therapeutic use of vaccines will strongly affect treatments for cancer, HIV/AIDS, and neurological diseases. Sharing of information among providers, intermediaries, and consumers will be necessary to achieve better efficiency and disease management. However, adoption of costly information technology will be driven by cost-benefit considerations.

Evidence-based medicine will play a growing role in the delivery of medical care that is both effective and cost-effective. Higher quality at lower cost can be achieved by reducing misuse and overuse based on clinical evidence. Hence, use of clinical practice guidelines that represent "best practices" and have been "proven" through clinical trials will become the standard for clinical care delivery.

Test Your Understanding

Terminology

cross-training
cultural competence
defined benefit plan
defined contribution plan
e-health plans
genometrics

high-deductible health
  plans
high-risk pools
HRA (health
  reimbursement
  arrangement)

HSA (health savings
  account)
managed competition
play-or-pay
single-payer health plan
xenotransplantation

Review Questions

1. Discuss the future direction of employer-based health insurance in the United States.
2. What are managed care's future challenges? How might MCOs address them?

3. What are some of the incremental changes in financing and insurance that the existing health care system might see?

4. What proposals might work in a universal access program in the United States, if and when the time comes to debate such proposals?

5. What main challenges regarding the future delivery of long-term care have been identified?

6. Discuss how the role of public health has been changing.

7. What challenges will the United States likely face in the future regarding the supply and demand of physicians and nurses?

8. What are some of the main reasons behind the deficits in geriatric training?

9. Discuss some of the changes in the areas of work organization in health care delivery.

10. Give an overview of what new technology might achieve in the delivery of health care.

11. What can be done to achieve greater adoption of evidence-based medicine in the delivery of health care?

REFERENCES

American Hospital Association. 1996. *American Hospital Association booklet*. Chicago.

Auerbach, D.I. et al. 2007. Better late than never: Workforce supply implications of later entry into nursing. *Health Affairs* 26, no. 1: 178–185.

Baker, E.L., and J.P. Koplan. 2002. Strengthening the nation's public health infrastructure: historic challenge, unprecedented opportunity. *Health Affairs* 21, no. 6: 15–27.

Biles, B. et al. 2004. Medicare advantage: Deja vu all over again? *Health Affairs Web Exclusive* 23, supplement 2: W4-586–W4-597.

Borger, C. et al. 2006. Health spending projections through 2015: Changes on the horizon. *Health Affairs Web Exclusive*, January–June 2006: W61–W73.

Buchmueller, T. et al. 2006. Trends in retiree health insurance, 1997–2003. *Health Affairs* 25, no. 6: 1507–1516.

Burke, S.P. et al. 2005. *Developing a better long-term care policy: A vision and strategy for America's future*. Washington, DC: National Academy of Social Insurance.

Catlin, A. at al. 2007. National health spending in 2005: The slowdown continues. *Health Affairs* 21, no. 1: 142–153.

CDC/Merck. 2004. *The state of aging and health in America, 2004*. Centers for Disease Control and Prevention/Merck Institute of Aging & Health. *http://www.cdc.gov/aging/*.

Christianson, J.B. et al. 2002. Defined-contribution health insurance products: Development and prospects. *Health Affairs* 21, no. 1: 49–64.

Claxton, G. et al. 2005a. *Employer health benefits: 2005 annual survey*. Washington, DC: The Kaiser Family Foundation and Health Research and Educational Trust.

Claxton, G. et al. 2005b. What high-deductible plans look like: Findings from a national survey of employers, 2005. *Health Affairs Web Exclusive* 24, Supplement 3: W5-434–W5-441.

Claxton, G. et al. 2006. *Employer health benefits: 2006 annual survey*. Washington, DC: The Kaiser Family Foundation and Health Research and Educational Trust.

Cohen, H.J. et al. 2002a. A controlled trial of inpatient and outpatient geriatric evaluation and management. *New England Journal of Medicine* 346, no. 12: 906–912.

Cohen, J.J. et al. 2002b. The case for diversity in the health care workforce. *Health Affairs* 21, no. 5: 90–102.

Coile, R.C. 2002. *Futurescan 2002: A forecast of healthcare trends*. Chicago: Health Administration Press.

Colwill, J.M., and J.M. Cultice. 2003. The future supply of family physicians: Implications for rural America. *Health Affairs* 22, no. 1: 190–198.

Congressional Budget Office (CBO). 1999. *CBO Memorandum: Projections of expenditures for long-term care services for the elderly*. Washington, DC.

Congressional Budget Office (CBO). 2004. *Financing long term care for the elderly*. Washington, DC: CBO.

Coughlin, T.A., and S. Zuckerman. 2005. Three years of state fiscal struggles: How did Medicaid and SCHIP fare? *Health Affairs Web Exclusive* 24, Supplement 3: W5-385–W5-398.

Crowley, J.S. 2006. *Medicaid long-term care services reforms in the Deficit Reduction Act*. Washington, DC: The Henry J. Kaiser Family Foundation.

D'Aunno, T. et al. 1996. Business as usual? Changes in health care's workforce and organization of work. *Hospital and Health Services Administration* 41, no. 1: 3–18.

Department of Health and Human Services. 2003. *The future supply of long-term care workers in relation to the aging baby boom generation, Report to Congress*. Washington, DC: Department of Health and Human Services.

Department of Health and Human Services. 2005. *Physician workforce policy guidelines for the United States, 2000–2020*. Washington, DC: Department of Health and Human Services.

Department of Health and Human Services (DHHS). 2006. *Health, United States, 2006*. Hyattsville, MD.

Eisenberg, B. 1997. Customer service in healthcare: A new era. *Hospital and Health Services Administration* 42, no. 1: 17–31.

Foundation for Accountability. 2001. *Portrait of the chronically ill in America, 2001*. Portland, OR: The Foundation for Accountability, and Princeton, NJ: The Robert Wood Johnson Foundation.

Friedland, R. 1996. The role of managed care in the future. *Generations* 20, no. 1: 37–41.

Galvin, R.S. et al. 2005. Has the Leapfrog Group had an impact on the health care market? *Health Affairs* 24, no. 1: 228–233.

Galvin, R.S., and S. Delbanco. 2006. Between a rock and a hard place: Understanding the employer mind-set. *Health Affairs* 25, no. 6: 1548–1555.

Gauthier, A. et al. 2006. *Toward a high performance health system for the United States*. New York: The Commonwealth Fund.

Gerrish, K. et al. 2007. Factors influencing the development of evidence-based practice: A research tool. *Journal of Advanced Nursing* 57, no. 3: 328–338.

Gilbert, M., and C. Counsell. 2000. Intensive care unit cross training: Saving dollars while retaining staff. *Journal of Nursing Administration* 30, no. 6: 308, 324.

Ginzberg, E. 1999. US health care: A look ahead to 2025. *Annual Review of Public Health* 20: 55–66. *http://biomedical.annual_reviews.org/cgi/content/full.*

Gold, M. 2006. Commercial health insurance: Smart or simply lucky? *Health Affairs* 25, no. 6: 1490–1493.

Gow, J. 2002. The HIV/AIDS epidemic in Africa: Implications for US policy. *Health Affairs* 21, no. 3: 57–69.

Halm, E.A. et al. 2007. Has evidence changed practice? Appropriateness of carotid endarterectomy after the clinical trials. *Neurology* 68, no. 3: 187–194.

The Henry J. Kaiser Family Foundation. 2006a. *Massachusetts health care reform plan.* April 2006. *http://www.kff.org.*

The Henry J. Kaiser Foundation. 2006b. *Health care in America 2006 survey.* October 2006. *http://www.kff.org.*

Holahan, J., and A. Cook. 2005. Changes in economic conditions and health insurance coverage, 2000–2004. *Health Affairs Web Exclusives* 24: w498–w508.

Haislmaier, E.F., and N. Owcharenko. 2006. The Massachusetts approach: A new way to restructure state health insurance markets and public programs. *Health Affairs* 25, no. 6: 1580–1590.

Institute for the Future. 2000. *Health and Health Care 2010: The forecast, the challenge.* San Francisco: Jossey-Bass Publishers.

Institute of Medicine. 1996. *2020 vision: Health in the 21st century.* Washington, DC: National Academy Press.

Issel, M., and R. Anderson. 1996. Take charge: Managing six transformations in health care delivery. *Nursing Economics* 14, no. 2: 78–85.

Kassalow, J.S. 2001. *Why health is important to US foreign policy.* New York: Council on Foreign Relations and Milbank Memorial Fund.

Keenan, P.S. et al. 2006. The "graying" of group health insurance. *Health Affairs* 25, no. 6: 1497–1506.

Kirby, J.B. et al. 2003. Has the increase in HMO enrollment within the Medicaid population changed the pattern of health service use and expenditures? *Medical Care* 41, (7 Supplement): III24–III34.

Kovner, C.T. et al. 2002. Who cares for older adults? Workforce implications of an aging society. *Health Affairs* 21, no. 5: 78–89.

Lamm, R.D., and R. H. Blank. 2005. The challenge of an aging society. *The Futurist,* July–August 2005: 23–27.

LAPSR (Los Angeles Physicians for Social Responsibility). 1996. *Health care reform: Information and commentary. http://www.labridge.com/psr.healthreform.html.*

Leape, L.L. et al. 2003. Adherence to practice guidelines: The role of specialty society guidelines. *American Heart Journal* 145, no. 1: 19–26.

May, J.H. et al. 2006. Hospitals' responses to nurse staffing shortages. *Health Affairs Web Exclusives* (January–June 2006): W316–W323.

Mays, G.P. et al. 2000. *Local public health practice: Trends and models.* Washington, DC: American Public Health Association.

McClellan, M., and K. Baicker. 2002. Reducing uninsurance through the nongroup market: Health insurance credits and purchasing groups. *Health Affairs Web Exclusives 2002:* W363–W366.

McKethan, A. et al. 2006. New directions for public health care purchasers? Responses to looming challenges. *Health Affairs* 25, no. 6: 1518–1528.

Miller, E.A., and V. Mor. 2006. *Out of the shadows: Envisioning a brighter future for long-term care in America.* Providence, RI: Brown University.

Milstien, J.B. et al. 2006. The impact of globalization on vaccine development and availability. *Health Affairs* 25, no. 4: 1061–1069.

National Association of County Health Officials. 1994. *Blueprint for a healthy community: A guide for local health departments.* Washington, DC.

Novick, L.F. 2001. Defining public health: Historical and contemporary developments. In *Public health administration: Principles for population-based management*, eds. L.F. Novick and G.P. Mays, 3–33. Gaithersburg, Maryland: Aspen Publishers Inc.

Oeyen, S. 2007. About protocols and guidelines: It's time to work in harmony! *Critical Care Medicine* 35, no. 1: 292–293.

Patel, V. 2002. Raising awareness of consumers' options in the individual health insurance market. *Health Affairs Web Exclusives 2002:* W367–W371.

RAND. 2005. *Future health and medical care spending of the elderly: Implications for Medicare.* Santa Monica, CA: RAND Corporation.

Robinson, W.D. et al. 2004. An interdisciplinary student-run diabetic clinic: Reflections on the collaborative training process. *Families, Systems, and Health* 22, no. 4: 490–496.

Sanofi-Aventis US. 2006. *Managed care digest series: Government digest.* Bridgewater, NJ: Sanofi-Aventis US.

Satcher, D. 2006. The prevention challenge and opportunity. *Health Affairs* 25, no. 4: 1009–1011.

Schaeffer, L.D., and D.E. McMurtry. 2004. When excuses run dry: Transforming the US health care system. *Health Affairs Web Exclusives* 2004: VAR117–VAR120.

Serota, S. 2002. The individual market: A delicate balance. *Health Affairs Web Exclusives 2002:* W377–W379.

Singh, D.A. 2005. *Effective management of long-term care facilities.* Sudbury, MA: Jones and Bartlett Publishers.

Slawson, D.C., and A.F. Shaughnessy. 2001. Using "medical poetry" to remove the inequities in health care delivery. *Journal of Family Medicine* 50, no. 1: 51–65.

Swartz, K. 2002. Government as reinsurer for very-high-cost persons in nongroup health insurance markets. *Health Affairs Web Exclusives 2002:* W380–W382.

US Census Bureau. 2001. *Statistical abstract of the United States, 2001.* Washington, DC: US Census Bureau.

White, B. 2001. The future of health care financing. *Family Practice Management* 8, no. 1: 31–36.

Whitmore, H. et al. 2006. Employers' views on incremental measures to expand health coverage. *Health Affairs* 25, no. 6: 1668–1678.

Wolff, J.L., and C. Boult. 2005. Moving beyond round pegs and square holes: Restructuring Medicare to improve chronic care. *Annals of Internal Medicine* 143, no. 6: 439–445.

Chapter 5
Douglas A. Singh, PhD, MBA

Overview of Long-Term Care

What You Will Learn

- Long-term care, as a distinct part of the health care delivery system, is best understood through 10 main dimensions that characterize long-term care as a set of varied services. The diverse services fulfill a variety of needs.

- The clients of long-term care are diverse in terms of age and clinical needs. The elderly, however, are the major users of long-term care services.

- Enabling technology reduces the need for long-term care services for many people. But, those who need assistance obtain long-term care services through three systems of care: informal, community based, and institutional.

- Informal care is the largest of the three systems of long-term care. Community-based services have four main objectives and can be classified into two groups: intramural and extramural. The institutional system forms its own continuum of care to accommodate clients whose clinical needs vary from simple to complex.

- Non-long-term care services are often needed by long-term care patients. The long-term care system cannot function without these services. Hence, the long-term care and non-long-term care systems of health care delivery must be rationally linked.

The Nature of Long-Term Care

Long-term care (LTC) is often associated with care provided in nursing homes, but that is a narrow view of LTC. Several types of noninstitutional LTC services are provided in a variety of community-based settings.

Family members and surrogates actually provide most of the long-term care that is unseen to outsiders and often unpaid. Another common misconception is that LTC services are meant only for the elderly. Many younger people, and even some children, require LTC services. The elderly, however, are the predominant users of these services, and most LTC services have been designed with the elderly client in mind.

There is no simple definition that can fully capture the nature of long-term care. This is because a broad range of clients and services are involved. Yet, certain characteristics are common to all LTC services, regardless of whether they are delivered in an institution or in a community-based setting. *Long-term care* can be defined as a variety of individualized and well-coordinated total care services that promote the maximum possible independence for people with functional limitations and that are provided over an extended period of time, using appropriate current technology and available evidence-based practices, in accordance with a holistic approach while maximizing both the quality of clinical care and the individual's quality of life. This comprehensive definition emphasizes 10 essential dimensions, which apply to both institutional and noninstitutional long-term care. An ideal LTC system will incorporate these 10 characteristics.

1. Variety of services.
2. Individualized services.
3. Well-coordinated total care.
4. Promotion of functional independence.
5. Extended period of care.
6. Use of current technology.
7. Use of evidence-based practices.
8. Holistic approach.
9. Maximizing quality of care.
10. Maximizing quality of life.

Variety of Services

The delivery of most types of medical services is based on what is called the *medical model*, according to which health is viewed as the absence of disease. When a patient suffers from some disorder, clinical interventions that are widely accepted by the medical profession are used to relieve the patient's symptoms. Prevention of disease and promotion of optimum health are relegated to a secondary status. By contrast, in long-term care, medical interventions are only a part of an individual's overall care. Emphasis is also placed on nonmedical factors such as social support and residential services.

Long-term care encompasses a variety of services for three main reasons: (1) to fit the needs of different individuals, (2) to address changing needs over time, and (3) to suit people's personal preferences. Needs vary greatly from one individual to another. Even the elderly, who are the predominant users of LTC services, are not a homogeneous group. For example, some people just require supportive housing, whereas others require intensive treatments. The type of services an individual requires is determined by the nature and degree of his or her functional disability and the presence of any other medical conditions and emotional needs that the individual may have.

Even for the same individual, the need for the various types of services generally changes over time. The change is not necessarily progressive, from lighter to more intensive levels of care. Depending on the change in condition and functioning, the individual may shift back and forth among the various levels and types of LTC services. For example, after hip surgery, a patient may require extensive rehabilitation therapy in a nursing facility for two or three weeks before returning home, where he or she receives continuing care from a home health care agency. After that, the individual may continue to live independently but require a daily meal from *Meals On Wheels*, a home-delivered meals service. Later, this same person may suffer a stroke and, after hospitalization, have to stay indefinitely in a LTC facility. Hospice care may become necessary at the end of a person's life.

People's personal preferences also play a role in the determination of where services are received. Experts generally agree that, to the extent possible, people should be able to live and receive services where they want. Almost always, people prefer to live in the community, the first choice being their own home. Home- and community-based services have increasingly become available so that people can age in the community. Severe declines in health, however, may necessitate institutional services, particularly for people who need care around the clock. Again, a variety of long-term care facilities are now available.

LTC services are an amalgam of five distinct types of services:

- Medical care.
- Mental health services.
- Social support.
- Residential amenities.
- Hospice services.

Understanding the distinctive features of these services is important. In actual practice, however, they should be appropriately integrated into the total package of care in accordance with individual needs.

Medical Care

Medical interventions in long-term care are primarily governed by the presence of two main health conditions that are closely related: chronic illness and comorbidity. First, as opposed to the care for acute conditions, LTC focuses on chronic ailments, particularly when they have already caused some physical or mental dysfunction. *Acute conditions* are episodic; require short-term but intensive medical interventions; generally respond to medical treatment; and are treated in hospitals, emergency departments, or outpatient clinical settings. *Chronic conditions*, on the other hand, persist over time and are generally irreversible, but must be kept under control. If not controlled, serious complications can develop. In order of their prevalence among the aged population, the most common chronic conditions are hypertension, arthritis, heart disease, cancers, and diabetes (Federal Interagency Forum, 2004). The mere presence of chronic conditions, however, does not indicate a need for long-term care. When chronic conditions are compounded by the presence of *comorbidity*—coexisting multiple health problems—they often become the leading cause of an individual's disability and erode that individual's ability to live without assistance. This is when LTC is needed. The prevalence of comorbidity and disability rise dramatically in aging populations.

Medical care in the LTC environment generally focuses on three main areas:

1. Continuity of care after treatment of acute episodes in hospitals.
2. Clinical management of chronic conditions and prevention of potential complications.
3. Hospitalization when necessary.

Continuity of Care after Hospitalization

Long-term care generally involves continuity of care after discharge from a hospital. Patients are hospitalized for acute episodes. Post-acute LTC often consists of *skilled nursing care*, which is physician-directed care provided by licensed nurses and therapists. Post-acute care may be provided in a patient's own home through home health care, or in a LTC facility. *Home health care* brings services such as nursing care and rehabilitation therapies to patients in their own homes because such patients do not need to be in an institution and yet are generally unable to leave their homes safely to get the care they need. A *long-term care facility* is an institution, commonly referred to as a nursing home, that is duly licensed to provide long-term care services.

Clinical Management and Prevention

Because chronic conditions cannot be cured, they must be managed. Left unmanaged, chronic conditions often lead to severe medical complications over time. For example, untreated diabetes can lead to heart problems, nerve damage, blindness, and kidney failure. The onset of complications arising from chronic conditions can be prevented or postponed through preventive medicine that includes adequate nutrition, therapeutic diets, hydration (fluid intake), ambulation (moving about), vaccination against pneumonia and influenza, and well-coordinated primary care services. Ongoing monitoring and timely interventions are generally necessary.

Hospitalization when Necessary

Onset of an acute episode requires medical evaluation and treatment in a hospital. Patients in LTC settings may encounter acute episodes, such as pneumonia, bone fracture, or stroke, and require admission to a general hospital. For the same medical conditions, the elderly are more prone to be hospitalized compared with people in younger age groups who may be treated as outpatients.

Mental Health Services

Long-term care patients frequently suffer from mental conditions, most notably depression, anxiety disorders, delirium, and dementia. Approximately two-thirds of nursing home residents suffer from mental disorders (Burns et al., 1993). Mental disorders range in severity from problematic, to disabling, to fatal. Research shows that depression, although common in nursing homes and assisted living facilities, often goes undetected (Smalbrugge et al., 2006; Watson et al., 2006). Under-diagnosis and under-treatment of depression is also a serious problem among community-dwelling older adults. The risk of depression in the elderly increases with other illnesses and when ability to function becomes limited (NIMH, 2007). *Dementia* is another common mental disorder. Characterized by memory loss, patients with dementia find it difficult to do things that they used to do with ease. Patients with dementia are also likely to become aggressive and undergo mood changes.

It is erroneous to believe that mental disorders are normal in older people or that older people cannot change or improve their mental health. But major barriers must be overcome in the delivery of mental health care. Efforts to prevent mental disorders among older adults have been inadequate because present knowledge about effective prevention techniques is not as extensive as our understanding of the diagnosis and treatment of physical disorders. On the other hand, treatment of many elderly people may be inadequate because assessment and diagnosis of mental disorders in older people can be particularly difficult: the elderly often focus on physical ailments rather than psychological problems (DHHS, 1999). Another drawback is that many elder care providers, including primary care physicians, are often not adequately trained in the diagnosis and treatment of mental health problems.

Mental health services are generally delivered by specialized providers in both outpatient and inpatient facilities. Because LTC facilities are responsible for a patient's total care, nursing home employees must be trained to recognize the need for mental health care, and the facility must arrange to obtain needed services from qualified providers in the community.

Social Support

Social support refers to a variety of assistive and counseling services to help people cope with situations that may cause stress, conflict, grief, or other emotional imbalances. The goal is to help people make adjustments to changing life events.

Various stressors commonly accompany the aging process itself and create such adverse effects as frailty, pain, increased medical needs, and the inability to do common things for oneself, such as obtaining needed information or running errands. Other stressors are event driven. Events that force an unexpected change in a person's lifestyle or emotional balance—such as moving to an institution, loss of a loved one, or experiencing social conflict—require coping with stress or grief. Even the thought of change brings on anxiety. Many people go through a period of "grieving" when coming to terms with change, which is a normal part of the transition process. Grieving may manifest in reactions such as anger, denial, confusion, fear, despondency, and depression (McLeod, 2002). Social support is needed to help buffer these adverse effects (Feld & George, 1994; Krause & Borawski-Clark, 1994).

Social support includes both concrete and emotional assistance provided by families, friends, neighbors, volunteers, staff members within an institution, organizations such as religious establishments and senior centers, or other private or public professional agencies. Such assistance may also include coordination of simple logistical problems that may otherwise become "hassles" of daily life, providing information, giving reminders, counseling, and offering spiritual guidance. Simply remaining connected with the outside world is an important aspect of social support for many people.

Residential Amenities

Supportive housing is a key component of LTC because certain functional and safety features must be carefully planned to compensate for people's disabilities to the maximum extent possible in order to promote independence. Some simple examples include access ramps that enable people to go outdoors, wide doorways and corridors that allow adequate room to navigate wheelchairs, railings in hallways to promote independent mobility, extra-large bathrooms that facilitate wheelchair negotiation, grab bars in bathrooms to prevent falls and promote unassisted toileting, raised toilets to make it easier to sit down and get up, and pull-cords in the living quarters to summon help in case of an emergency.

Congregate housing—multi-unit housing with support services—is an option for seniors and disabled adults. *Support services* are basic assistive services. They may include meals, transportation, housekeeping, building security, social activities, and outings. However, not all housing arrangements provide all of these services.

In LTC institutions, adequate space, privacy, safety, comfort, and cleanliness are basic residential amenities. In addition, the institutional environment must feel home like, it must encourage social activities, it must promote recreational pursuits, and the décor must be both pleasing and therapeutic.

Hospice Services

Hospice services, also called end-of-life care, are regarded as a component of long-term care. The focus of hospice, however, differs considerably from other LTC services. *Hospice* incorporates a cluster of special services for the terminally ill with a life expectancy of six months or less. It blends medical, spiritual, legal, financial, and family support services. However, the emphasis is on comfort, palliative care, and social support over medical treatment. *Palliation* refers to medical care that is focused on relieving unpleasant symptoms such as pain, discomfort, and nausea.

The hospice philosophy also regards the patient and family together as one unit of care. The option to use hospice means that temporary measures to prolong life will be suspended. The emphasis is on maintaining the quality of life and letting the patient die with dignity. Psychological services focus on relieving mental anguish. Social and legal services help with arranging final affairs. Counseling and spiritual support are provided to help the patient deal with his or her death. After the patient's death, bereavement counseling is offered to the family or surrogates.

The services are generally brought to the patient, although a patient may choose to go to a freestanding hospice center if one is available. Hospice care can be directed from a hospital, home health agency, nursing home, or freestanding hospice.

Individualized Services

Long-term care services are tailored to the needs of the individual patient. Those needs are determined by an assessment of the individual's current physical, mental, and emotional condition. Other factors used for this purpose include past history of the patient's medical and psychosocial conditions; a social history of family relationships, former occupation, community involvement, and leisure activities; and cultural factors such as racial or ethnic background, language, and religion. An individualized plan of care is developed so that each type of need can be appropriately addressed through customized interventions.

Well-Coordinated Total Care

Long-term care providers are responsible for managing the total health care needs of an individual client. *Total care* means that any health care need is recognized, evaluated, and addressed by appropriate clinical professionals. Coordination of care with various medical providers such as the attending physicians, dentists, optometrists, podiatrists, dermatologists, or audiologists is often necessary to prevent complications or to deal with the onset of impairments at an early stage. The need for total care coordination can also be triggered by changes in basic needs or occurrence of episodes. Transfer to an acute care hospital or treatment for mental or behavioral disorders may become necessary. Hence, long-term care must interface with non-LTC services.

Promotion of Functional Independence

LTC becomes necessary when there is a remarkable decline in an individual's ability to independently perform certain common tasks of daily living. Among children, disabilities can result from birth defects, brain damage, or mental retardation. Younger adults may lose functional capacity as a result of an accident or a crippling disease such as multiple sclerosis.

The goal of LTC is to enable the individual to maintain functional independence to the maximum level practicable. Restoration of function may be possible to some extent through appropriate rehabilitation therapy, but, in most cases, a full restoration of normal function is an unrealistic expectation. The individual must be taught to use adaptive equipment such as wheelchairs, walkers, special eating utensils, or portable oxygen devices. Staff members must render care and assistance whenever the patient is either unable to do things for him- or herself or absolutely refuses to do so.

In keeping with the goal of maximizing functional independence for the patient, nursing home staff members should concentrate on maintaining whatever ability to function the patient still has and on preventing further decline of that ability. For example, a patient may be unable to walk independently but may be able to take a few steps with the help of trained staff members. Assistance with mobility helps maintain residual functioning. Progressive functional decline may be slowed by appropriate assistance and ongoing maintenance therapy, such as assisted walking, range of motion exercises, bowel and bladder training, and cognitive reality orientation. However, in spite of these efforts, it is reasonable to expect a gradual decline in an individual's functional ability over time. As this happens, services must be modified in accordance with the changing condition. In other words, LTC must "fill-in" for all functions that can no longer be carried out independently. For instance, a comatose patient who is totally confined to bed presents an extreme case in which full assistance from employees is required. In most other instances, staff members motivate and help the patient do as much as possible for him- or herself.

Extended Period of Care

For most LTC patients, the delivery of various services extends over a relatively long period because most recipients of care will at least require ongoing monitoring to note any deterioration in their health and to address any emerging needs. Certain types of services—such as professional rehabilitation therapies, post-acute convalescence, or stabilization—may be needed for a relatively short duration, generally less than 90 days. In other instances, LTC may be needed for years, perhaps indefinitely. In either situation, the period during which care is given is much longer than it is for acute care services, which generally last only for a few days. Because patients stay in nursing care facilities over an extended time, holistic care and quality of life (discussed later) must be integrated into every aspect of LTC delivery.

Use of Current Technology

Use of technology varies according to the type of LTC setting. Certain types of safety technologies, such as nonslip footwear and hip protectors that protect the hip from injury during a fall, can be used in almost all settings. Other technologies, such as call systems to summon assistance, bathing systems, and wander management systems, are designed for specific applications. Chapter 7 covers LTC technology in greater detail.

Use of Evidence-Based Practices

Evidence-based care relies on the use of best practices that have been established through clinical research. Increasingly, clinical processes that have been proven to provide improved therapies are being standardized into *clinical practice guidelines*. These guidelines become evidence-based standardized protocols that are indicated for the treatment of specific health conditions. They have been developed to assist practitioners in delivering appropriate health care for specific clinical circumstances. An increasing number of standard guidelines have been developed for use in nursing homes. Some of these same guidelines can also be used in other LTC settings such as home health and assisted living.

Holistic Approach

In sharp contrast to the medical model, the *holistic model* of health proposes that health care delivery should focus not merely on a person's physical and mental needs, but should also emphasize well-being in every aspect of what makes a person whole and complete. In this integrated model, a patient's mental, social, and spiritual needs and preferences should be incorporated into medical care delivery and all aspects of daily living.

By its very nature, effective LTC is holistic. Once the need for LTC has been established, a holistic approach must be used in the delivery of care. The following are brief descriptions of the four aspects of holistic caregiving:

1. *Physical.* This refers to the technical aspects of care, such as medical examination, nursing care, medications, diet, rehabilitation treatments, etc. It also includes comfort factors such as appropriate temperature and cozy furnishings, cleanliness, and safety in home and institutional environments.

2. *Mental.* The emphasis is on the total mental and emotional well-being of each individual. It may include treatment of mental and behavioral problems when necessary.

3. *Social.* Almost everyone enjoys warm friendships and social relationships. Visits from family, friends, or volunteers provide numerous opportunities for socializing. The social aspects of health care include housing, transportation services, information, counseling, and recreation.

4. *Spiritual.* The spiritual dimension operates at an individual level. It includes personal beliefs, values, and commitments in a religious and faith context. Spirituality and spiritual pursuits are very personal matters, but for most people they also require continuing interaction with other members of the faith community.

Maximizing Quality of Care

Quality of care is maximized when desirable clinical- and satisfaction-related outcomes have been achieved. Maximization of quality is an ongoing pursuit, and is never fully achieved. Hence, maximizing quality requires a culture of continuous improvement. It requires a focus on the other nine dimensions encompassing the nature of LTC discussed in this section. It requires emphasis on both clinical and interpersonal aspects of caregiving. To improve quality, standards such as regulatory standards and evidence-based clinical practice guidelines must be implemented. Quality must be evaluated or measured to discover areas needing improvement, and processes should be changed as necessary. This becomes an ongoing effort.

Maximizing Quality of Life

Quality of life refers to the total living experience, which results in overall satisfaction with one's life. Technology that enables people to live independently generally enhances the quality of life. Quality of life is a multifaceted concept that recognizes at least five factors: lifestyle pursuits, living environment, clinical palliation, human factors, and personal choices. Quality of life can be enhanced by integrating these five factors into the delivery of care.

1. Lifestyle factors are associated with personal enrichment and making one's life meaningful through activities one enjoys. For example, almost everyone enjoys warm friendships and social relationships. Elderly people's faces often light up when they see children. Many residents in institutional settings may still enjoy pursuing their former leisure activities, such as woodworking, crocheting, knitting, gardening, and fishing. Many residents would like to engage in spiritual pursuits or spend some time alone. Even patients whose functioning has decreased to a vegetative or comatose state can be creatively engaged in something that promotes sensory awakening through visual, auditory, and tactile stimulation.

2. The living environment must be comfortable, safe, and appealing to the senses. Cleanliness, décor, furnishings, and other aesthetic features are critical.

3. Palliation should be available for relief from unpleasant symptoms such as pain or nausea.

4. Human factors refer to caregiver attitudes and practices that emphasize caring, compassion, and preservation of human dignity in the delivery of care. Institutionalized patients generally find it disconcerting to have lost their autonomy and independence. Quality of life is enhanced when residents have some latitude to govern their own lives. Residents also desire an environment that promotes privacy. For example, one field study of nursing home residents found that dignity and privacy issues were foremost in residents' minds, overshadowing concerns for clinical quality (Health Care Financing Administration, 1996).

5. As pointed out earlier, people overwhelmingly choose to be independent. However, even institutions should make every effort to accommodate patients' personal choices. For example, food is often the primary area of discontentment, which can be addressed by offering a selective menu. Many elderly resent being awakened early in the morning when nursing home staff begin their responsibilities to care for patients' hygiene, bathing, and grooming. Patient privacy is compromised when a facility can offer

only semi-private accommodations. But, in that case, the facility can at least give the patients some choice in deciding who their roommates would be.

Clients of Long-Term Care

More than 10 million Americans are estimated to need LTC services. The majority (58%) are elderly, but a significant proportion (42%) are under the age of 65. Among those who need LTC, 14% are in nursing homes and 86% reside in the community (Kaiser, 2007).

LTC clients can be classified into five main categories:

1. Older adults.
2. Children and adolescents.
3. Young adults.
4. People with HIV/AIDS.
5. People needing subacute or high-tech care.

Older Adults

The elderly, people 65 years of age or older, are the primary clients of long-term care. Most of the elderly, however, are in good health. According to household interviews of the elderly civilian noninstitutionalized population, only 25% described their health as fair or poor (DHHS, 2008a). It is reasonable to assume that the segment of the elderly population in fair-to-poor overall health is likely to require LTC at some point. Even for those in good or excellent health, short-term LTC (needed for 90 days or less) may become necessary after an accident, surgery, or acute illness. Also, important differences in health exist according to population characteristics. Those in fair or poor health are more likely

to be black, Hispanic, or American Indian rather than white or Asian; financially poor or near poor; and rural rather than urban residents.

A person's age, or the presence of chronic conditions, by itself does not predict the need for long-term care. However, as a person ages, chronic ailments, comorbidity, disability, and dependency tend to follow each other. This progression is associated with increased probability that a person would need long-term care (Figure 5–1). In 2007, approximately 7% of civilian, noninstitutionalized elderly in the United States needed help with personal care from other individuals (DHHS, 2008b).

Disability is commonly assessed in terms of a person's ability to perform certain key everyday activities. Although chronic mental impairments are often assumed to eventually manifest in physical dysfunction, that is not always the case. Individuals with certain chronic mental illnesses may be able to perform most everyday activities but may require supervision and monitoring. Severe dementias, on the other hand, which are mostly confined to older people, are commonly accompanied by physical functional limitations.

Two standard measures are available to determine a person's level of dependency. The first, the *activities of daily living (ADL)* scale, is used to determine whether an individual needs assistance in performing six basic activities: eating, bathing, dressing, using the toilet, maintaining continence, and transferring into or out of a bed or chair. Grooming and walking a distance of eight feet are sometimes added to evaluate self-care and mobility. The ADL scale is the most relevant measure for determining the need for assistance in a long-term care facility. Therefore, ADLs are a key input in determining a facil-

Figure 5–1 Progressive Steps Toward the Need for Long-Term Care Among the Elderly

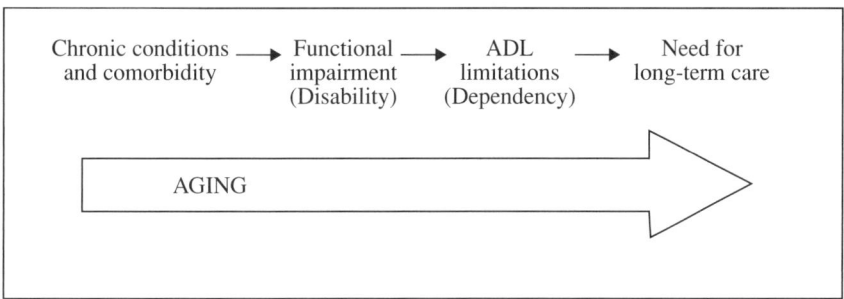

ity's aggregate patient acuity level. *Acuity* is a term used to denote the level of severity of a patient's condition and, consequently, the amount of care the patient would require.

The second commonly used measure is called *instrumental activities of daily living (IADL)*. This measure focuses on a variety of activities that are necessary for independent living. Examples of IADLs include doing housework, cooking, doing laundry, grocery shopping, taking medication, using the telephone, managing money, and moving around outside the home (Lawton & Brody, 1969). The measure is most helpful when a nursing home patient is being discharged for community-based LTC or independent liv-

ing. It helps in assessing how well the individual is likely to adapt to living independently and what type of support services may be most appropriate to ensure that the person can live independently.

Children and Adolescents

In children, functional impairments are often birth related, such as brain damage that can occur before or during childbirth (Figure 5–2). Examples of birth-related disorders include cerebral palsy, autism, spina bifida, and epilepsy. These children grow up with physical disability and need help with ADLs. The term *developmental disability* describes the

Figure 5–2 Common Conditions Creating the Need for Long-Term Care Among the Nonelderly

Children/adolescents (ages birth to 17):	Birth defects Brain damage Mental retardation
Young adults (ages 18–64):	Major injury Serious illness AIDS Complications from surgery

general physical incapacity such children may face at a very early age. Those who acquire such dysfunctions are referred to as developmentally disabled, or DD for short. *Mental retardation*, that is, below-average intellectual functioning, also leads to developmental disability in most cases. The close association between the two is reflected in the term MR/DD, which is short for mentally retarded/developmentally disabled. Thus, some children and adolescents can have the need for LTC services that are generally available in special pediatric long-term care and MR/DD facilities.

Young Adults

Permanent disability among young adults commonly stems from neurological malfunctions, degenerative conditions, traumatic injury, or surgical complications. For example, multiple sclerosis is potentially the most common cause of neurological disability in young adults (Compston & Coles, 2002). Severe injury to the head, spinal cord, or limbs can occur in victims of vehicle crashes, sports mishaps, or industrial accidents. Other serious diseases, injuries, and respiratory or heart problems following surgery can make it difficult, or even impossible, for a patient to breathe naturally. Such individuals, who cannot breathe (or ventilate) on their own, require a ventilator. A *ventilator* is a small machine that takes over the breathing function by automatically moving air into and out of the patient's lungs. Ventilator-dependent patients also require total assistance with their ADLs.

Many MR/DD victims are entering adulthood. The aging process begins earlier in people with mental retardation, and the age of 50 has been suggested to demarcate the elderly segment in this population (Altman, 1995). An increasing number of people with MR/DD are now living beyond the age of 50. Hence, this population will manifest not only severe mental and physical impairments but also the effects of chronic conditions and comorbidity.

Evidence suggests that MR/DD patients may function better in community-based residential settings than in traditional nursing homes. Studies of patients who had moved out of nursing homes to community settings demonstrated that these patients had higher levels of adaptive behavior, lifestyle satisfaction, and community integration than residents who remained in nursing homes (Heller et al., 1998; Spreat et al., 1998). Opportunity to make choices, small facility size, attractive physical environment, and family involvement were associated with higher levels of adaptive behavior and community integration (Heller et al., 1999; Heller et al., 2002).

People with HIV/AIDS

When it first gained national attention in the early 1980s, AIDS was a fatal disease that resulted in a relatively painful death shortly after HIV infection. Since then, the introduction of protease inhibitors, antiretroviral therapy, and antibiotics for the treatment of AIDS-related infections has vastly improved the health condition of HIV/AIDS patients. Consequently, AIDS has evolved from an end-stage terminal illness into a chronic condition. With reduced mortality, the prevalence of HIV in the population has actually increased, including among the elderly.

Over a period of time, people with AIDS are subject to a number of debilitating conditions, which create the need for assistance. Hence, the demand for LTC services is increasing, particularly because at least 25% of all known people with HIV/AIDS are age 50 and older (New York City Department of

Health and Mental Hygiene, 2004) and mortality rates from HIV/AIDS have decreased.

Care of HIV/AIDS patients presents special challenges, especially because this population has characteristics that are quite dissimilar to the rest of the LTC population. HIV/AIDS patients have a significantly higher prevalence of depression, other psychiatric disorders, and dementia associated with AIDS. HIV/AIDS patients also have a significantly higher prevalence of weight loss and incontinence of bladder and bowel (Shin et al., 2002).

People Requiring Subacute or High-Tech Care

A growing number of nursing facilities have developed subacute and technology-intensive services. The term *subacute care* applies to post-acute services for people who require convalescence from acute illnesses or surgical episodes. These patients may be recovering but are still subject to complications while in recovery. They require more nursing intervention than what is typically included in skilled nursing care. The patients are transferred from the hospital to a nursing home after the acute condition has been treated, or after surgery. Some common orthopedic episodes include hip and knee replacement. Other subacute and high-tech services are needed for patients who require ventilator care, head trauma victims, comatose patients, and those with progressive Alzheimer's disease.

The Long-Term Care Delivery System

The LTC system is sometimes referred to as the *continuum of long-term care*, which means the full range of long-term care services that increase in the level of acuity and complexity from one end to the other—from informal and community-based services at one end of the continuum to the institutional system at the other end.

The long-term care delivery system has three major components:

- The informal system.
- The community-based system.
- The institutional system.

The first component, informal care, is the largest, but it generally goes unrecognized. For the most part, it is not financed by insurance and public programs, but it includes private-duty nursing arrangements between private individuals. The other two components have formalized payment mechanisms to pay for services, but payment is not available for every type of community-based and institutional service. In many situations, people receiving these services must pay for them out of their personal resources.

Although institutional management is the focus of this book, the other two components, informal care and community-based service, also have important implications for administrators who manage LTC institutions. The community-based services and informal systems compete with the institutional system in some ways, but are also complementary.

The three subsystems that form the LTC continuum are illustrated in Figure 5–3. The patients' levels of acuity and the complexity of services they need increase from one end of the continuum to the other, for the most part. Informal care provided mainly by family members or friends involves basic assistance and is at one extreme of the continuum. Next on the continuum are the various community-based in-home services and

Figure 5–3 The Continuum of Long-Term Care

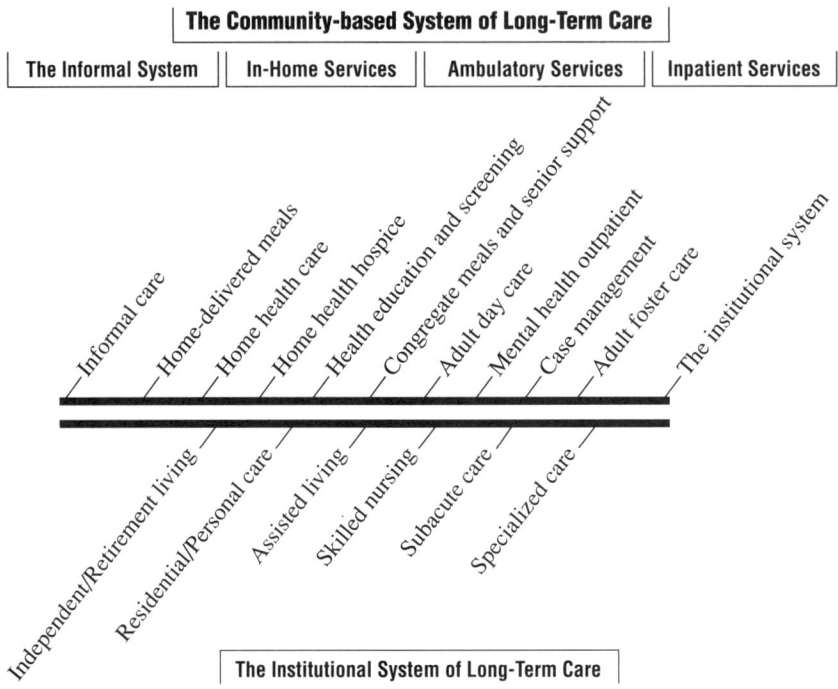

ambulatory services. Finally, there are different levels of institutional settings.

Given the complexity of the LTC system, case management (also called care management) fills in a key role. *Case management* is a centralized coordinating function in which the special needs of older adults are identified and a trained professional determines which services would be most appropriate, determines eligibility for those services, makes referrals, arranges for financing, and coordinates and monitors delivery of care to ensure that clients are receiving the prescribed services. Case management helps link, manage, and coordinate services to meet the varied and changing health care needs of elderly clients. Case management provides a single entry point for obtaining information about and accessing services. The extent of disability and personal needs primarily determine

which services on the continuum may be best suited for an individual. However, client preferences, availability of community-based services, and ability to pay for services also play a significant role.

In recent years, numerous public and private health care organizations have proliferated—organizations that offer information to consumers on how to care for someone at home, how to find and pay for community-based services, and how to find an appropriate institutional setting.

The Informal System

The informal long-term care system is very large. An accurate estimate of its size is difficult, mainly because the system is not formally organized and it cannot even be called a system in the true sense. However, there are perhaps more than 7 million Americans who provide care to more than 4 million elderly persons with functional limitations. The economic value of such care may be as high as $96 billion a year (O'Keeffe & Siebenaler, 2006). For the most part, services rendered are believed to be basic, such as general supervision and monitoring, running errands, dispensing medications, cooking meals, assistance with eating, grooming and dressing, and, to a lesser extent, assistance with mobility and transfer.

The extent of informal care that an individual receives is highly dependent on the extent of the social support network the individual has. People with close family, friends, neighbors, or surrogates (such as members of a religious community) can often continue to live independently much longer than those who have little or no social support. For those who do not have an adequate informal support network, community-based services can become an important resource for allowing an individual to continue to live independently.

The Community-Based System

Community-based LTC consists of formal services provided by various health care agencies. These services can be categorized as intramural and extramural. Community-based LTC services have a fourfold objective:

1. To deliver LTC in the most economical and least restrictive setting whenever appropriate for the patient's health care needs.

2. To supplement informal caregiving when more advanced skills are needed than what family members or surrogates can provide to address the patients' needs.

3. To provide temporary respite to family members from caregiving stress.

4. To delay or prevent institutionalization.

Intramural Services

Intramural services are taken to patients who live in their own homes, either alone or with family. The most common intramural services include home health care and Meals On Wheels. Limited support programs that provide services such as homemaker, chores and errands, and handyman assistance also exist, but the funding to pay for such services is not well established and varies from community to community.

Extramural Services

Extramural services are community-based services that are delivered outside a patient's home. They require that patients come and receive the services at a community-based location. This category mainly includes ambulatory services, such as adult day care, mental health outpatient clinics, and congregate meals provided at senior centers. Respite care is another type of service that can be classified as extramural.

Adult day care enables a person to live with family but receive professional services in a daytime program in which nursing care, rehabilitation therapies, supervision, and social activities are available. Adult day care centers generally operate programs during normal business hours five days a week. Some programs also offer services in the evenings and on weekends. *Senior centers* are local community centers where seniors can congregate and socialize. Many centers offer a daily meal. Others sponsor wellness programs, health education, counseling services, information and referral, and some limited health care services. ***Respite care*** can include any kind of LTC service (adult day care, home health, or temporary institutionalization) when it allows family caregivers to take time off while the patient's care is taken over by the respite care provider. It allows family members to get away for a vacation or deal with other personal situations without neglecting the patient.

The Institutional System

A variety of LTC institutions form the institutional continuum, with facilities ranging from independent living facilities or retirement centers at one extreme to subacute care and specialized care facilities at the other extreme (see the lower section of Figure 5–3). On the basis of the level of services they provide, institutional LTC facilities may be classified under six distinct categories:

- Independent or retirement living.
- Residential or personal care.
- Assisted living.
- Skilled nursing.
- Subacute care.
- Specialized care.

For most people, the array of facilities that often go by different names can be remarkably confusing. This is particularly true because distinctions between some of them can be blurry. For example, what is defined as board-and-care (i.e., residential and personal care) in one state may be called assisted living in another. This is because services provided by these facilities can overlap. Brief descriptions of these facilities follow. Additional details are found in Chapter 7.

Independent or Retirement Housing

Independent housing units and retirement living centers are not LTC institutions in the true sense because they are meant for people who can manage their own care. These residences do not deliver clinical care but emphasize privacy, security, and independence. Their special features and amenities are designed to create a physically supportive environment to promote an independent lifestyle. For example, the living quarters are equipped with emergency call systems. Bathrooms have safety grab bars. Rooms are furnished with kitchenettes. Congregate housing units have handrails in the hallways for stability while walking. Other housing units offer detached cottages with individual garages that allow residents to come and go as they please. ***Hotel services*** such as meals, housekeeping, and laundry may or may not be available.

Residential or Personal Care Homes

Facilities in this category go by different names such as domiciliary care facilities, adult care facilities, board-and-care homes, and foster care homes. In addition to providing a physically supportive environment, these facilities generally provide light assistive care such as medication use management and assistance with bathing and grooming. Other basic services such as meals, housekeeping, laundry, and social and recreational activities are also generally included. Because personal care homes are located in residential neighborhoods, they are sometimes regarded as a community-based rather than an institutional service.

Assisted Living Facilities

An ***assisted living facility*** can be described as a residential setting that provides personal care services, 24-hour supervision, scheduled and unscheduled assistance, social activities, and some nursing care services (Citro & Hermanson, 1999). The services are specially designed for people who cannot function without assistance and therefore cannot be accommodated in a retirement living or residential care facility.

The range of services in assisted living facilities is similar to that in personal care homes, except that the level of frailty among the residents is generally higher. Hence, assistance with some ADLs is often furnished. Common types of ADL help include assistance with eating, bathing, dressing, toileting, and ambulation. Most residents also require help with medications.

Skilled Nursing Facilities

These are the typical nursing homes at the higher end of the institutional continuum. Compared with the types of residences discussed earlier, the environment in skilled nursing facilities is more institutionalized and clinical. Yet, many facilities have implemented creative ideas in layout and design to make their living environments as pleasant and homelike as practicable. Some of these innovations are discussed in Chapter 8.

These facilities employ full-time administrators who must understand the varied concepts of clinical and social care and have been trained in management and leadership skills. The facility must be adequately equipped to care for patients who require a high level of nursing services and medical oversight, yet the quality of life must be maximized. A variety of disabilities—including problems with ambulation, incontinence, and behavioral episodes—often coexist among a relatively large number of patients. Compared with other types of facilities, nursing homes have a

significant number of patients who are cognitively impaired, suffer from other mental ailments such as depression, and have physical disabilities and conditions that often require professional intervention. The social functioning of many of these patients has also severely declined. Hence, the nursing home setting presents quite a challenge to administrators in the integration of the four service domains discussed earlier—medical care, mental health services, social support, and residential amenities.

Subacute Care Facilities

Subacute care, defined earlier, has become a substitute for services that were previously provided in acute care hospitals. It has grown because it is a cheaper alternative to hospital stay. Early discharge from acute care hospitals has resulted in a population that has greater medical needs than what skilled care facilities were earlier able to provide.

Specialized Care Facilities

By their very nature, both subacute care and specialized care place high emphasis on medical and professional nursing services. Some nursing homes have opened specialized care units for patients requiring ventilator care, treatment of Alzheimer's disease, intensive rehabilitation, or closed head trauma care. Other specialized facilities include intermediate care facilities for the mentally retarded (ICF/MR). The key distinguishing feature of the latter institutions is specialized programming and care modules for patients suffering from mental retardation and associated disabilities. Another type of specialized facility provides pediatric LTC to children with developmental disabilities.

The Non-Long-Term Health Care System

Health care services described in this section are complementary to long-term care. Even though these services fall outside the LTC domain, they are often needed by long-term care patients. Hence, ideally, the two systems—long-term care and non–long-term care—should be rationally linked. The following are the main non-LTC services that are complementary to long-term care:

- *Primary care*, which is defined as medical care that is basic, routine, coordinated, and continuous over time. It is delivered mainly by community-based physicians. It can also be rendered by mid-level providers such as physician's assistants or nurse practitioners. Primary care is brought to the patients who reside in nursing homes, whereas those residing in less institutionalized settings such as retirement living communities or personal care homes commonly visit the primary care physician's office.

- Mental health care delivered by community-based mental-health outpatient clinics and psychiatric inpatient hospitals.

- Specialty care delivered by community-based physicians in specialty practices, such as cardiology, ophthalmology, dermatology, or oncology. Certain services are also delivered by freestanding chemotherapy, radiation, and dialysis centers. Other services are provided by dentists, optometrists, opticians, podiatrists, chiropractors, and audiologists in community-based clinics or mobile units that can be brought to a long-term care facility.

- Acute care delivered by hospitals and outpatient surgery centers. Acute episodes in a LTC setting require transfer of the patient to a hospital by ambulance.

- Diagnostic and health screening services offered by hospitals, community-based clinics, or mobile medical services. Some common types of services brought to LTC facilities include preventive dentistry, X-ray, and optometric care.

Rational Integration of Long-Term Care and Complementary Services

The LTC delivery system cannot function independently of other health care services. Hence, the LTC system must be rationally linked to the rest of the health care delivery system (Figure 5–4). In a well-integrated system, patients should be able to move with relative ease between needed services. At least some streamlining and coordination of services can be achieved through information technology, such as electronic health records.

Types of services comprising the broader health care continuum are summarized in Table 5–1. Long-term care patients, regardless of where they may be residing, frequently require a variety of services along the health care continuum, dictated by the changes in the patient's condition and episodes that occur over time. As an example, a person living at home may undergo partial mastectomy for breast cancer, return home under the care of a home health agency, require hip surgery after a fall in the home, and subsequently be admitted to a skilled nursing facility for rehabilitation. This individual will need recuperation, physical therapy, chemotherapy, and follow-up visits to the oncologist. Once she is able to walk with assistance and her overall condition is stabilized, she may wish to be

Figure 5–4 Key Characteristics of a Well-Designed LTC System

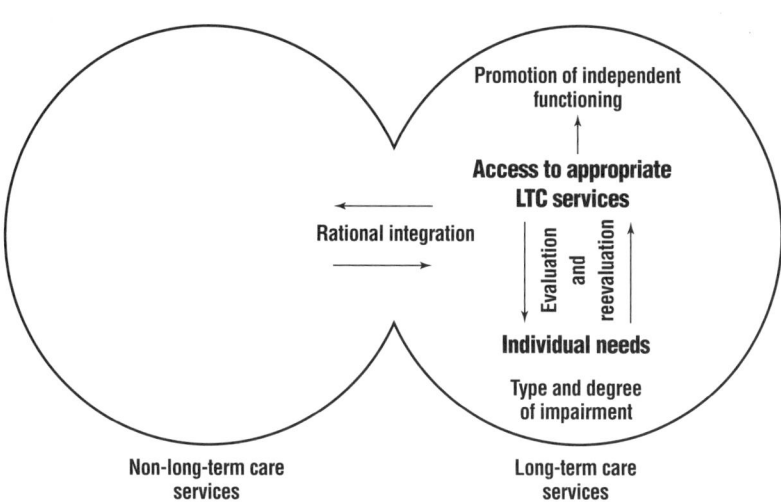

moved to an assisted living facility. To adequately meet the changing needs of such a patient, the system requires rational integration, but the flow of care is not always as smooth as it should be. Integrated care also requires an evaluation of the patient's needs in accordance with the type and degree of impairment and a reevaluation as conditions change. Depending on the change in condition and functioning, the patient may move between the various levels and types of LTC services and may also need transferring between LTC and non-LTC services.

Table 5–1 The Continuum of Health Care Services

Types of Health Services	Delivery Settings
Preventive care	Public health programs
	Community programs
	Personal lifestyles
Primary care	Physician's office or clinic
	Self-care
	Alternative medicine
Specialized care	Specialist provider clinics
Chronic care	Primary care settings
	Specialist provider clinics
	Home health
	Long-term care facilities
	Self-care
	Alternative medicine
Long-term care	Long-term care facilities
	Home health
Subacute care	Special subacute units (hospitals, long-term care facilities)
	Home health
	Outpatient surgical centers
Acute care	Hospitals
Rehabilitative care	Rehabilitation departments (hospitals, long-term care facilities)
	Home health
	Outpatient rehabilitation centers
End-of-life care	Hospice services provided in a variety of settings

For Further Thought

1. How does long-term care differ from other types of medical services?

2. How can a nursing home facilitate the delivery of total care?

3. Why is it important that caregivers in long-term care settings not perform every task of daily living for the patient? How much should caregivers do for patients who have functional impairments?

4. For nursing home residents, dignity and privacy issues are often more important than clinical quality. Identify some staff practices that will promote each individual's privacy and dignity.

For Further Learning

Administration on Aging: A federal agency established under the Older Americans Act.

www.aoa.gov/

Family Caregiver Alliance: A nonprofit organization set up to provide information and resources to address the needs of families and friends providing long-term care at home.

http://www.caregiver.org

The George Washington Institute for Spirituality and Health: Affiliated with the George Washington University, the Institute is a leading organization on educational and clinical issues related to spirituality and health.

http://www.gwish.org/

The Meals On Wheels Association of America: This organization represents those who provide congregate and home-delivered meal services to people in need.

http://www.mowaa.org/index.asp

National Council on Aging: A private, nonprofit organization providing information, training, technical assistance, advocacy, and leadership in all aspects of care for the elderly. It provides information on training programs and in-home services for older people. Publications are available on topics such as lifelong learning, senior center services, adult day care, long-term care, financial issues, senior housing, rural issues, intergenerational programs, and volunteers serving the aged.

www.ncoa.org

National Mental Health Association: The country's oldest and largest nonprofit organization that addresses all aspects of mental health and mental illness.

www.nmha.org

REFERENCES

Altman, B.M. 1995, July. *Elderly Persons with Developmental Disabilities in Long-Term Care Facilities*. AHCPR Pub. No. 95-0084. Rockville, MD: Agency for Health Care Policy and Research (now Agency for Healthcare Research and Quality).

Burns, B. et al. 1993. Mental health service use by the elderly in nursing homes. *American Journal of Public Health* 83: 331–337.

Citro, J., & Hermanson, S. 1999. Fact sheet: Assisted living in the United States. Washington, DC: American Association of Retired Persons.

Compston, A., & Coles, A. 2002. Multiple sclerosis. *Lancet* 359, no. 9313: 1221–1231.

DHHS. 1999. Mental health: A report of the Surgeon General. Rockville, MD: U.S. Department of Health and Human Services.

DHHS. 2008a. Trends in health and aging. Respondent-assessed health by age, sex, and race/ethnicity: United States, 1982–2006. Available at: http://205.207.175.93/aging/TableViewer/tableView .aspx (accessed September 2008).

DHHS. 2008b. Early release of selected estimates based on data from the 2007 National Health Interview Survey. Available at: http://www.cdc.gov/nchs/data/nhis/earlyrelease/earlyrelease 200806.pdf (accessed September 2008).

Federal Interagency Forum on Aging-Related Statistics. 2004. *Older Americans 2004: Key Indicators of Well-Being*. Washington, DC: U.S. Government Printing Office.

Feld, S., & George, L.K. 1994. Moderating effects of prior social resources on the hospitalizations of elders who become widowed. *Journal of Aging and Health* 6: 275–295.

Health Care Financing Administration. 1996. Nursing home quality of life study spotlights residents' concerns. *Health Care Financing Review* 17, no. 3: 324.

Heller, T., et al. 1998. Impact of age and transitions out of nursing homes for adults with developmental disabilities. *American Journal of Mental Retardation* 103, no. 3: 236–248.

Heller, T., et al. 1999. Autonomy in residential facilities and community functioning of adults with mental retardation. *Mental Retardation* 37, no. 6: 449–457.

Heller, T., et al. 2002. Eight-year follow-up of the impact of environmental characteristics on well-being of adults with developmental disabilities. *Mental Retardation* 40, no. 5: 366–378.

Kaiser (Kaiser Commission on Medicaid and the Uninsured). 2007. *Medicaid Facts*. The Henry J. Kaiser Family Foundation. Available at: http://www.kff.org/medicaid/upload/2186_05.pdf (accessed September 2008).

Krause, N., & Borawski-Clark, E. 1994. Clarifying the functions of social support in later life. *Research on Aging* 16: 251–279.

Lawton, M.P., & Brody, E.M. 1969. Assessment of older people: Self-maintaining and instrumental activities of daily living. *Gerontology* 9: 179–186.

McLeod, B.W. 2002. *And Thou Shalt Honor: A Caregiver's Companion*. Wiland-Bell Productions, distributed by Rodale at www.rodalestore.com.

New York City Department of Health and Mental Hygiene. 2004. *HIV Surveillance and Epidemiology Program Quarterly Report*, 2, no. 1. New York: New York City Department of Health and Mental Hygiene.

NIMH (National Institute of Mental Health). 2007. *Older Adults: Depression and Suicide Facts*. Available at: http://www.nimh.nih.gov/health/publications/older-adults-depression-and-suicide-facts.shtml (accessed September 2008).

O'Keeffe, J. & Siebenaler, K. 2006. *Adult Day Services: A Key Community Service for Older Adults*. Washington, DC: U.S. Department of Health and Human Services.

Shin, J.K. et al. 2002. Quality of care measurement in nursing home AIDS care: A pilot study. *Journal of the Association of Nurses in AIDS Care* 13, no. 2: 70–76.

Smalbrugge, M., et al. 2006. The impact of depression and anxiety on well-being, disability and use of health care services in nursing home patients. *International Journal of Geriatric Psychiatry* 21, no. 4: 325–332.

Spreat, S., et al. 1998. Improve quality in nursing homes or institute community placement? Implementation of OBRA for individuals with mental retardation. *Research in Developmental Disabilities* 19, no. 6: 507–518.

Watson, L.C., et al. 2006. Depression in assisted living is common and related to physical burden. *American Journal of Geriatric Psychiatry* 14, no. 10: 876–883.

Chapter 6

Douglas A. Singh, PhD, MBA

Long-Term Care Policy: Past, Present, and Future

What You Will Learn

- Public policy can take many different forms and can come from different governmental sources.

- There is no single process or model that can describe how policies are made, except that legislative policymaking follows a well-defined process.

- Policies do not always achieve their intended objectives and sometimes produce unintended side effects that can be positive or negative.

- In the United States, long-term care policy and general welfare have been closely intertwined. The Social Security Act of 1935 and the creation of Medicare and Medicaid in 1965 were landmark policies that indirectly started the nursing home industry. Regulation of the industry soon followed.

- Quality of care issues in nursing homes took center stage during the 1980s. The Nursing Home Reform Act of 1987 provides current nursing home regulations dealing with patient care, but the regulations also have some serious drawbacks.

- Most of the current activity in long-term care policy is at the state level. Community-based services and purchase of private insurance are receiving various degrees of state-level attention.

- The complex interaction of financing, access, utilization, and expenditures is critical to current and future long-term care policy.

- Future policy initiatives are necessary in the areas of prevention, financing, workforce development, health information systems, mental health, and evidence-based practices.

Policy Overview

Long-term care (LTC) policy is specifically crafted to address issues pertaining to access, financing, delivery, quality, and efficiency of LTC services. Long-term care policy is a subset of broader health policies that fall within the domain of public policy.

Public policy refers to decisions made and actions taken by the government that are intended to address current and potential issues that the government believes are in the best interest of the public. As with other types of decisions, policy is intended to accomplish certain defined purposes. However, the intended objectives of public policy are not always achieved. On the other hand, public policy can produce some unintended consequences, even though such unintended results are not always bad.

When the intended goals of public policy pertain to health care, the government's decisions and actions are referred to as **health policy**. Health policies pertain to health care in all aspects, including production, delivery, and financing of health care services. Health policies affect groups or classes of individuals, such as physicians, the poor, the elderly, or children. They can also affect various types of organizations, such as medical schools, managed care organizations, nursing homes, manufacturers of medical technology, or employers in the American industry. Health policy can have a major effect on access to services, shifts in utilization, market competition, availability of an adequate and qualified workforce, and development and use of technology.

Long-term care policies particularly affect the recipients of services such as the elderly or disabled; provider organizations such as nursing homes, home health agencies, and senior centers; caregivers such as physicians and certified nursing assistants; managers such as nursing home administrators; manufacturers and purveyors of technology and medical supplies; and, sometimes, potential consumers of long-term care. For example, favorable tax policies adopted by many states are intended to provide financial incentives so that more consumers can buy long-term care insurance to enable them to cover high LTC expenses later on. However, research shows that tax incentives have not induced the purchase of LTC insurance any more than other factors such as income, health status, and family support (Nixon, 2007). This is one example in which public policy may not produce the intended effects.

The term *policy* is sometimes also used in the context of private policy. More appropriately, however, private policies are strategic decisions that various private organizations make to better serve their markets. In the health care sector, public policy is often an important consideration when private organizations make strategic decisions. For example, a strategic decision by a skilled nursing facility to convert some of its beds to deliver subacute care may be driven by a public policy to increase reimbursement for subacute care. This would be an important consideration in addition to market demand factors.

Forms and Sources of Policy

Commonly, policy takes the form of laws passed by legislative bodies such as the U.S. Congress or state legislatures. Administrative bodies, such as the Centers for Medicare and Medicaid Services (CMS) or state health boards, interpret the legislation and formulate rules and regulations to implement the laws. In the process of interpretation and implementation, the administrative bodies also end up creating public policy. The term ***policymakers*** is generally applied to legislators and decision makers in regulatory agencies who become actively involved in crafting laws and regulations to address health care issues. The two sources of policymaking just mentioned are the most common. Less frequently, certain decisions rendered by the courts and executive orders issued by the President of the United States or state governors also become public policy. The president often plays an important role in policymaking by generating support of his agenda in Congress, by appealing to the American people as to why certain issues are important, and by proposing legislation. Hence, all three branches of government—legislative, judicial, and executive—can make policy. The executive and legislative branches can establish health policies; the judicial branch can uphold, strike down, or modify existing laws affecting health and health care. Examples in all three areas follow. (1) Legislation contained in the Balanced Budget Act of 1997 required Medicare to develop a prospective payment system (PPS) to reimburse skilled nursing facilities. This legislative policy triggered several rounds of policymaking. First, the Health Care Financing Administration (now called Centers for Medicare and Medicaid Services) developed and implemented a new payment methodology in 1998. Subsequently, to address concerns from nursing home operators, Congress instituted a series of temporary payment increases through two pieces of legislation—the Balanced Budget Refinement Act of 1999 and the Medicare, Medicaid, and SCHIP Benefits Improvement and Protection Act of 2000 (MedPAC, 2002). (2) A 1999 decision by the U.S. Supreme Court in *Olmstead v. L.C.* directed states to provide community-based services for persons with disabilities—including persons with developmental disabilities, persons with physical disabilities, persons with mental illness, and the elderly—when such services were determined to be appropriate by professionals responsible for rendering health care to these people. (3) The 2004 Executive Order 13335 provided incentives for the use of health information technology (HIT) and established the position of a National Health Information Technology Coordinator. One of the main objectives of this executive order was to develop a nationwide HIT infrastructure that would allow a patient's electronic health records to be portable and available to different health care providers (i.e., make electronic health records ***interoperable***). The LTC profession has been actively participating to ensure that it is included in this national policy. These examples also illustrate that public policy can take many different forms that can have far-reaching consequences. When policies require that certain individuals or organizations perform or behave in a certain manner, the policies carry the force of law. Violations can result in various kinds of penalties that can include monetary fines, expulsion from participation in public programs, and prison terms for criminal offences.

Health policy may be made at the national, state, or local level of government. For example, national building and fire safety codes govern the construction, design, and safety features for LTC facilities. State policies govern licensure of facilities and health care professionals. States also establish guidelines that insurance companies must follow in the design and sale of LTC insurance. Local governments establish zoning laws specifying where LTC facilities may be built. Local governments may also decide on the availability of certain community-based services on the basis of budget constraints.

Policymaking

There is no single process or model that can describe how policies are made because there are different sources of policy. Hence, policymaking is difficult to describe, and the process can be obscure (Cockrel, 1997). On the other hand, policymaking does not occur in a vacuum. In a representative democracy, the policymaking process must insure that all relevant viewpoints are heard and that the rights of individuals are protected. The larger and more diverse the constituency, the more difficult policymaking becomes (MRSC, 1999).

The formation and implementation of legislative policy generally occurs in a policy cycle that has six main stages: (1) issue raising, (2) policy design, (3) building of public support, (4) building of policy support, (5) legislative decision making, and (6) policy implementation. The enactment of a new policy is generally preceded by a variety of actions that first create a widespread sense that a problem exists and that it must be addressed. The actions are intended to bring issues to the forefront with some degree of importance and urgency. At the second stage, specific policy proposals are designed in the form of a *bill*, which is simply a proposed piece of legislation. If the bill is crafted at the federal level, the proposal is reviewed by various committees and subcommittees in Congress. Amendments may be added. At the third stage, to build public support, policy proposals are sent to organizations and interest groups that may be affected by them. *Interest groups* are an organized sector of society—such as a business association, citizen group, labor union, or professional association—whose main purpose is to protect its members' interests through active participation in the policymaking process.

Hearings are held and testimonies, both in favor of and in opposition to the proposed policy, are given by citizens, business representatives, labor groups, interest groups, professional associations, and experts in the field. At the fourth stage, internal support of the policy becomes critical for it to pass. Influential members of Congress meet with members of their own party, influential leaders from the opposition, and with the president in an effort to gain support. At the fifth stage, the issues are debated on the congressional floor. In the end, a majority vote is needed, and subsequently the bill becomes law if the president signs it. At the sixth stage, once legislation has been signed into law, it is forwarded to the appropriate administrative agency, such as the CMS, for implementation. The agency publishes proposed regulations in the *Federal Register* and holds hearings on how the law would be implemented.

Policymaking can be triggered by events such as natural disasters, growing social problems such as crime, severe economic shocks such as the Great Depression (started in 1929 and ended in the late 1930s), increasing burden on taxpayers such as the rising cost of health care services, demand from consumers such as product safety, etc. For example, the Social Security Act of 1935 was passed during the Great Depression. Widely reported events such as fires and cases of food poisoning in nursing homes during the early 1970s prompted development of nursing home regulations in 1974.

Policy and Politics

Policymaking and politics are often closely intertwined because most policymakers are politicians. The danger is that policymaking often becomes highly politicized and becomes hostage to the ideologies of a political party. The primary concern of politicians is to get elected or reelected. Hence, certain public policies are driven by the desire to keep campaign promises or to please some powerful constituent group. For example, politicians pay attention to powerful organizations, such as the AARP, that represent the growing population of the elderly. It was in this political context that the Medicare Prescription Drug, Improvement, and Modernization Act of 2003 was passed. Going against the wishes of the elderly would have been political suicide for some.

The policy-for-politics approach generally does not ask for or consider the cost benefit of a proposed policy. It is pushed through mainly for ensuring votes. For example, no one cared to inquire what impact the new prescription drug program would have on reducing future disability among the elderly.

Long-Term Care Policy: Historical Perspectives

Policy evolution in the United States did not progress according to some planned design. This follows the general pattern of American health policymaking. Health care policymaking has followed an ad hoc approach to incrementally address issues as they have cropped up.

Welfare Policies and Long-Term Care

The history of LTC policy in the United States goes back to the building of poorhouses (or almshouses) in the late 17th century. A *poorhouse* was a government-operated institution during colonial and post-colonial times where the destitute of society, including the elder-

ly, the homeless, the orphan, the ill, and the disabled, were given food and shelter, and conditions were often squalid. The first poorhouse in the United States is recorded to have opened in 1660 in Boston (Wagner, 2005, p. 10). The poorhouse program was adopted from the Elizabethan system of public charity based on English Poor Laws. In the United States, cities, counties, and states operated these facilities, which were often located on farms and, hence, referred to as poor farms. The poorhouses were part of a very limited public relief system that was financed mainly by local governments. These facilities admitted poor and needy persons of all kinds, including those released from prison, and the ill who did not have family or relatives to take care of them. In response to the growing concerns about abuse and squalid living conditions, some states created state-run Boards of Charities in the mid-1800s to oversee and report on the local poorhouse operations. The Boards' efforts led to some improvement in living conditions and to separation of the insane from the sane and the dependent elderly from the able bodied (Stevenson, 2007). The tireless efforts of Dorothea Lynde Dix (1802–1887), a social reformer, were particularly instrumental in convincing Massachusetts' legislature to pass laws that would put the mentally ill in separate facilities. These reform efforts spread to other states and even abroad to Canada and Europe.

Passage of the Social Security Act in 1935 was a landmark piece of legislation. The elderly were particularly hard hit during the Great Depression as many of them saw their lifetime savings disappear. Hence, the federal government specifically addressed the needs of America's elderly. Simultaneously, deplorable conditions in the poorhouses fueled a reform movement that favored community-based care over institutionalization.

An Old Age Assistance (OAA) program was included in the Social Security Act. However, instead of providing direct community-based services, the OAA program made federal money available to the states to provide financial assistance to needy elderly persons. The Social Security program, even though it left out a relatively large number of Americans (including many elderly and disabled people) was instrumental in putting an end to the poorhouse system (Wagner, 2005, pp. 132–133). For the fiscal year that ended on June 30, 1936, Congress authorized the sum of $49,750,000 under Title I of the Act in the form of matching grants, meaning the states participating in the program would share in the total cost of the program (Social Security Administration, undated). Prior to this, several states had their own old age assistance programs. The new law purposely prohibited payments to anyone living in a public institution (i.e., a poorhouse). An unintended side effect of this policy was that it started a private nursing home industry in the United States because many elderly now were able to pay for services in homes for the aged and boarding homes (Eustis et al., 1984, p. 17).

The Hospital Survey and Construction Act of 1946, commonly known as the Hill-Burton Act, provided federal funds to states for the construction of new hospital beds. An unplanned result of the Hill-Burton legislation was that many of the old hospitals that were being replaced were converted to nursing homes (Stevenson, 2007).

Policies during the 1950s provided federal funds for the construction of nursing homes while, at the same time, OAA payments were increased, and a 1950 Social Security Amendment required payments for medical care to be made directly to nursing homes rather than to the recipients of care. Nursing homes could now contract directly with the state governments and get reimbursed for services delivered to the elderly poor. Also, at this time, nursing homes were required to be licensed by the states. The legislation contained no specific standards for licensure; hence, each state set its own standards (Phillips, 1996).

Financing and Growth of Nursing Homes

The creation of Medicare and Medicaid in 1965 as Title 18 and Title 19 amendments, respectively, to the Social Security Act brought about the most transforming changes on the American health care landscape. Medicare and Medicaid are two major public insurance programs. *Medicare* covers health care services for the elderly, certain disabled people, and those who have end-stage renal disease (kidney failure). *Medicaid* covers health care services for the poor. These programs are more fully discussed in Chapter 7.

With the creation of Medicare and Medicaid, LTC became a part of the health care delivery system in the United States. Also, the federal and state governments became the largest payers for LTC services, and the politics of long-term nursing home care took roots. Medicare and Medicaid funding for nursing homes also attracted Wall Street investors and real estate developers to a fast-growing nursing home industry dominated by chains—that is, multifacility systems that own and operate nursing homes in several states (Hawes et al., 2007). Medicare and Medicaid policies favored payments to nursing homes that lawmakers could regulate rather than payments for community-based services that would be difficult to regulate. These policies led to the institutionalization of a large number of people, many of whom did not belong in nursing homes.

Nursing home utilization and government expenditures exploded shortly after Medicare and Medicaid went into effect. The massive infusion of dollars into the nursing home industry, which had already acquired a tarnished image, prompted regulations to hold individual nursing homes accountable for meeting minimum standards of care. In 1968, Congress passed legislation, commonly known as the Moss Amendments (named after Senator Frank Moss), that paved the way for comprehensive regulations to improve care in the nation's nursing homes. It was not until 1974, however, that final regulations for skilled nursing facilities were promulgated, and their enforcement began in earnest. Compliance with standards such as staffing levels, staff qualifications, fire safety, and delivery of services now became a requirement for participation in the Medicare and Medicaid programs. Later, these regulations were widely criticized that they concentrated on a facility's capacity to give care, not on the quality of services actually delivered (DHEW, 1975).

Interestingly, licensing of health care professionals and hospitals was initiated by the professionals themselves and by the institutional providers, respectively. In contrast, licensing of nursing homes and of nursing home administrators (NHAs) came about through federal laws. As mentioned earlier, the 1950 amendments to the Social Security Act required that states license nursing homes in order to participate in the OAA program. Licensing of NHAs was a major exception to the general trend of requests from professionals that anyone practicing in their respective professions be licensed. The demand for qualified persons to manage nursing homes was not initiated by the industry, but came

about as a result of public outcry over fraud and abuse. As a result, the 1967 amendments to the Social Security Act included a provision that, for states to participate in the Medicaid program, they had to pass laws to govern the licensing of NHAs. In contrast, hospital administrators were not required to be licensed. One key characteristic of licensure is that it is a responsibility of each state, not the federal government. Licensure by the state permits an institution to begin and continue operations and health care professionals to begin and continue to practice (Eustis et al., 1984, pp. 143–145).

Financing of Community-Based Services

Social Security amendments in 1974 authorized federal grants to states for various types of social services. These programs included protective services, homemaker services, transportation services, adult day care, training for employment, information and referral, nutrition assistance, and health support (Lee, 2004). The Social Security Amendment of 1975 created Title 20, which consolidated the federal assistance to states for social services into a single grant. Under Title 20, one of the goals for the states was to prevent or reduce "inappropriate institutional care by providing for community-based care, home-based care, or other forms of less intensive care."[1] In 1981, Title 20 was amended to create Social Services Block Grants. The single block grants actually reduced federal funding to the states for social services. Also, Title 20 covered services for all ages, not just the elderly. Consequently, block grants have provided relatively little money for LTC services.

---

[1]Title XX appears in the United States Code as §§1397-1397f, subchapter XX, chapter 7, Title 42.

Also in 1981, the Home and Community Based Services waiver program was enacted under Section 1915(c) of the Social Security Act. The 1915(c) waivers, as they are commonly referred to, allow states to offer LTC services that are not otherwise available through the Medicaid program, which had authorized payments for institutional care only. The waivers have been particularly successful, and states have increasingly used them to expand community-based LTC services, thus saving money on institutional care. Today, all states provide waiver services to the elderly, working-age people with disabilities, and those with developmental disabilities. Some states also serve people with AIDS and those with serious mental health problems (Miller et al., 2006). Between 1987 and 1997, spending on waiver programs soared from $451 million to $8.1 billion (Coleman, 1999), an increase of 1,696%. By 2006, there were 329 waivers, and the expenditures amounted to $25.6 billion in state and federal Medicaid dollars (Acosta & Hendrickson, 2008).

Deregulation Averted

In the early 1980s, nursing home regulations came under the broader sweep to deregulate industry and downsize the federal bureaucracy. Rumors leaked out that a task force on regulatory reform in the Reagan administration was planning to downgrade sanitation standards, eliminate staff development requirements, reduce physician visits, delete medical director requirements, reduce social work programs, and ignore certain staff qualifications (Trocchio, 1984). Various interest groups such as consumer advocates and professional associations representing medical directors, social workers, and activity personnel lobbied Congress. In the end, interest

group politics and congressional opposition derailed any attempts to deregulate the nursing home industry.

Efforts to Address Quality Issues

The nursing home industry remained fraught with scandals about severely substandard quality of care and an ineffective regulatory system to enforce compliance with standards. At the request of Congress, the Institute of Medicine (IOM) conducted a comprehensive study that culminated in a scathing report on the state of nursing homes in the United States. The study found that residents of nursing homes were being abused, neglected, and given inadequate care. Sweeping reforms were proposed (IOM, 1986). The IOM's prestige lent scientific credibility to its recommendations, and the report triggered the most comprehensive revision of the federal standards, inspection process, and enforcement system for nursing homes since the creation of Medicare and Medicaid in 1965 (Hawes et al., 2007). National organizations representing consumers, nursing homes, and health care professionals worked together to create consensus positions on major nursing home issues and supported them before Congress. Their consensus positions on most IOM recommendations laid the foundation for a new federal law (Turnham, 2001). Although the IOM report has been widely credited to be the impetus for the Nursing Home Reform Act of 1987, it has also been observed that the *Estate of Smith v. Heckler* (1984) class-action lawsuit in Colorado may have played a role. The suit was brought on behalf of all the Medicaid beneficiaries in the state's nursing homes. In essence, the suit charged that the constitutional rights of the nursing home residents were violated because the federal and state governments failed to enforce its laws and regulations. The district court judge, Richard T. Matsch, ruled against the plaintiffs, but his decision was later overturned on appeal. The appeals court ruled that the Secretary of the Department of Health and Human Services (DHHS) did have a duty to establish a system that could determine whether a nursing facility was providing the high-quality care required by the Social Security Act (Phillips, 1996, pp. 10–14).

In 1987, President Reagan signed into law the Omnibus Budget Reconciliation Act of 1987 (OBRA-87), which contained the Nursing Home Reform Act. OBRA-87 brought enormous changes to nursing home operations. The most important provisions of the law are summarized (Castle, 2001; Turnham, 2001) as follows:

- Emphasis on a resident's quality of life as well as quality of care.

- New expectations that each resident's ability to walk, bathe, and perform other activities of daily living will be maintained or improved absent medical reasons.

- A resident assessment process leading to development of an individualized care plan.

- 75 hours of training and testing of paraprofessional staff, such as nursing assistants.

- Right to remain in the nursing home absent nonpayment, dangerous resident behaviors, or significant changes in a resident's medical condition.

- New opportunities for services inside and outside a nursing home to address the needs of residents with mental retardation or mental illnesses.

- Right to safely maintain or bank personal funds with the nursing home.

- Right to return to the nursing home after a hospital stay or an overnight visit with family and friends.

- Right to choose a personal physician and to access medical records.

- Right to organize and participate in a resident or family council.

- Access to an ombudsman to resolve disputes and grievances.

- Right to be free of unnecessary and inappropriate physical and chemical restraints.

- New remedies to be applied to certified nursing homes that fail to meet minimum federal standards.

OBRA-87 also changed the way state inspectors approached nursing home inspections. Inspectors were to no longer spend their time exclusively with staff or with facility records, as was the case in the past. Conversations with residents and families and observation of dining and medication administration became critical steps in the inspection process (Turnham, 2001).

Ironically, OBRA-87 reforms were nearly repealed in 1995 as part of a larger attempt to reform Medicaid. This time, part of the nursing home industry supported repeal of the OBRA reforms, particularly the enforcement provisions. But consumer advocates, aided by researchers, were able to use empirical evidence about the positive effects of OBRA provisions to effectively oppose the dilution of federal regulations. Once consumer advocates redefined the issue as one of quality of care, Congress opposed the repeal of the Nursing Home Reform Act (Hawes et al., 2007).

OBRA-87 altered the regulatory landscape in a significant way. Even though substantial funds were allocated to carry out the legislative mandate, it was a complex piece of legislation, and numerous hurdles were encountered in developing regulations. The final rules were published at the end of 1994 to be effective in July 1995, more than eight years after the law had been passed (Phillips, 1996, p. 35).

Oversight for Other Services

It is interesting to note that while the nursing home industry has been under the spotlight from federal policymakers for more than half a century now, the same policymakers have shown little interest in the assisted living industry. The latter has been one of the fastest growing areas of LTC delivery in recent years, and the aging-in-place philosophy has raised the level of clinical acuity of residents in these facilities. The absence of direct federal reimbursement to assisted living facilities is perhaps the reason any federal regulatory oversight is unlikely, unless at some point crises and failure of care similar to those encountered during the long history of nursing homes become apparent (Edelman, 2003). Most regulatory efforts for assisted living facilities have occurred at the state level. Similar variations in state regulations exist for adult day care centers. Medicaid-funded adult day care services must meet applicable state licensing and regulatory requirements such as minimum staff-to-participant ratios. The majority of states have instituted inspections (O'Keeffe & Siebenaler, 2006).

A 1988 court ruling on a class-action lawsuit, *Duggan v. Bowen*, opened up broad access to Medicare-covered home health services, and for some time, home health had become the fastest growing health care service in the United States. In August 1997, Congress enacted the Balanced Budget Act (BBA) of 1997, which mandated that Medicare's cost-based, retrospective reimbursement policy for home health agencies as well as skilled nursing facilities be replaced by a prospective payment system (PPS). This policy was part of a broader financial reform to slow down the growth of Medicare spending. A prospective reimbursement method for skilled nursing facilities was implemented in July 1998 and a home health PPS reimbursement was implemented in October 2000.

Current State of Long-Term Care Policy

The national stage for LTC policy has been largely silent as other pressing issues preoccupy politicians. Long-term care is not expected to see any major changes in the near future. States, on the other hand, continue to forge incremental policy initiatives to expand the purchase of private LTC insurance and reduce the level of institutional care in favor of community-based services. Both initiatives are intended to curtail the states' burden of nursing home expenditures and to save money overall in the LTC delivery system. A third area of state-level policymaking encompasses ongoing efforts to license alternative housing and care facilities. The institutional continuum of LTC includes various types of living and care arrangements other than traditional nursing homes.

Public policy in long-term care has evolved in three main directions: financing, utilization, and quality. Almost all health care policy can be classified into these categories.

Financing, access, and utilization go hand in hand. *Utilization* is the actual use of health care occurs when people needing services have access to them. *Access* is the ability of a person needing services to obtain those services. Two main factors drive access: financing and availability of services. If *financing* (i.e., the ability to pay for services) is adequate but availability is limited, the services get rationed and access is restricted. On the other hand, if services are available but financing is not, access becomes restricted for those who cannot afford the services. Also, increased utilization negatively affects financing. Increased utilization makes total expenditures rise, and financing becomes constrained.

Financing

Financing is the means by which patients pay for the services they receive. Financing varies by the type of service, and there can be different sources of financing even for the same service. For example, care in a skilled nursing facility can be financed through Medicaid, Medicare, private insurance, Veterans Health Administration, or one's own personal funds. Hence, LTC financing is quite fragmented because no single source can be tapped on to pay for services. Consequently, access and utilization become uneven. People face financial obstacles in a system that is complex and nonintegrated. Complexities arise when people have to move from one type of service to another, such as from nursing home to the community or vice versa, or even when they have to stay within one LTC sector. For example, many who require nursing home care for a long period of time can face a financing nightmare. Medicare pays only for post-acute short-term stays, and Medicaid requires people to exhaust their financial resources to become eligible. Many elders who do not qualify for either program have to pay on a private basis either through private LTC insurance or out of personal savings. In 2005, 44% of the financing for nursing home care was derived from Medicaid, and only 16% came from Medicare. Private out-of-pocket payments financed 26%, and 7% was paid through privately purchased LTC insurance. The remainder was paid through miscellaneous private and public sources (Kaiser, 2007).

Expansion of Community-Based Services

Medicaid remains the largest source of funding for LTC services. It finances 41% of the total spending for LTC services of all types. Spending on Medicaid home- and community-based services (HCBS) has been growing, but states vary greatly in financing HCBS. In 2006, spending on HCBS accounted for 41% ($44.9 billion) of total Medicaid LTC services spending, up from 13% in 1990 (Kaiser, 2007). As mentioned earlier, lawsuits such as *Duggan v. Bowen* and *Olmstead v. L.C.* played an important role in shifting utilization from institution-based care to community-based services. More recently, the Deficit Reduction Act of 2005 provided federal funding to states to expand community-based care. As part of this legislation, Congress granted $1.8 billion over five years for states to provide 12 months of LTC services in a community setting to individuals who currently receive Medicaid services in nursing homes (Kasper & O'Malley, 2006). This legislation may be a turning point in national LTC policy because it makes rebalancing between institutional and community-based services a national priority (Mor et al., 2007) under a federal–state joint initiative referred to as Money Follows the Person. Under this program, when a person transfers from a nursing home to the community, funds that had previously paid for nursing home care are transferred to community-based services for that person.

HCBC has been viewed as a potentially more cost-effective option than nursing home care, but research evidence remains inconclusive that expanding community-based care lowers overall LTC spending (Grabowski, 2006; Long et al., 2005). It reduces expenditures for nursing home services, but opens up access to HCBS for many who previously did not have access. On the other hand, studies do show that community-based services significantly improve the quality of life of clients. People prefer less restrictive noninstitutional settings over services received in LTC facilities.

Reimbursement to Providers

Other policy issues related to financing surround the levels of reimbursement to providers from Medicare and Medicaid. Nursing home operators have long contended that payments from public payers have been inadequate to support quality services. Independent experts have also voiced opinions that reimbursement levels should be raised. However, Medicaid and Medicare administrators have been concerned about rising expenditures, while the public is not inclined to pay more in taxes. The paradox is that, unlike many other industries, nursing home care is highly labor intensive because caregivers have to render services one on one. Hence, few options are available to increase productivity or slash operating costs.

Incentives for Private Insurance

Coverage for nursing home care from private LTC insurance has increased slightly in recent years, but fewer than 10% of people 50 years of age and older have purchased private insurance for long-term care (Seff, 2003). The elderly population most likely to benefit from private LTC coverage also has a lower average income than the general population.

Hence, LTC insurance is difficult to market because premiums must be high enough to cover costs but low enough to attract clients. Insurance is based on the principle of adequately spreading risk among a large segment of the population. However, younger healthy groups have shown little interest in buying LTC insurance because they see the need for LTC only as a remote possibility.

A few states offer tax deductions or credits for purchasing private insurance, but the incentives appear to be too small to induce many people to purchase LTC plans (Wiener et al., 2000). Another state-based policy initiative that is designed to increase the number of middle-income people who buy private insurance is the Partnership for Long-Term Care program. The program was designed by the Robert Wood Johnson Foundation, a private nonprofit organization, through a demonstration project in California, Connecticut, Indiana, and New York. Currently, about half the states have implemented the program. The Partnership program encourages individuals to purchase insurance, and, if these individuals require LTC services, they can apply for Medicaid after their insurance benefits have been exhausted. To qualify for Medicaid, these individuals would be allowed to keep all or some of their financial assets. Otherwise, under Medicaid policy, people have to first use up their income and assets before they can qualify for benefits. Under the Partnership program, exceptions are made to this rule. States have been permitted to do this under the Deficit Reduction Act of 2005. Some experts believe that the Partnership program has made progress toward meeting its goals. For example, the original four states have been modestly successful in promoting quality insurance products. As of mid-2006, about 240,000 Partnership insurance plans had been sold, and about 194,000 were being used to obtain services. There are critics, but the program was not intended to be a comprehensive solution to all LTC needs; it was designed to fill a financial gap (Alliance for Health Reform, 2007).

Another area in which progress has been made is information to consumers. Long-term care, with its many service and financing options, is confusing for most people. People have also assumed that the government will somehow pay for their LTC needs. Government resources, however, have been shrinking and it is unlikely that public resources will be enough to meet the needs of a burgeoning elderly population. The DHHS has created the National Clearinghouse for Long-Term Care Information (see For Further Learning). The website is designed to help people understand why planning for LTC is important and how they can plan for it.

Utilization

Table 6–1 provides capacity and utilization data for nursing homes. During the 1990s, nursing home beds in the United States continued to increase while their utilization continued to decrease. Between 2000 and 2006, both the number of nursing homes and beds decreased. As a result, there was some improvement in capacity utilization as reflected in the occupancy rates. On the other hand, the utilization of nursing homes by the population, as reflected in the resident rates, has continued to decline at a rather dramatic rate.

During the 1980s, nursing homes entered the subacute and rehabilitation markets, mainly as a result of the DRG-based (diagnosis-related group) prospective payment system implemented in hospitals, which created incentives for early discharge of patients from hospitals. The trend accelerated during the 1990s because the proliferation of managed care put further pressures on reducing the length of stay in hospitals. While these trends should have increased nursing home utilization, other factors in play since the 1980s promoted the use of alternative settings such as home health care, other community-based LTC services, and assisted living facilities.

It is estimated that 5 to 12% of residents in nursing homes require low levels of care according to their functional and clinical characteristics (Mor et al., 2007). Their needs

Table 6–1 Nursing Home Utilization (Selected Years)

	1992	1995	2000	2006
Number of nursing homes	15,846	16,389	16,886	15,899
Number of beds	1,692,123	1,751,302	1,795,388	1,716,102
Occupancy rates[a]	86.0%	84.5%	82.4%	83.5%
Resident rates[b]	444.4	404.5	349.1	270.6

Sources: Data from *Health, United States* 1996–97, p. 248; *Health, United States* 2007, pp. 370–371.

[a]Percent of beds occupied (number of residents per 100 available beds).

[b]Number of nursing home residents of all ages per 1,000 population 85 years of age and over.

could be met with appropriate community-based LTC services. However, HCBS programs, being part of the state-administered Medicaid programs, have not developed uniformly across states. Also, states vary in their enthusiasm for nursing home transition programs. Some states, for example, have transitioned residents to assisted living facilities instead of home- and community-based services. Motivation of individuals and their families and the availability of a community support system to supplement formal services are viewed as key factors in determining who transitions back to the community from nursing homes. Logistical barriers may also hamper transitions. For example, hospital discharge planners find it easier to move patients from the hospital to nursing homes. Arranging for appropriate community-based services is generally time consuming and complex because it requires coordination and determination of how services will be financed. Other obstacles include shortage of housing alternatives (Mor et al., 2007) and waiting lists for community-based care in some states (Kasper & O'Malley, 2006).

Some efforts are being made at the state level to carry out evaluations of HCBS to improve the programs. In the meantime, policymakers are hesitant to broadly implement new initiatives because they have not been validated for quality and evaluated for how much they would end up costing (Acosta & Hendrickson, 2008).

Private paying patients have found the residential and social lifestyles in assisted living facilities to be much more appealing than those in skilled nursing facilities. Many people have figured that they might as well spend their personal savings in an upscale assisted living home and later apply for Medicaid if they need care in a skilled nursing facility.

Quality

Quality has been a well-recognized issue in LTC for some time. Because Medicare and Medicaid finance more than half of the nation's nursing home care, government regulations play a major role in establishing standards to ensure at least the minimum level of quality. Research has demonstrated that the overall effects of this regulation have been positive. On the other hand, little has been done to ensure quality of care in assisted living facilities and for community-based services.

From the standpoint of quality of care delivered to nursing home residents, OBRA-87 was revolutionary. For example, the sharp decline in the use of physical and chemical restraints has been attributed to the requirements of OBRA-87. Other positive care practices since the implementation of OBRA-87 standards include improved staffing levels, more accurate medical records, comprehensive care planning, increased use of incontinence training programs and a decrease in the use of urinary catheters, and increased participation of residents in activity programs (Hawes et al., 1997; Marek et al., 1996; Teno et al., 1997; Zhang & Grabowski, 2004). OBRA-87 also mandated a comprehensive patient assessment process, which led to the development of a standardized Resident Assessment Instrument (RAI). The assessment protocols are designed to help nursing homes identify and treat or manage chronic conditions, the onset of acute illnesses, adverse effects of medications, or other factors that caused or contributed to a clinical problem (Hawes, 2003).

Although substantial progress has been made, OBRA-87 remains controversial for several reasons:

- In 2006, nearly one-fifth of the facilities were cited for violations that caused harm or presented immediate jeopardy to residents. Improvements appear to have reached a plateau (Wiener et al., 2007).

- Regulations continue to be inconsistently applied both within and across regions (Miller & Mor, 2006). Over a decade ago, Phillips (1996) had pointed out that there were significant differences in how inspectors applied the regulations and gave citations for noncompliance with the regulations. The oversight process is reliable only for assessing aggregate results, but inspectors frequently disagree on the scope and severity of problems uncovered (Lee et al., 2006).

- Phillips (1996) concluded that only 16% of the OBRA-87 regulations actually focused on clinical care and therefore did not primarily focus on high-quality care.

- Enforcement of OBRA-87 regulations takes on a punitive rather than a remedial tone. Nonflagrant violations can be better addressed with a focus on improvement rather than punishment (Willging,[2] 2008).

- Staffing levels have been relatively stable for many years, despite the increased clinical acuity in the patient population (Wiener et al., 2007).

- There is practically no available quantitative data on quality of life, which is an important component of LTC (Wiener et al., 2007).

----

[2]Dr. Willging was president of the American Health Care Association (AHCA) at the time OBRA-87 was passed. The AHCA was heavily involved in representing the for-profit nursing home sector, which supported the legislation.

Policy for the Future

The future of LTC will be shaped by both policy and innovation, but policy will continue to play the dominant role. Long-term care faces many serious challenges ahead. Much will depend on (1) the health status of Americans and the prevalence of disability in the population; (2) birth and mortality rates; (3) quality of education for the younger generation, innovations that generate national wealth, and quality of immigration that would be necessary for a strong economy; and (4) availability of financial resources as well as priorities for their use. These factors are critical from a broad policy perspective. The future need for LTC services is just one part of the equation; much will depend on the nation's ability to actually finance and deliver the needed services. For example, if the infrastructure for delivery (such as a skilled workforce) is inadequate, many people may have to do without the services they may otherwise need.

The complex interaction among financing, access, and utilization for LTC services would play out within a broader context of health policy for two main reasons: (1) The aging of the population will have far-reaching repercussions beyond LTC, with spillover effects for retirement, Social Security, primary health care, acute care in hospitals, and numerous other health care services. With aging, the utilization for all types of health care services increases, not just the need for LTC. (2) Financing for LTC services is an integral part of the Medicare and Medicaid programs, which also cover various types of other health care services.

Life expectancy for a newborn in the United States has risen from 68.2 years in

1950 to 78.1 years in 2006, the highest ever recorded (Heron et al., 2008). During the same time period, birth rates[3] dwindled from 24.1 to 14.2 (Martin et al., 2009). More than 75 million baby boomers are about to enter retirement age in 2011 and beyond. Between 2005 and 2050, the nation's elderly population is projected to more than double, while the number of working-age Americans and children will grow more slowly than the elderly population (Passel & Cohn, 2008).

Future growth of one population group at the expense of another group (in this case, growth of the elderly population while at the same time a contraction of the working population) is called the ***demographic imperative***. It has potentially serious consequences at two main fronts: (1) With fewer working people and a burgeoning elderly population, the financial burden for LTC on future generations is expected to be enormous. This is an impending dilemma that policymakers have been reluctant to bring up for public policy debates. (2) A labor force crisis for LTC delivery is already beginning to emerge because a smaller proportion of people from a shrinking pool of new workers are choosing employment in health care delivery settings (Stone & Wiener, 2001). Commissions have been organized at both federal and state levels to recommend solutions to address the issue of labor shortages (Friedland, 2004).

The future need for LTC will be closely associated with health and disability trends in an aging population. Actually, some research has shown that there are positive trends in the health of older Americans, thanks to advances in medical treatments. The bad news, however, is that obesity and diabetes have both increased among older people as it has in the younger age groups, and hypertension has increased in older women (Kramarow et al., 2007). Nevertheless, at least according to one source, the rise in the number of people with activity limitations is expected to moderate over time. Acosta and Hendrickson (2008) projected the number of people with activity limitations to rise 14% between 2010 and 2020, but the rate of increase would moderate to 10.5, 7.9, and 5.8%, respectively, during the subsequent 10-year periods between 2020 and 2050. Even according to this scenario, the aging demographic lends urgency to how best to restructure federal and state budgets to pay for more than 12 million older Americans who will probably need LTC services starting in 2010 (Acosta & Hendrickson, 2008). On the other hand, policymakers will continue to explore new ways for providing cost-effective LTC services without turning LTC into an expanded social program because both Medicare and Medicaid face serious cost challenges in the future. As part of these efforts, funding for community alternatives will continue, but many recipients of care in the home- and community-based settings will eventually need to be institutionalized. In addition to policies that promote community-based care, other policies can help strengthen the LTC system.

Prevention

LTC policy issues tend to focus on receiving and delivering care, rather than on actions that can prevent or delay the need for care. Enhancing community environments that can promote walking—such as repairing or building sidewalks, ensuring safety from traffic, protecting older adults from crime, and promoting leisure activities—can improve physical activity and promote better health. Other

---

[3]Birth rate is number of live births per 1,000 population.

preventive measures include a balanced diet, obesity control, smoking cessation, and vaccinations against influenza and pneumonia. Both community-based and institution-based fall prevention programs are critical because they result in high medical costs, disability, functional limitations, and diminished quality of life (CDC/Merck, 2007).

Financing

Currently, most middle-class families are unprepared to meet LTC expenses. Most people think that Medicare would pay for their LTC needs, but Medicare covers only short-term post-acute care after discharge from a hospital. Less than 10% of the elderly have private LTC insurance (Burke et al., 2005). Without a strong reliance on private LTC insurance coverage, the public sector will see its expenditures grow rapidly. Purchasing LTC insurance is both expensive and confusing. Also, current tax policies provide greater incentives to business owners and older adults than to younger people when they purchase LTC insurance. The Congressional Budget Office (CBO, 2004) recommended improving the way private markets for LTC insurance currently function, but policy initiatives are needed to expand purchase of private insurance.

Workforce

It is estimated that between 2000 and 2010 alone, when the baby boomers are about to reach retirement age, an additional 1.9 million direct care workers would be needed in LTC settings (DHHS, 2003). Stone (2003) believes that shortage of a stable and qualified workforce may be the most important and most neglected policy concern. The infra-

structure can be severely restricted in its capacity to provide services without an adequate number of qualified workers. Experts in LTC rate workforce issues at par with the aging of the population itself (Miller et al., 2008). An inadequate supply of qualified workers hinders recruitment efforts. Once recruited, retention becomes equally challenging. Some health care workers have low preferences about caring for elderly people who have physical and mental incapacities. Hard work without adequate pay is another factor that makes people leave employment in the LTC sector.

Another issue that must be addressed is training deficits in geriatrics among physicians, nurses, therapists, social workers, and pharmacists. Ironically, all 125 U.S. medical schools have a pediatrics department, but only three have a geriatrics department. Evidence shows that care of older adults by health care professionals prepared in geriatrics yields better physical and mental outcomes without increasing costs (Cohen et al., 2002). It is estimated that only about 9,000 practicing physicians in the United States (2.5 geriatricians per 10,000 elderly) have formal training in geriatrics. This number is expected to drop down to 6,000 in the near future. Among nurses, less than 0.05% have advanced certification in geriatrics (CDC/Merck, 2004).

There are also not enough well-trained administrators to provide leadership in the LTC field. Recruitment and retention of NHAs is a growing problem nationwide (Maine Department of Professional and Financial Regulation, 2004). Lack of appropriate educational standards as a requirement for licensure of NHAs no doubt contributes to the problem. In turn, the shortage of NHAs prevents the raising of national educational standards to a minimum of a bachelor's degree in health care administration.

Health Information Technology

Leaders in the LTC field tend to look to the government for direction in health information technology (HIT) adoption (Hudak & Sharkey, 2007). Interoperable HIT can enable providers to track patients' care across hospitals, nursing homes, home health agencies, pharmacies, and physicians' offices. Interoperability is essential for an integrated system of health care that interfaces with LTC services. Long-term care needs to be fully represented in all future interoperable electronic health records. Such systems are particularly critical because the elderly frequently make transitions between LTC and non-LTC settings. Currently, such transitions rarely occur smoothly because of high rates of missing or inaccurate information (Miller & Mor, 2006). HIT can also help reduce isolation among seniors and caregivers through electronically enabled social networks and online training for caregivers (Martin et al., 2007). HIT applications can also improve staff efficiency, interface with quality measures, reduce billing errors, improve clinical accuracy, and improve communication among providers.

Mental Health

The quality of mental health services in LTC settings remains a challenge. There are concerns that patients are not receiving the mental health care they need or that they are receiving inappropriate, and sometimes unnecessary, mental health services. Even though certain aspects of mental health and psychiatric care are addressed in the OBRA-87 legislation, outcome evaluations have presented challenges (Streim et al., 2002).

Evidence-Based Practices

As pointed out earlier, quality improvement in LTC has come to a standstill. Also, there is little evidence that merely increasing the amount of spending improves quality. To the contrary, quality improvement often reduces costs. Evidence-based practices will drive the future of quality improvement in all types of health care delivery settings. Best practices in the form of clinical practice guidelines have been developed for long-term care. However, no policy initiatives have emerged to provide incentives for their use.

For Further Thought

1. Why is it important for administrators in the long-term care field to understand policy and policymaking?
2. What lessons in U.S. policymaking can be learned from the passage of the Nursing Home Reform Act in 1987 and its near-repeal in 1995?
3. Do interest groups help or hinder the policymaking process?
4. Should policy be made only after due consideration of its cost-benefit?

For Further Learning

Clearinghouse for the Community Living Exchange Collaborative: A joint effort of the Institute for Rehabilitation and Research and Rutgers Center for State Health Policy. The Exchange is a vital hub of information collection, sharing, and dissemination.

http://www.hcbs.org

National Clearinghouse for Long-Term Care Information. U.S. Department of Health and Human Services

http://www.longtermcare.gov/LTC/Main_Site/index.aspx

Overview of the Nursing Home Reform Act

http://www.ltcombudsman.org/uploads/OBRA87summary.pdf

REFERENCES

Acosta, P., & Hendrickson, L. 2008. *Discussion Brief: Advancing Medicaid HCBS Policy: From Capped Consumer to Consumer-Directed*. Rutgers Center for State Health Policy. Retrieved September 2008 from http://www.hcbs.org/files/136/6774/ConsumerChoice.pdf.

Alliance for Health Reform. 2007. *Long-Term Care Partnerships: An Update*. Washington, DC: Alliance for Health Reform.

Burke, S.P., et al. 2005. *Developing a Better Long-Term Care Policy: A Vision and Strategy for America's Future*. Washington, DC: National Academy of Social Insurance.

Castle, N.G. 2001. Citations and compliance with the Nursing Home Reform Act of 1987. *Journal of Health and Social Policy* 13, no. 1: 73–95.

CBO. 2004. *Financing Long Term Care for the Elderly*. Washington, DC: Congressional Budget Office.

CDC/Merck. 2004. *The State of Aging and Health in America, 2004*. Centers for Disease Control and Prevention and Merck Company Foundation. Retrieved October 2008 from http://www.cdc.gov/aging/pdf/State_of_Aging_and_Health_in_America_2004.pdf.

CDC/Merck. 2007. *The State of Aging and Health in America*. Centers for Disease Control and Prevention and Merck Company Foundation. Retrieved October 2008 from http://www.cdc.gov/aging/pdf/saha_2007.pdf.

Cockrel, J. 1997. *Public Policymaking in America*. Retrieved September 2008 from http://www.ca.uky.edu/agc/pubs/ip/ip19/ip19.pdf.

Cohen, H.J., et al. 2002. A controlled trial of inpatient and outpatient geriatric evaluation and management. *New England Journal of Medicine* 346, no. 12: 906–912.

Coleman, B. 1999. *Trends in Medicaid Long-Term Care Spending*. Research report, AARP Public Policy Institute. Retrieved September 2008 from http://www.aarp.org/research/assistance/medicaid/aresearch-import-646-DD38.html#community.

DHEW (Department of Health, Education, and Welfare). 1975. *Long Term Care Facility Improvement Study: Introductory Report*. Washington, DC: Department of Health, Education, and Welfare.

DHHS (Department of Health and Human Services). 2003. *The Future Supply of Long-Term Care Workers in Relation to the Aging Baby Boom Generation, Report to Congress.* Washington, DC: Department of Health and Human Services.

Edelman, T.S. 2003. Enforcement in the assisted living industry: Dispelling the Industry's Myths. *NAELA Quarterly* 3, no. 2: 9–12.

Eustis, N., et al. 1984. *Long-Term Care for Older Persons: A Policy Perspective.* Monterey, CA: Brooks/Cole Publishing.

Friedland, R.B. 2004. *Caregivers and Long-Term Care Needs in the 21st Century: Will Public Policy Meet the Challenge.* Washington, DC: Health Policy Institute, Georgetown University.

Grabowski, D.C. 2006. The cost-effectiveness of noninstitutional long-term care services: Review and synthesis of the most recent evidence. *Medical Care Research and Review* 63, no. 1: 3–28.

Hawes, C. 2003. Ensuring quality in long-term care settings. In D. Blumenthal et al. (eds.). *Long-term Care and Medicare Policy: Can We Improve the Continuity of Care?* (pp. 131–143). Washington, DC: National Academy of Social Insurance.

Hawes, C., et al. 1997. The impact of OBRA-87 and the RAI on indicators of process quality in nursing homes. *Journal of the American Geriatrics Society* 45, no. 8: 977–985.

Hawes, C., et al. 2007. *The RAI and the Politics of Long-Term Care: The Convergence of Science and Politics in U.S. Nursing Home Policy.* Report published by the Milbank Memorial Fund. Retrieved September 2008 from http://www.milbank.org/reports/footnotes/US.html.

Heron, M.P., et al. 2008. Deaths: Preliminary data for 2006. *National Vital Statistics Reports*, Vol. 56, no. 16. Hyattsville, MD: National Center for Health Statistics.

Hudak, S., & Sharkey, S. 2007. *Health Information Technology: Are Long Term Care Providers Ready?* Oakland, CA: California HealthCare Foundation.

IOM. 1986. *Improving the Quality of Care in Nursing Homes.* Washington, DC: National Academy Press, Institute of Medicine.

Kaiser (Kaiser Commission on Medicaid and the Uninsured). 2007. *Medicaid Facts.* The Henry J. Kaiser Family Foundation. Retrieved September 2008 from http://www.kff.org/medicaid/upload/2186_05.pdf.

Kasper, J., &. O'Malley, M. 2006. *Nursing Home Transition Programs: Perspectives of State Medicaid Officials.* Kaiser Commission on Medicaid and the Uninsured. Retrieved September 2008 from http://www.kff.org/medicaid/upload/7484.pdf.

Kramarow, E., et al. 2007. Trends in the health of older Americans, 1970–2005. *Health Affairs* 26, no. 5: 1417–1425.

Lee, J. 2004. *Aging Policy and Policy in U.S.* Center for Human Resource Research, Ohio State University (PowerPoint slides, June 2004). Retrieved September 2008 from www.kspa.org/multy_board/bbs_files/20060406041206.ppt.

Lee, R.H., et al. 2006. Reliability of the nursing home survey process: A simultaneous survey approach. *The Gerontologist* 46, no. 6: 772–780.

Long, S.K., et al. 2005. Getting by in the community: Lessons from frail elders. *Journal of Aging and Social Policy* 17, no. 1: 19–44.

Maine Department of Professional and Financial Regulation. 2004. Report of the Board of Nursing Home Administrators. Retrieved February 2009 from http://www.maine.gov/pfr/legislative/documents/nursingh.pdf.

Marek, K.D., et al. 1996. OBRA '87: Has it resulted in positive change in nursing homes? *Journal of Gerontological Nursing* 22, no. 12: 32–40.

Martin, J.A., et al. 2009. Births: Final data for 2006. *National Vital Statistics Reports*, Vol. 57, no. 7. Hyattsville, MD: National Center for Health Statistics.

Martin, R.D., et al. 2007. *Essential but Not Sufficient: Information Technology in Long-Term Care as an Enabler of Consumer Independence and Quality Improvement.* Report to the National Commission for Quality Long-Term Care. Mclean, VA: BearingPoint Management and Technology Consultants.

MedPAC. 2002. *Report to Congress: Medicare Payment Policy.* Washington, DC: Medicare Payment Advisory Commission.

Miller, E.A., & Mor, V. 2006. *Out of the Shadows: Envisioning a Brighter Future for Long-Term Care in America.* Providence, RI: Brown University.

Miller, E.A., et al. 2008. Assessing experts' views of the future of long-term care. *Research on Aging* 30, no. 4: 450–473.

Miller, N.A., et al. 2006. Strengthening home and community-based care through Medicaid waivers. *Journal of Aging and Social Policy* 18, no. 1: 1–16.

Mor, V., et al. 2007. Prospects of transferring nursing home residents to the community. *Health Affairs* 26, no. 6: 1762–1771.

MRSC. 1999. *Local Government Policy-Making Process* (Report No. 45). Seattle, WA: The Municipal Research Services Center of Washington.

Nixon, D.C. 2007. *State Programs to Encourage Long Term Care Insurance: Worthwhile or Wasted?* Paper presented at the annual meeting of the Midwest Political Science Association. Palmer House Hotel, Chicago, April 12, 2007. Retrieved September 2008 from http://www.allacademic.com/meta/p198586_index.html.

O'Keeffe, J., & Siebenaler, K. 2006. *Adult Day Services: A Key Community Service for Older Adults.* Washington, DC: U.S. Department of Health and Human Services.

Passel, J.S., & Cohn, D. 2008. *U.S. Population Projections: 2005–2050.* Washington, DC: Pew Research Center.

Phillips, R.E. 1996. *Crises in the Regulation of Long-Term Care.* Doctoral dissertation: Western Michigan University, April 1996.

Seff, M.K. 2003. Clearing up health care myths. *Golden Lifestyles* (Jan. Feb. Mar.): 7.

Social Security Administration. Undated. Legislative history: Social Security Act of 1935. Retrieved September 2008 from http://www.ssa.gov/history/35acti.html.

Stevenson, K. 2007. *History of Long-Term Care.* Retrieved September 2008 from http://www.elderweb.com/home/main.

Stone, R. 2003. Reality of caring for the long-term care population. In *Long-term Care and Medicare Policy: Can We Improve the Continuity of Care?*, D. Blumenthal et al. (eds.) (pp. 40–47). Washington, DC: National Academy of Social Insurance.

Stone, R., & Wiener, J. 2001. *Who Will Care for Us? Addressing the Long-term Care Workforce Crisis.* Washington, DC: Urban Institute and the American Association of Homes and Services for the Aging.

Streim, J.E., et al. 2002. Regulatory oversight, payment policy, and quality improvement in mental health care in nursing homes. *Psychiatric Services* 53, no. 11: 1414–1418.

Teno, J., et al. 1997. The early impact of the Patient Self-Determination Act in long-term care facilities: Results from a ten-state sample. *Journal of the American Geriatrics Society* 45, no. 8: 939–944.

Trocchio, J. 1984. Nursing home deregulation: Regulatory reform efforts. *Nursing Economics* 2, no. 3: 185–189.

Turnham, H. 2001. *Federal Nursing Home Reform Act from the Omnibus Budget Reconciliation Act of 1987*. National Long Term Care Ombudsman Resource Center. Retrieved September 2008 from http://www.ltcombudsman.org/ombpublic/49_346_1023.cfm.

Wagner, D. 2005. *The Poorhouse: America's Forgotten Institution*. Lanham, MD: Rowman & Littlefield Publishers.

Wiener, J.M., et al. 2000. Federal and state initiatives to jump start the market for private long-term care insurance. *Elder Law Journal* 8, no. 1: 57–102.

Wiener, J.M., et al. 2007. *Nursing Home Care Quality: Twenty Years After the Omnibus Budget Reconciliation Act of 1987*. Menlo Park, CA: The Henry J. Kaiser Family Foundation.

Willging, P. 2008. Personal electronic communication. September 23, 2008.

Zhang, X., & Grabowski, D.C. 2004. Nursing home staffing and quality under the Nursing Home Reform Act. *The Gerontologist* 44, no. 1: 13–23.

Chapter 7

Douglas A. Singh, PhD, MBA

The Long-Term Care Industry

What You Will Learn

- The primary component of the long-term care industry consists of various providers in community-based settings, quasi-institutions, and institutional facilities. The industry cannot function without other key partners.

- Home health care is a prime example of community-based long-term care providers. Others include homemaker and personal care service providers, adult day care providers, and hospice service providers.

- Independent living and retirement centers and custodial care providers such as adult foster care facilities can be referred to as quasi-institutions.

- Institutional providers are the most visible sector of the long-term care industry. They range from assisted living facilities to a variety of providers that are commonly referred to as nursing homes. Some institutional long-term care services are based in hospitals.

- Commercial insurance companies and managed care organizations play a critical role in the financing of long-term care services.

- A variety of health care personnel are involved in the delivery of long-term care. They can be classified as administrative professionals, clinicians, paraprofessional caregivers, ancillary personnel, and social support professionals.

- The ancillary sector includes case management agencies that assist clients with identifying and obtaining appropriate long-term care services, long-term care pharmacies that provide drug management and pharmaceuticals to facilities, and developers of long-term care technology.

Scope of the Industry

Efficient delivery of services to a nation's population necessitates a long-term care (LTC) industry. The industry in the United States has been shaped primarily by LTC policy. But, the government's role has been mainly indirect—as a financier and regulator. The government plays a very small role in the direct delivery of LTC services. The LTC industry mainly consists of providers of services other than informal caregivers and government agencies that deliver social services. Among the providers are hospital-based LTC services that emerged in the late 1980s. Hospice services provide end-of-life care and are regarded as a component of long-term care. The industry cannot function without other key partners. These partners include the insurance industry, managed care organizations, professionals employed in the LTC industry, case management agencies, long-term care pharmacies, and developers of technology.

The Provider Sector

Providers are organizations or individuals that deliver LTC services and get paid for the services delivered. The health care industry is replete with examples of providers, including hospitals, nursing homes, home health agencies, hospices, physicians, pharmacists, and laboratories. Various private organizations and facilities, both for-profit and non-profit, are part of the LTC industry. Most of these organizations deliver institutional care, but the private sector that delivers community-based services has also grown. A prime example is home health care, which

has been a growing industry in itself. The LTC industry is predominantly funded by the government, and certain sectors of the industry are more stringently regulated than others.

Community-Based Service Providers

Four main types of providers constitute the community-based sector of the LTC industry: (1) certified home health providers, (2) homemaker and personal care service providers, (3) adult day care providers, and (4) hospice service providers.

Certified Home Health Providers

Home health care is consistent with the philosophy of maintaining people in the least restrictive environment possible. Without the availability of skilled nursing care and rehabilitation services in patients' own homes, the patients would have to be in hospitals or nursing homes to receive the same services at a much higher expense.

As pointed out in Chapter 6, the 1988 class-action lawsuit of *Duggan v. Bowen* was instrumental in expanding home health benefits under Medicare. The new rules that took effect in 1989 (1) removed the requirement of a three-day hospital stay before home health visits would be covered under Medicare, (2) abolished the maximum limit of 100 visits, and (3) included coverage for skilled observation with stable health needs rather than expectations of improvement, as the former criterion had specified. In spite of these changes, Medicare criteria continue to focus on recovery from acute illness, not long-term maintenance or assistance with functional disability (Hughes & Renehan, 2005). Although visits continue until the client's plan of care is addressed, this period is short, often a few weeks in length for most clients (Dieckmann, 2005).

Between 1990 and 1996 alone, the number of home health care providers grew from 5,800 to 9,900 (Liu et al., 1999). In 2007, there were 9,284 Medicare-certified home health agencies. Of these, 17% were affiliated with an institution such as a hospital or nursing facility and 83% were freestanding (NAHC, 2008). Medicare is the largest single payer for home health services. For Medicaid beneficiaries, states pay for the same services that Medicare does. Private insurance also includes skilled home care benefits.

In addition to Medicare-certified agencies, there are numerous noncertified home care agencies, home care aide organizations, and hospices. Often, such agencies do not provide the breadth of services that Medicare requires. For example, home health aide organizations do not provide skilled nursing care (NAHC, 2008).

Homemaker and Personal Care Service Providers

Various private agencies offer services for in-home assistance. Some of these agencies are also Medicare-certified to deliver skilled nursing and rehabilitation care. Homemaker and personal care services, however, are not covered under the Medicare program. To varying degrees, states pay for homemaker and personal care for Medicaid beneficiaries. Personal funds are used to pay for these services by those who do not qualify for Medicaid. Homemaker and personal services include assistance with personal hygiene (such as bathing), light housework, laundry, meal preparation, transportation, and grocery shopping.

Adult Day Care Providers

Adult day care is a nonresidential, community-based extramural service. It enables people to live with their families and fulfills family caregivers' need for respite so they can go to work during the day. These centers may be located in senior centers, nursing facilities, churches or synagogues, or hospitals. Many centers also provide transportation from home to the center and back. On the other hand, lack of transportation and the high cost of transportation are also major impediments to the use of adult day services (O'Keeffe & Siebenaler, 2006).

Based on their focus, there are three main models of adult day services (NADSA, 2008): (1) the social model emphasizes recreation and furnishes meals and some basic health-related services; (2) the medical/health model provides nursing care and rehabilitation therapies in addition to social activities; and (3) the specialized model provides services only to specific care recipients, such as those with dementia or developmental disabilities. Many programs combine the first two models. Among those using adult day services nationwide, 52% have some cognitive impairment and are the largest users of this type of service. Other users are frail elderly who need supervision and those with mental retardation/developmental disabilities (PIC, 2003).

In 2002, more than 3,400 adult day centers were operating in the United States, and they provided care to 150,000 adults each day (PIC, 2003). The vast majority were operated by a parent organization, such as a hospital or nursing facility, on a nonprofit basis. Adult day care has become a growth industry because of rising demand, and an increasing number of for-profit centers are being opened.

The national average for adult day care cost is around $56 per day (Feldstein, 2008). Costs often vary by the type of service, particularly the extent of health care services the participant requires. Medicare does not pay for adult day care, but expenses can be covered through a variety of other sources. Under the home- and community-based services (HCBS) waiver program, introduced in Chapter 6, Medicaid is the leading source of payment for adult day care. Other sources of funding include Title III of the Older Americans Act, Veterans Health Administration, private long-term care insurance, and private out-of-pocket funds. Some rehabilitation therapies may be covered under Medicare.

Hospice Service Providers

Medicare added hospice benefits in 1983, 10 years after the first hospice opened in the United States. For a patient to receive hospice benefits, a physician must certify that the patient is terminally ill and that the patient's life expectancy is six months or less. Benefit payments by Medicare, however, are not limited to six months. The patient must also agree to waive the right to benefits for the medical treatment of the terminal illness.

People most commonly served by hospice have cancer, heart disease, unspecified debility, dementia, or lung disease. Cancer accounts for approximately 41% of all diagnoses. In 2007, 39% of all deaths in the United States occurred in hospices (NHPCO, 2008).

Hospice can be a part of home health care when the services are provided in the patient's home. In other instances, services are taken to patients in nursing homes, retirement centers, or hospitals. Services can be organized out of a hospital, nursing home, freestanding hospice facility, or home health agency. In

2007, there were roughly 4,700 hospice providers located in all 50 states, the District of Columbia, Puerto Rico, Guam, and the U.S. Virgin Islands. The majority of hospices are independent, freestanding agencies (Figure 7–1).These hospices served 1.4 million patients in 2007 (NHPCO, 2008).

Medicare is the primary source of payment (83.6% in 2007) for hospice care (NHPCO, 2008). Other sources include private insurance and Medicaid.

Quasi-Institutional Providers

As noted in Chapter 5, the institutional continuum of LTC includes a range of facilities that often do not have clear-cut distinctions. Yet, these facilities can be classified into three main categories: (1) independent living

Figure 7–1 Types of Hospice Agencies, 2007

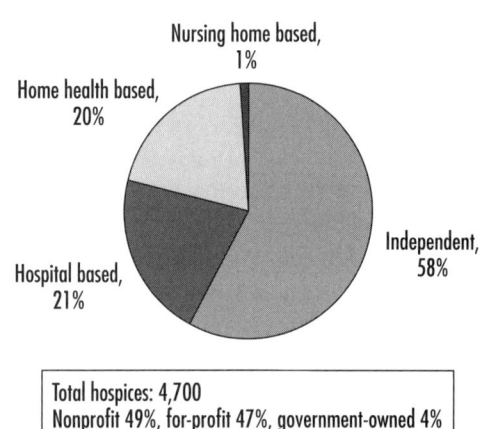

Total hospices: 4,700
Nonprofit 49%, for-profit 47%, government-owned 4%

Sources: Data from National Hospice and Palliative Care Organization, 2008; and *NHPCO Facts and Figures: Hospice Care in America,* retrieved October 2008 from http://www.nhpco.org/files/public/Statistics_Research/NHPCO_facts-and-figures_2008.pdf.

facilities, which are not truly institutions because they do not generally deliver health care; (2) custodial care providers that limit their services to social support and personal care; and (3) assisted living facilities and nursing homes. Here, the first two categories are referred to as quasi-institutions because clinically oriented services are either nonexistent or minimum in these facilities.

Independent Living and Retirement Centers

The variety of community-based LTC services that are now available have enabled many older and disabled adults to live independently in supportive housing units. The residents can come and go as they please. Facilities include designated parking spaces.

The two main independent living categories are (1) government-assisted housing and (2) private-pay housing. These dwellings differ from other institutional settings in that staff are generally not present 24 hours a day. A business manager generally maintains office hours five days a week and may be available on-call for emergencies.

Government-Assisted Housing

The U.S. Department of Housing and Urban Development (HUD) administers three different housing programs:

1. Under the Public Housing program, HUD administers federal aid to local housing agencies that manage the housing for low-income residents at rents they can afford. Anyone with low income, including the elderly and disabled persons, can apply for the program.

2. The Section 8 program offers vouchers or certificates that allow people to choose any housing in the private market that meets certain requirements and apply the voucher or certificate toward rent. Section 8 program is also managed by local public housing agencies.

3. The Section 202 Supportive Housing for the Elderly program is specifically meant for low-income people who are at least 62 years old at the time of initial occupancy.

HUD provides interest-free capital advances to private, nonprofit sponsors to finance the development of supportive housing for the elderly. HUD also provides rent subsidies for the projects to help make them affordable. The capital advance does not have to be repaid for 40 years as long as the project serves very-low-income elderly persons. A similar program is Section 811 Supportive Housing for Persons with Disabilities. Additional supportive services such as Meals On Wheels, homemaker services, and transportation are arranged from community-based providers.

Private-Pay Housing

Many upscale retirement centers abound, in which one can expect to pay a fairly substantial entrance fee plus a monthly rental or maintenance fee. These complexes have various types of recreational facilities and social programs. The fees often include the evening meal. Cleaning services, transportation, and other types of basic assistance may be provided at an extra charge. Many of these facilities provide monthly blood pressure and vision screenings, and many organize local outings for shopping and entertainment. Nursing or rehabilitation services, when needed, can be arranged with a local home health agency.

Custodial Care Providers

Custodial care is nonmedical care that includes routine assistance with the activities of daily living (ADLs), but does not include active nursing or rehabilitative treatments. Such care is provided to maintain function because the person's overall condition is not likely to improve. It is the focus of residential or personal care. Custodial services are rendered by *paraprofessionals*, such as aides, rather than licensed nurses or therapists. The facilities in this sector go by various names: adult foster care homes, board-and-care homes, personal care homes, sheltered care homes, and domiciliary care homes. Each state has established its own standards to license these facilities. Funding typically comes from Medicaid, private insurance, and personal sources. Medicare does not pay for custodial care alone. Depending on temporary needs, home health care can be called in to deliver skilled nursing and rehabilitation services.

Adult foster care (AFC) homes (also called adult family homes or adult family care) are family-run homes that provide room, board, supervision, and custodial care. The homes are modified to accommodate people with disabilities and prevent unsupervised wandering because many residents have some degree of dementia or psychiatric diagnosis. There is 24-hour supervision in the homes. Typically, the caregiving family resides in part of the home. To maintain the family environment, most states license fewer than 10 beds per family unit. However, many people have made a business of AFC by buying several houses and hiring families to live in them and care for the residents. A skeleton staff is employed to provide assistance with ADLs, to clean, and to cook meals.

Some states are trying to boost capacity of custodial care providers. Under the Money Follows the Person program, states see a greater need for quasi-institutional alternatives. However, in some states, such facilities are declining in numbers. Low reimbursement rates relative to assisted living are seen as one factor in the declining number of persons willing to be AFC providers (Mollica et al., 2008).

Institutional Providers

Institutional providers are the most visible sector of the LTC industry. Most people equate LTC with long-term care institutions. Institutional care generally connotes some degree of confinement to an institution because of a relatively high level dependency.

Assisted Living Facilities

For lack of clear-cut distinctions, there can be considerable overlap among personal care, custodial care, and assisted living. Here, assisted living facilities are regarded as those facilities that provide services that range between custodial care and skilled nursing care. Most assisted living residents require assistance with some ADLs, such as bathing, dressing, and toileting, but do not need intensive medical and nursing care. Flexible services that meet residents' scheduled and unscheduled needs and allow residents to age in place are key elements of the philosophy of assisted living (Hawes, 2001).

Assisted living has been the fastest growing type of LTC institution in the United States. These facilities generally have a skeleton staff of licensed nurses, mostly licensed practical (or vocational) nurses, who perform admission assessments and deliver basic nursing care. Advanced nursing care and rehabilitation therapies can be arranged through a home health agency.

There are an estimated 39,500 assisted living facilities serving more than 900,000 residents in the United States (AAHSA, 2008). Assisted living is paid for on a private basis for the most part. The average monthly charges are approximately $3,200, which is about half of what a private room would cost in a skilled nursing facility (Prudential, 2008). Costs, however, vary considerably among states. Costs also vary according to amenities, room size and type (e.g., shared versus private), and the services required by the resident. Most facilities charge a basic monthly rate that covers rent, board, and utilities. Additional fees are charged for nursing and personal care services. Many facilities also charge a one-time entrance fee, which may be equal to one month's basic rent. In some states, assisted living care may be covered under the Medicaid program for the recipients of Supplemental Security Income (SSI) or may be funded through Title XX Social Services Block Grants or 1915(c) HCBS waivers. The main purpose of these grants and waivers is to extend Medicaid services to people who otherwise would have to reside in nursing homes at a much higher cost to the Medicaid program. Upscale facilities, however, do not participate in public payment programs.

Although most states license assisted living facilities, the trend is toward increasing the regulatory oversight of these facilities. This is mainly because there is a general trend for assisted living providers to expand services to keep their residents as long as they are able to stay. For example, many assisted living facilities are providing specialized care for the elderly who have dementia

and Alzheimer's disease. On the other hand, moderate to severe cognitive impairment and behavioral problems in particular are often the most common reason for discharging a resident from an assisted living facility (Mead et al., 2005).

Nursing Homes

In the minds of many people, long-term care is synonymous with nursing homes. The appellation "nursing home," however, has no specific meaning. In health care literature, the term "nursing home" is generally used for facilities that are licensed as nursing homes and are often certified by the federal government. Licensing of nursing homes is mandatory in every state. In addition to licensing, certification enables a nursing home to participate in the Medicare and Medicaid programs. Details on licensure and certification of nursing homes are covered in Chapter 5.

Skilled Nursing Facilities

A skilled nursing facility (SNF) provides a full range of clinical LTC services, from skilled nursing care to rehabilitation to assistance with all ADLs. ***Skilled nursing care*** is medically oriented care provided by a licensed nurse. Examples of skilled nursing care include monitoring of unstable conditions; clinical assessment of needs; and treatments such as intravenous feeding, wound care, dressing changes, or clearing of air passages. Examples of skilled rehabilitation include post-surgical orthopedic care after knee or hip replacement, cardiopulmonary rehabilitation that is necessary after heart surgery or heart catheterization, and improvement of physical strength and balance. A variety of disabilities—including problems with ambulation, incontinence, and behavior—often coexist among a relatively large number of patients in need of skilled care. Compared with other types of facilities, nursing homes have a significant number of patients who are cognitively impaired because of depression, delirium, or dementia. The social functioning of many of the patients is also severely impaired.

A physician must authorize the need for skilled care. An attending physician must approve the plan of treatment. Delivery of care is also periodically monitored by the attending physician who makes rounds and follows up on the course of various treatments being given. Rehabilitation services are provided by registered therapists—physical therapists, occupational therapists, and speech/language pathologists—who may be employed in-house or contracted from a therapy services provider. The majority of direct care with ADLs is delivered by paraprofessionals, such as certified nursing assistants and therapy assistants, but under the supervision of licensed nurses and therapists.

In June 2006, there were 15,899 nursing homes in the United States (National Center for Health Statistics, 2007). According to a 2008 industry survey, 17% of skilled nursing facilities had an assisted living unit or wing and 30% had an Alzheimer's unit or wing (MetLife, 2008). Between 1995 and 2006, the number of nursing home beds declined by 2%, and the number of residents receiving care in these facilities declined by 3% (see Table 6–1 in Chapter 6). This is mainly because government policy has increasingly supported utilization of community-based LTC alternatives. On the other hand, there is some evidence that occupancy rates in nursing homes may be gradually creeping up (Kramer, 2003). This trend is expected to continue as the community-based LTC industry matures. A growing population with chronic

conditions, comorbidities, and subsequent disability along with increased lifespans will eventually need nursing home care.

The nursing home industry in the United States is dominated by private, for-profit nursing home chains that operate a group of nursing homes under one corporate ownership. Approximately 54% of all nursing home beds in the United States are chain affiliated because chains have acquired an increasing number of independent facilities. In 2007, the 10 largest nursing home chains operated at least 100 nursing homes each (Sanofi-Aventis, 2008a). About 62% of all nursing home beds are operated by proprietary (for-profit) nursing homes, and 29% are operated by private nonprofit entities (U.S. Census Bureau, 2008, Table 183). The remaining 9% are government owned (most of which are owned and operated by local counties; approximately 135 are operated by the Veterans Health Administration). The average size of a nursing home (108 beds) has changed little over time.

Although the charges for services vary quite substantially among states, the national average for a private room in 2008 was $217 per day (Prudential, 2008). Medicaid is the largest single source of payment for nursing home services. Coverage under Medicare is for a short duration subsequent to a hospital stay. Less than 8% of institutional LTC services are paid through private insurance. Some LTC insurance policies may cover only a portion of the total expenses—especially when care in a nursing home is needed over several years.

Subacute Care Facilities

Subacute care includes post-acute services for people who require convalescence from acute illnesses or surgical episodes. These patients may be recovering but are still subject to complications while in recovery. They require more nursing intervention than what is typically included in skilled nursing care. According to the National Association of Subacute/Post Acute Care (NASPAC), the severity of a patient's condition often requires active physician contact, professional nursing care, involvement of an interdisciplinary team in total care management, and complex medical or rehabilitative care (NASPAC, 2005). The patients may still have an unstable condition that requires active monitoring and treatment, or they may require technically complex nursing treatments such as wound care, intravenous therapy, blood transfusion, dialysis, ventilator care, or AIDS care.

Subacute services are generally found in three types of locations:

1. ***Transitional care units (TCUs)***, which are skilled nursing units located within hospitals. Hospitals entered into this service after they started facing severe occupancy declines because of payment restrictions from the government, starting in the mid-1980s. They generally have higher staff-to-patient ratios and can provide more intensive rehabilitation and nursing therapies than freestanding skilled care facilities.

2. Unlike TCUs that are certified as skilled nursing facilities, long-term care hospitals (LTCHs) are certified as acute care hospitals. Here, LTCHs are classified as nursing homes because they compete with other types of LTC institutions. LTCHs treat patients with subacute or multiple chronic problems requiring long-term, hospital-level care. Many LTCH patients are admitted directly from short-stay acute-care

hospital intensive care units with complex medical needs. Not surprisingly, LTCHs are the most expensive of the three types of subacute settings. Skilled nursing facilities are often a more cost-effective alternative, and at least some physicians think that the level and intensity of care in the two settings is comparable. LTCHs play an important role in providing high-level continuity of care to Medicare patients. Nationwide, the number of LTCHs has grown rapidly from 105 facilities in 1993 to 392 in 2006 (MedPAC, 2004, 2008).

3. Many skilled nursing facilities have developed subacute units by offering technology intensive services and by raising the staff skill-mix by hiring additional registered nurses and having therapists on staff. Some subacute type services are also rendered by community-based home health agencies.

Specialized Facilities

Specialized facilities generally provide special services for individuals with distinct medical needs. For example, inpatient rehabilitation facilities (IRFs) provide intense therapies, an intermediate care facility for the mentally retarded (ICF/MR) has specialized programs for the mentally retarded and/or developmentally disabled populations, and Alzheimer's facilities have developed a specialized niche within the institutional continuum of LTC.

Inpatient Rehabilitation Facilities

IRFs are either freestanding facilities, sometimes called rehabilitation hospitals, or they may be rehabilitation units located within acute care hospitals. These specialized facilities provide intensive rehabilitation therapies that can last three hours or more per day, five days per week. The most common rehabilitation diagnoses include spinal cord and traumatic brain injuries, orthopedic conditions, stroke, and complex arthritis-related conditions.

Intermediate Care Facilities for the Mentally Retarded

Federal regulations provide a separate certification category for LTC facilities classified as ICF/MRs. In 1971, Public Law 92–223 authorized Medicaid coverage for care in ICF/MR facilities. States have been required by federal law to provide appropriate services to each person with MR/DD in an ICF/MR or in a community-based setting outside of institutional care (see *Olmstead v. L.C.* in Chapter 6). However, all 50 states have at least one ICF/MR facility for those who cannot be housed in community settings. This program serves approximately 129,000 people with mental retardation and other related conditions. Most have other disabilities in additional to mental retardation. Many of the individuals are nonambulatory and have seizure disorders, behavior problems, mental illness, visual or hearing impairments, or a combination of these. All beneficiaries must qualify for Medicaid assistance financially (CMS, 2006).

Alzheimer's Facilities

Alzheimer's disease is a progressive degenerative disease of the brain, producing memory loss, confusion, irritability, and severe functional decline. The disease becomes progressively worse and eventually results in death. Alzheimer's facilities provide special programming and have special security features because the residents tend to wander.

Carefully designed lighting, color, and signage are used to orient the residents (Skaggs & Hawkins, 1994).

Continuing Care Retirement Communities

Full-service continuing care retirement communities (CCRCs)—also called life-care communities—integrate and coordinate the independent living and other institution-based components of the LTC continuum. Different levels of services are generally housed in separate buildings, all located on one campus. The range of services is based on the concept of *aging-in-place*, which accommodates the changing needs of older adults while living in familiar surroundings. The range of services includes housing, health care, social services, and health and wellness programs. The residents' independence is preserved, but assistance and nursing care are available when needed. Approximately 1,900 CCRCs operate in the United States (AAHSA, 2008).

The CCRC living option is directed at middle- and upper-middle-income clientele. Communities are operated by both for-profit and nonprofit organizations. Residents typically choose to enter these communities when they are in their late 70s and are still relatively healthy. A CCRC commonly has the following levels of LTC services available:

- Independent living units may be in the form of cottages or apartments. Generally, various size options are available from studio apartments to two- or three-bedroom apartments.

- Custodial care and assisted living are available in an adjoining facility.

- A skilled nursing facility is located in a separate building. Residents of the CCRC receive priority in admission.

CCRCs, for the most part, require private financing, with the exception of services delivered in a Medicare-certified SNF. To become a resident in a CCRC, customarily the client must pay an entrance fee that can range between $60,000 and $120,000 (AAHSA, 2008). In addition, a monthly accommodation fee is charged (average monthly cost is about $2,700). The monthly charges are adjusted when a resident needs personal or nursing care. A contract, called a continuing care agreement, which lasts for more than one year and that describes the service obligations of the CCRC and the financial obligations of the resident, must be signed. The contract often has a cancellation clause that specifies the amount of refund a resident may be entitled to upon leaving the community.

Three types of CCRC contracts are common in the industry: extensive, modified, and fee-for-service. Extensive contracts include a complete package of services and a commitment to provide unlimited future LTC services when needed. A modified contract promises to offer future LTC services at a discounted fee. The fee-for-service contract has the lowest entrance fee, but future LTC services are billed at the full rates applicable at the time.

The Insurance Sector

The insurance sector plays an important role in the financing of LTC services. It includes numerous commercial insurance companies. Companies that have the largest market share are Genworth Life Insurance Company, John Hancock, and Metropolitan Life Insurance Company, although there are many others that offer LTC insurance. These companies offer individual and group LTC insurance. Employees of the federal government can purchase LTC insurance at group rates through the Federal Long-Term Care Insurance Program.

Individual insurance is purchased by people directly through insurance companies or insurance brokers very much like they would purchase auto insurance or home insurance. *Group insurance* is made available to individuals through their employers, unions, professional organizations, or consumer organizations such as the AARP. Generally, group premiums are lower than those for individually purchased insurance because a large number of people band together to purchase insurance through a group sponsor. Managed care organizations (MCOs) are also involved in LTC insurance.

Commercial Insurance

Approximately 8 million Americans have LTC insurance; 400,000 people obtained coverage in 2007 alone. In 2007, 180,000 individuals received insurance benefits, and the insurance industry paid out $3.5 billion in claims for the three main types of covered LTC services (Figure 7–2). Alzheimer's is the primary reason for claim payment; 27% of Alzheimer's-related claims are paid for nursing home care and 18% for home health care.

Half the people who apply to purchase insurance are between the ages of 55 and 64; the average age is 57 (American Association for Long-Term Care Insurance, 2008). Purchase of insurance becomes increasingly unaffordable later in life, and the denial rates of people applying to purchase insurance increase because of the presence of chronic conditions. Besides a person's age, premium costs also vary according to the type of coverage and the state in which a person resides. A typical plan may offer $150 in daily benefits with a 5% compounded increase in benefits each

Figure 7–2 Claims For Services Paid Under Long-Term Care Insurance Coverage, 2007

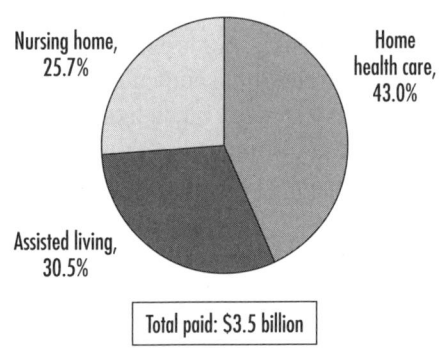

Nursing home, 25.7%

Home health care, 43.0%

Assisted living, 30.5%

Total paid: $3.5 billion

Sources: Data from American Association for Long-Term Care Insurance. 2008; and *The 2008 Sourcebook for Long-Term Care Insurance Information.* Westlake Village, CA: AALTCI.

year, a coverage period of 36 months, and a 90-day *elimination period*, which is the initial waiting period during which LTC services are used but not covered by insurance.

Commercial insurance companies are risk underwriters. They determine the level of premiums necessary to cover potential claims in the future. They collect premiums and pay claims arising from the utilization of LTC services when the covered beneficiaries use the services in accordance with the insurance contract. Commercial insurance companies, however, do not select the providers of services. That choice is left to the beneficiaries.

Managed Care

Managed care is an approach to delivering a comprehensive array of health care services to a defined group of enrolled members through efficient management of service utilization and payment to providers. The most common type of MCO that is active in the delivery of LTC services is health mainte-

nance organizations (HMOs). HMOs enter into financial contracts with Medicaid and Medicare to deliver health care services to the beneficiaries enrolled in these programs.

HMOs are also insurance entities that underwrite risk. In contrast with commercial insurance companies, however, HMOs select the providers of services. The selected providers are those with whom the HMO has payment contracts. Under the Medicaid program, the Balanced Budget Act of 1997 gave states the authority to enter into contracts with two broad types of managed care entities: HMOs and Prepaid Health Plans (PHPs). HMOs take the responsibility to provide a comprehensive package of health care services included in the Medicaid benefits. PHPs offer a less comprehensive package of Medicaid benefits. For example, a PHP may only deliver services covered under an HCBS waiver program.

Both HMOs and PHPs employ a utilization management function in which a primary care physician or some other managing entity authorizes medically necessary services before care is delivered. Beneficiaries must use approved providers for receiving various health care services.

In 2007, all states except Alaska, Mississippi, and Wyoming had Medicaid recipients enrolled in HMOs. Approximately 15 states had 80% or more of their Medicaid beneficiaries enrolled in HMOs. Of all Medicaid beneficiaries nationwide, 63.5% received health care services through HMOs in 2007 (Sanofi-Aventis, 2008b).

The Balanced Budget Act of 1997 also authorized the Medicare+Choice program, which was renamed Medicare Advantage in 2003. Medicare gives its beneficiaries the choice to either remain in the traditional Medicare program or enroll in Medicare

Advantage, in which services are provided through various MCOs. In 2007, almost 20% of the beneficiaries were enrolled in Medicare Advantage (Sanofi-Aventis, 2008b).

Long-Term Care Professionals

A variety of health care professionals are involved in the delivery of long-term care. They can be classified as (1) administrative professionals, (2) clinicians, (3) paraprofessional caregivers, (4) ancillary personnel, and (5) social support professionals. The types of personnel involved vary according to the level of LTC services delivered in a given setting. For example, independent living and retirement centers may employ one or two administrative professionals and a small staff of ancillary personnel. A nursing home has all five categories of LTC professionals. Certain clinicians may be found only in specialized facilities. Growth of the LTC industry will continue to create jobs in all areas, many of which already have critical shortages.

Administrative Professionals

Every agency or organization requires at least one administrative professional to manage the organization. The number and types of administrative professionals increase with the organization's size and complexity.

Administrators

Administrators are needed to manage the organization. They must also oversee compliance with federal and state regulations and ensure that services are delivered in accordance with the organization's policies and established standards. Administrators must have a good understanding of financing and reimbursement systems pertinent to their organization. They must be knowledgeable about legal and ethical constraints. Administrators who manage larger organizations must also be skilled in managing human resources, marketing the facility's services, and overseeing the facility's quality improvement program. Leadership, communication, financial management, and problem-solving skills are also essential for effective management of LTC organizations.

The title for the administrator's position may vary, such as administrator, executive director, director, manager, or general manager. This section mainly focuses on administrators of home health agencies, assisted living facilities, and nursing homes.

Home Health Agency Administrators

According to Medicare Conditions of Participation for home health agencies, the administrator must either be a licensed physician, a registered nurse, or someone who has training and experience in health services administration and at least one year of supervisory or administrative experience in home health care or related health programs (CMS, 2005). Agencies often employ a registered nurse or someone with a business degree as administrator.

Assisted Living Administrators

A number of states now require administrators of assisted living facilities to be licensed. Education, experience, and examination requirements vary from state to state. On the other hand, the National Association of Long Term Care Administrator Boards (NAB) has established requirements for licensure as a residential care/assisted living (RC/AL) administrator. To be licensed, individuals must complete a 40-hour state-approved course covering the domains of practice and pass the NAB's licensure examination. To take the NAB's licensure exam, an individual must have a combination of education and experience (NAB, 2007): (1) a high school diploma and two years of experience in assisted living, including one year in a management position; or (2) an associate's degree and one year of experience in assisted living, including six months in a management position, or (3) a bachelor's degree and six months of management experience in assisted living. The NAB examination for RC/AL covers five main areas, referred to as the domains of practice: resident care management, human resource management, organizational management, physical environment management, and business/financial management. A state may also require working experience with a trained preceptor. A *preceptor* is a nursing home or assisted living administrator who meets prescribed qualifications and has been certified to mentor interns in an administrator-in-training (AIT) program. Generally, licensed nursing home administrators are allowed to manage assisted living facilities without any further training. Continuing education requirements are also becoming common for license renewal.

Nursing Home Administrators

A nursing home administrator (NHA) must be licensed by the state. Qualifications required for licensure vary widely from one state to another. The first step toward becoming a licensed NHA is to contact the particular state's licensing agency and obtain a copy of the state's licensure requirements. The prospective administrator must meet the min-

imum educational qualifications. Most states require a college degree; some states also require completion of a short course in long-term care. A common requirement by all states is passing the national examination administered by the NAB. In addition to the NAB examination, candidates must pass a shorter examination on state nursing home regulations. Some states may also require an internship with a state-certified preceptor who is also a practicing NHA. Many states have reciprocity agreements, meaning that an administrator licensed in one state can obtain a license in another state if that state has a reciprocity agreement with the other state.

Nursing homes are complex organizations to manage and have been the target of much regulatory oversight and public criticism. The NHA position is, in many respects, similar to that of a general manager in a complex human services delivery organization. The NHA must have a 24/7 commitment to an organization that must meet the patients' clinical needs, ensure their social and emotional well-being, preserve their individual rights, promote human dignity, and improve their quality of life. The NHA must have adequate understanding of the clinical, social, and residential aspects of care delivery.

The nursing home must also operate as an efficient business. The NHA must manage staff relations, budgets and finances, marketing, and quality. Hence, NHAs typically have a broad range of managerial responsibilities and are closely involved in day-to-day operational details.

Nursing home administration entails much more than overseeing the various functions in an organization or following set routines. Over time, effectively managed nursing facilities achieve acceptable levels of organizational stability and have predictable outcomes in patient care quality and financial performance. In the long run, success is achieved by managing six critical areas:

1. The community must come to view the nursing home as a vital service organization. One of the NHA's primary roles should be to serve the community in partnership with other public and private health agencies and care delivery organizations.

2. NHAs must understand and operate within the confines of what reimbursement will allow.

3. The LTC industry has evolved over time, and it will continue to change. The NHA must adapt to new trends and new demands as they become established.

4. Compliance with legal and regulatory requirements is essentials. The organization must also be managed according to the highest standards of ethical conduct.

5. The internal operations must be streamlined to deliver services in a seamless fashion.

6. NHAs must manage the operation through effective leadership, human resource development, strategic marketing, financial control, and data-driven quality improvement.

Risk taking and innovation will mark successful administrators of the future. Being an NHA is a rewarding career, both financially and professionally. The psychological rewards that can come from delivering quality care to patients, helping family members, supporting community initiatives, coaching the staff, and building excellence into the organization often exceed the financial rewards.

Department Directors

Department directors constitute the middle-management stratum of a nursing home. The organization of nursing homes is well established. The main department directors include the director of nursing, food service director or dietary manager, social worker or director of social services, activity director, business office manager, housekeeping/laundry supervisor, and maintenance supervisor. They report to the administrator and carry out supervisory functions in their respective departments. Their main role is to ensure adequate staffing, availability of supplies and materials, and coordination of service delivery that complies with established standards. Required qualifications are established by state nursing home regulations. Qualifications for the various department directors are covered in Part III of the book.

Other Administrative Personnel

Depending on the size and type of organization, administrative personnel may include assistant administrators, office managers, bookkeepers, and receptionists. Very large LTC organizations may also employ human resource or personnel directors, admissions coordinators, and marketing directors. At a minimum, most organizations need (1) a receptionist to greet visitors, provide information, and handle basic office tasks and (2) a bookkeeper whose main responsibility is to handle all billings and collections. Additional help is generally needed for payroll and accounts payable functions.

Clinicians

Various types of clinicians are employed in home health agencies, nursing homes, and assisted living facilities. They mainly include physicians, nurses, rehabilitation professionals, dietitians, and assistants and technicians who work under the direction of these professionals. With the exception of nurses, most others are generally contracted.

Physicians

Only very large and specialized facilities can afford to employ a full-time physician. Most organizations contract with a physician in the capacity of a medical director, which is typically a part-time position. It is not uncommon for the medical director to also provide medical services to many of the patients in nursing homes. The patient, however, has the right to choose his or her attending physician provided that the physician is willing to follow up on the patient's medical care while he or she is in the nursing home. The patient's physician is also involved in the plan of care for services provided by a home health agency. Admission to a nursing facility or care by a home health agency is also authorized by a physician. Physicians play a central role in the medical care of patients. Other clinicians follow physicians' orders for prescribed medical, nursing, rehabilitation, and dietary interventions. Most physicians practicing in the LTC field are generalists or family practitioners rather than specialists.

All states require physicians to be licensed in order to practice. The licensure requirements include graduation from an accredited medical school that awards a doctor of medicine (MD) or doctor of osteopathic medicine (DO) degree, successful completion of a licensing examination governed by either the National Board of Medical Examiners or the National Board of Osteopathic Medical Examiners, and completion of a supervised internship/residency program. Residency is graduate medical education in a specialty that takes the form of paid on-the-job training. Most physicians serve a one-year rotating internship after graduation from medical school and before entering a residency program. Both MDs and DOs use traditionally accepted methods of treatment, including drugs and surgery. The two differ mainly in their philosophies and approach to medical treatment. *Osteopathic medicine*, practiced by DOs, emphasizes the musculoskeletal system of the body such as correction of joints or tissues. In their treatment plans, DOs emphasize preventive medicine such as diet and the environment as factors that might influence natural resistance. MDs are trained in *allopathic medicine*, which views medical treatment as active intervention to produce a counteracting reaction in an attempt to neutralize the effects of disease. MDs trained as generalists may also use preventive medicine along with allopathic treatments (Shi & Singh, 2008).

Nurses

The two main categories of nurses in LTC settings are registered nurses (RNs) and licensed practical (or vocational) nurses (LPNs or LVNs). All nurses must be licensed by the state in which they practice. The two main educational programs today for RNs are associate's degree (ADN) programs offered by community colleges and bachelor of science degree (BSN) programs offered by four-year colleges and universities. Regulations require the delivery of skilled nursing services to be under the supervision of RNs. In LTC settings, RNs compose only a small percentage of the workforce. They mostly hold administrative and supervisory positions such as director of nursing or head nurse. A number of studies have shown that an adequate number of RNs in nursing homes positively affects quality outcomes.

The majority of nurses in LTC settings are LPNs/LVNs who are graduates of one-year practical nursing programs offered at community colleges or vocational technical schools. LPNs/LVNs render treatments and administer medications. LPNs also function as charge nurses and team leaders and supervise the work of paraprofessional caregivers.

Nonphysician Practitioners

Nonphysician practitioners (NPPs) are clinical professionals who practice in many of the areas in which physicians practice but who do not have an MD or DO degree. The two main types of NPPs who practice in LTC settings are nurse practitioners and physician assistants.

Nurse practitioners (NPs) are advanced practice nurses who provide health care services similar to those of primary care physicians. They can diagnose and treat a wide range of health problems. Some physicians employ NPs to follow up on the medical care of their patients. Studies of NPs in nursing homes suggest that they enhance the medical services available to residents and prevent unnecessary hospital admissions (IFAS, 2005). NPs receive advanced graduate-level education and clinical training beyond what is required for RN preparation. Most have master's degrees; some specialize in geriatrics (American Academy of Nurse Practitioners, 2007).

Physician assistants (PAs) are increasingly employed to provide LTC services under the direction of a physician. Both NPs and PAs are sometimes referred to as physician extenders because they enable physicians to see more patients and make better use of their

skills and time. Admission to a PA training program requires roughly two years of science-based college coursework. After enrolling in a PA program, students study the basic medical sciences and physical examination techniques, followed by clinical training that includes classroom instruction and clinical rotations in primary care and several medical and surgical specialties. Overall, the PA student completes more than 2,000 hours of supervised clinical practice prior to graduation. The didactic and clinical training takes an average of 26 months. Their scope of practice includes performing physical examinations, diagnosing and treating illnesses, ordering and interpreting laboratory tests, and making rounds at LTC facilities (American Academy of Physician Assistants, 2007). Both NPs and PAs can prescribe drugs when authorized to do so under state law. Their generalist training and emphasis on patient relationships make them particularly valuable in LTC caregiving.

Rehabilitation Professionals

Rehabilitation therapies enable patients to regain lost functioning and improve current functioning. The most common rehabilitation services are provided by physical therapists, occupational therapists, and speech/language pathologists. Certain treatments can be provided by assistants under the direction and supervision of therapists. Services of a physiatrist are common in facilities that provide intensive rehabilitation.

Physiatrists

A *physiatrist* is a physician who has specialized in physical medicine and rehabilitation. Physiatrists can treat a variety of problems from pain to work- and sports-related injuries.

Diagnoses may include severe arthritis, brain injury, spinal cord injury, stroke, multiple sclerosis, amputations, and various conditions requiring post-surgical recovery. Physiatrists may prescribe drugs or assistive devices and direct therapists to carry out various types of treatments to help restore, improve, or maintain function.

Physical Therapists and Assistants

Physical therapists (PTs) specialize in the treatment of musculoskeletal disorders (loss of function associated with bones, joints, spine, and soft tissue), neuromuscular disorders (loss of function associated with the brain and nervous system, such as stroke), patients recovering from cardiopulmonary problems, and severe wounds. They specialize in the restoration of various ADL functions.

PTs need a master's degree from a physical therapy program accredited by the Commission on Accreditation in Physical Therapy Education. Of the 209 accredited physical therapy programs in 2007, 43 offered master's degrees and 166 offered doctoral degrees. Master's degree programs typically last two years, and doctoral degree programs last three years. In the future, a doctoral degree might be the required entry-level degree. All states require PTs to pass national and state licensure exams before they can practice (BLS, 2007). The Federation of State Boards of Physical Therapy develops and administers the national examinations for both PTs and physical therapy assistants (PTAs).

PTAs can provide part of a patient's treatment under the direction and supervision of a PT. In many states, PTAs are required by law to have at least an associate's degree (BLS, 2007). Most states also require PTAs to be licensed.

Occupational Therapists and Assistants

Occupational therapists (OTs) are involved in a broad range of therapies that help patients recover or maintain the daily living and work skills. Their goal is to help patients achieve independence and satisfaction in all facets of their lives. For example, OTs can help patients learn how to use a computer or care for their daily needs such as dressing, cooking, and eating.

A master's degree or higher in occupational therapy is the minimum requirement for entry into the field. In 2007, 124 master's degree programs offered entry-level education, 66 programs offered a combined bachelor's and master's degree, and 5 offered an entry-level doctoral degree. OTs must be licensed to practice. To obtain a license, applicants must graduate from an accredited educational program and pass a national certification examination. Those who pass the examination are awarded the title "Occupational Therapist, Registered (OTR)" (BLS, 2007). OTR is a registered trademark of the National Board for Certification in Occupational Therapy (NBCOT), which administers the national certification examination.

Occupational therapy assistants help patients with rehabilitative activities and exercises outlined in a treatment plan developed in collaboration with an OT. An associate's degree or a certificate from an accredited community college or technical school is generally required to qualify as an occupational therapy assistant. To be licensed in most states, occupational therapy assistants must pass a national certification examination administered by NBCOT after they graduate. Those who pass the examination are awarded the title "Certified Occupational Therapy Assistant (COTA)" (BLS, 2007).

Speech/Language Pathologists

Speech/language pathologists (SLPs)—informally referred to as speech therapists—assess, diagnose, and treat speech, language, and cognitive disorders. ***Dysphagia***, that is, swallowing difficulty, is another common problem that SLPs are called upon to treat in LTC settings.

A master's degree is commonly required for licensure in most states; it is mandatory for receiving the Certificate of Clinical Competence from the Council of Clinical Certification of the American Speech-Language-Hearing Association (ASHA). In 2007, more than 230 colleges and universities offered graduate programs in speech/language pathology accredited by the Council on Academic Accreditation in Audiology and Speech-Language Pathology of ASHA (BLS, 2007).

Clinical Dietitians and Technicians

Clinical ***dietitians***, sometimes referred to as nutritionists, provide nutritional information and diet-related services to patients. They assess patients' nutritional needs, develop and implement nutrition programs, and evaluate the results. They also confer with physicians and other health care professionals to coordinate medical and nutritional needs. Clinical dietitians often develop diet plans for patients who have renal problems, diabetes, heart disease, and weight loss or weight gain issues.

Minimum qualifications for clinical dietitians include a bachelor's degree from a program approved by the Commission on Accreditation for Dietetics Education (CADE) of the American Dietetic Association (ADA), completion of a CADE-accredited and super-vised practicum at a health care facility that can be 6 to 12 months in length, and passing a national examination administered by the Commission on Dietetic Registration (CDR) of the ADA (ADA, 1997a). Those who complete these requirements are awarded the title "Registered Dietitian (RD)." As of 2007, there were 281 bachelor's degree programs and 22 master's degree programs approved by CADE (BLS, 2007).

Dietetic technicians assist dietitians in the delivery of food service in accordance with nutritional guidelines. Under the supervision of dietitians, they may plan and produce meals based on established guidelines, teach principles of food and nutrition, or counsel individuals. Becoming a Dietetic Technician, Registered (DTR), requires completion of at least a two-year associate's degree from a program accredited or approved by CADE, completion of 450 hours of supervised practicum, and passing a national examination administered by CDR (ADA, 1997b).

Paraprofessional Caregivers

Long-term care services heavily rely on paraprofessional caregivers, who give most of the hands-on personal care and assist patients with all ADLs. They also change bed linens and serve meals to patients. These paraprofessionals include certified nursing assistants (CNAs), therapy aides, personal care attendants, and home health aides. They constitute the largest group of health care workers in the LTC industry. Paraprofessional positions are at the bottom of the organizational hierarchy. These workers typically carry heavy workloads, are poorly paid, and are often treated with little respect.

In most LTC organizations, such as nursing homes, assisted living facilities, and home health agencies, paraprofessionals work under the direction of licensed nurses. CNAs are also trained to take vital signs; watch for and report any changes in the patients' condition to nurses; and do simple urine tests for sugar, acetone, and albumin. The 1987 Nursing Home Reform Act mandated that CNAs receive a minimum of 75 hours of training. The training program must include 16 hours of hands-on training in which the trainee demonstrates knowledge while performing tasks for an individual under the direct supervision of a nurse. CNA students must also pass a state certification exam and skills test, and subsequently complete 12 hours of in-service or continuing education each year (Wright, 2006). CNAs can received further training to become rehabilitation aides who provide basic therapies such as walking and range of motion exercises under the supervision of licensed therapists and nurses. CNAs can also become medication aides after further training to safely give medications to patients.

Ancillary Personnel

A variety of ancillary personnel provide hotel services such as meals, cleaning, laundry, and maintenance of physical plant and equipment in LTC facilities. Food service personnel such as cooks and cook's helpers prepare meals. Dietary aides wash dishes and cooking utensils. Building cleaning workers include janitors and housekeepers. Laundry washers sort and wash linens. Others fold, store, and deliver clean linens to patient care areas. Maintenance personnel handle basic repairs and groundskeeping.

Social Support Professionals

Social support professionals include social workers and activity professionals. In LTC settings, social workers engage in diagnostic assessment of patients' cognitive, behavioral, and emotional status; counseling; and conflict resolution. They help people cope with various types of issues in their everyday lives. They also have community resource expertise that is often called upon to obtain professional services available in the community. A bachelor's degree in social work (BSW) is the minimum requirement for social work positions in nursing homes and assisted living facilities. The Council on Social Work Education accredits educational programs in social work. In 2008, there were 463 accredited bachelor's degree programs and 191 accredited master's social work programs (Council on Social Work Education, 2008).

Activity professionals provide a variety of recreational programs for groups and individuals to improve and maintain the patients' physical, mental, and emotional well-being. Programs include arts and crafts, games, music, movies, dance and movement, social celebrations, and community outings. Passive activities such as reading and working with puzzles are prescribed for those who prefer solitude. Although no specific degrees are specified for activity professionals, the National Certification Council for Activity Professionals (NCCAP) offers four different tracks, based on education and experience, for the credential, Activity Director, Certified (ADC). NCCAP also offers three different tracks for the credential, Activity Assistant, Certified (AAC). Another organization, the National Council for Therapeutic Recreation Certification (NCTRC) offers the Certified Therapeutic Recreation Specialist (CTRS) credential based on education, experience, and a certification examination.

The Ancillary Sector

The ancillary sector produces services and products that help people locate the right kind of services, facilitate caregiving, improve people's quality of life, or improve organizational efficiencies.

Case Management Agencies

The myriad LTC services can present daunting challenges for most people who either need services for themselves or for those who need to help family or friends find appropriate services. Case management agencies do not provide actual LTC services. They assist clients in navigating the system by assessing client needs, identifying sources of payment, matching client needs with available services that are likely to best address those needs, making referrals to appropriate services, and providing ongoing follow-up and coordination as circumstances change over time. Services are often coordinated both within and outside the LTC system.

Case management agencies employ experienced nurses and social workers as case managers. These professionals have specialized training in patient need assessment and a comprehensive knowledge of both financing and service resources.

Long-Term Care Pharmacies

Historically, LTC facilities have experienced numerous challenges in providing pharmaceutical services to their residents. Medication errors, preventable adverse drug events, and delivery of pharmaceutical services, in general, have posed the main challenges (Stevenson et al., 2007). The Omnibus Budget Reconciliation Act of 1990 required pharmacies to review Medicaid recipients' entire drug profile and to evaluate therapeutic duplication, drug-disease contraindications, drug interactions, incorrect dosage, duration of drug treatment, drug–allergy interactions, and evidence of clinical abuse or misuse. In part because of this regulatory requirement, certain pharmacy providers have specialized in LTC pharmacy practice. Through their consultant pharmacists, LTC pharmacies offer comprehensive drug management services and often coordinate related quality improvement activities (Stevenson et al., 2007). Such comprehensive services, round-the-clock attention to critical and emergency medications, and dispensing of intravenous medication solutions are generally not available through retail community pharmacists.

Long-term care pharmacies are estimated to serve three out of every five residents in LTC facilities (LTCPA, 2006). In 2007, there were 1,125 LTC pharmacies in the United States that derived at least half of their revenue from LTC facilities (Sanofi-Aventis, 2008a).

Long-Term Care Technology

Technology has been playing an increasing role in all aspects of health care delivery. Adoption of technology for LTC use has been slow, but it will continue to grow in homes, other residential settings, and LTC institutions. Innovative products are being brought to the market all the time. For example, various types of **domotics** technology, that is, "smart home" technology, can enable a growing number of elderly people live in their own homes. Long-term care technology can be classified into seven main categories:

1. *Enabling technology.* Also referred to as assistive technology, this includes various devices and equipment that enable people to do things independently despite functional impairments. Examples include hearing aids, simple self-feeding aids such as specially designed eating utensils, and custom-fitted mobility scooters that improve people's quality of life regardless of whether they are living independently in their own homes or in LTC institutions. Some newer technologies enable people to live independently. These technologies include reminder systems that are particularly useful for those with mild cognitive impairments. Automatic enunciators remind people of tasks they must do that day, such as keeping a doctor's appointment. Enunciators are also being integrated with medication administration systems to remind people when certain medications must be taken. Talking blood sugar monitors, thermometers, blood pressure monitors, and automated pill dispensers are now available for use in the home (Cheek et al., 2005). The National Association of Home Builders has developed an aging-in-place certification specialist program. A Certified Aging-in-Place Specialist (CAPS) has specialized skills in home remodeling solutions to enable older adults live in their own homes as they age. Various products

and devices are used to promote accessibility and safety in the bathroom, bedroom, or kitchen. For example, clapper lighting systems turn on the lights at the sound of clapping.

2. *Safety technology.* Personal emergency response systems (PERS) are now widely available for people living alone to summon help in an emergency. Technology that uses signals, alarms, and wireless transmitters can be installed in nursing facilities to notify staff when a wandering patient opens a door to go out. Wireless sensors to ensure patient safety are also being developed. Fall detection devices can signal the staff when an at-risk resident attempts to leave a bed, wheelchair, or toilet unattended.

3. *Caregiving technology.* Feeding and nutritional therapies—such as enteral and parenteral feeding—have been around for a long time. Other technologies such as in-home dialyzers for people with kidney failure are more recent. Caregivers are now increasingly using automated medication dispensing systems that improve accuracy and efficiency. A variety of beds and overlays are available to reduce pressure to promote healing of pressure ulcers. Ultrasound bladder scanners are used for the management of urinary incontinence. Barcode technology has been adopted to verify patient identification and dispense medications. **Home telehealth systems** use telecommunication technology for the distance monitoring of patients and delivery of health care with or without the use of video technology. They have the potential to improve

access and reduce costs by minimizing the need for the patient to make trips to physicians' offices or for home health nurses to make frequent visits to the patient's home. Interactive technology enables "virtual visits" between clinicians and patients. It enables distance monitoring of the patient and promotes self-management of chronic conditions. Remote patient monitoring systems collect data on vital signs and blood pressure and allow a nurse to also observe any behavior changes.

4. *Labor-saving technology.* Introduction of labor-saving technology is designed to improve worker efficiency and reduce physical injuries by decreasing the need for heavy transfers and lifting. Electrically operated ceiling-suspended dining tables can convert a dining room to a multipurpose room at the flip of a switch. Ceiling-mounted patient lifting and transfer equipment and labor-saving bathing systems are other examples of labor-saving technology. Computerized medical records that replace handwritten charting can save caregivers time that can be spent in delivering patient care.

5. *Environmental technology.* Products and fibers that have greater fire resistance; improved fabrics for upholstered furniture that resist soil and fluid absorption; new fibers for carpeting that resist soil, stains, and odors; and nonskid floor coverings are some examples that enhance the aesthetics and safety of living environments. Computerized controls for hot water systems are designed to save energy and prevent the supply of overheated water that can cause severe burns. Sensorial signals, such as color and textured materials, are employed to support orientation of cognitively impaired individuals in their own homes and in institutions (Cheek et al., 2005).

6. *Staff training technology.* Interactive tools, CD-ROMs, and remote video teleconferencing are available to provide training and continuing education on a large variety of topics.

7. *Information technology.* Information technology (IT) deals with the transformation of data into useful information. IT is a broad area. In health care organizations, application of IT falls into four main categories:

- *Clinical information systems* are designed to be used by various clinicians to support the delivery of patient care. Electronic medical records, for example, can provide quick and reliable information necessary to guide clinical decision making and to produce timely reports on quality of care delivered. Computerized provider order entry (CPOE) systems enable electronic transmission of medication orders to the pharmacy and help reduce errors. Clinical information systems also support patient assessment, care planning, and clinical documentation. These systems can be integrated with other applications such as administrative and financial systems, menu planning, and food ordering.

- *Administrative information systems* are designed to assist in carrying out financial and administrative support activities such as payroll, patient accounting, billing, accounts receivable, materials management, budgeting and cost control, and management of residents' personal funds.

• *Decision support systems* provide information and analytical tools that support effective management. For example, the system can help analyze performance indicators, staffing adequacy, staff productivity, rates of infections and patient incidents such as falls, and staff injuries.

• *The Internet*, or the Web as it is commonly called, is now widely used by clients and providers to access information. A vast amount of clinical and caregiving information can be accessed online. Various IT applications, however, have also become Web-based. In this manner, updated software applications can be accessed and used on the Internet at all times. Various LTC providers increasingly use the Web for advertising their services and provide other client-related information.

For Further Thought

1. In what ways is the long-term care industry likely to evolve in the future?
2. Are hospitals likely to play a bigger role in the future delivery of long-term care?

For Further Learning

Assisted Living Federation of America: A group that offers basic consumer-oriented information on assisted living and gives a directory of assisted living facilities. This trade organization represents assisted living and other senior housing facilities.

www.alfa.org

Home Care Research Initiative: This organization supports research projects to address issues in long-term care. Research articles and fact sheets can be downloaded.

http://www.vnsny.org/hcri/index.html

Hospice Foundation of America: A nonprofit organization that provides leadership in the development and application of hospice and its philosophy of care.

http://www.hospicefoundation.org

National Adult Day Services Association: This organization represents the adult day care industry and also furnishes consumer information.

http://www.nadsa.org

National Association for Home Care and Hospice: The nation's largest trade association representing the interests and concerns of home care agencies, hospices, home care aide organizations, and medical equipment suppliers.

http://www.nahc.org

National Association of Long Term Care Administrator Boards (NAB). This organization administers the national licensure examinations for assisted living and nursing home administrators. It has publications available to prepare for the examination. The website also provides links to the licensing agencies in all states.

http://www.nabweb.org

National Association of Subacute and Post-Acute Care. The association was formed in 1995 through a consolidation of the International Subacute Healthcare Association and the American Subacute Care Association.

http://www.naspac.net/faq.asp

National Hospice Foundation: A nonprofit, charitable organization affiliated with the National Hospice and Palliative Care Organization that provides support and information about hospice care options.

www.nationalhospicefoundation.org

REFERENCES

American Academy of Nurse Practitioners. 2007. *Frequently Asked Questions: Why Choose a Nurse Practitioner as Your Healthcare Provider*. Retrieved November 2008 from http://www.npfinder .com/faq.pdf.

American Academy of Physician Assistants. 2007. *Physician Assistant Practice in Long-Term Care Facilities*. Retrieved November 2008 from http://www.aapa.org/gandp/issuebrief/long-term-care.htm.

AAHSA. 2008. *Aging Services: The Facts*. American Association of Homes and Services for the Aging. Retrieved December 2008 from http://www.aahsa.org/article.aspx?id=74#GeneralFacts.

American Association for Long-Term Care Insurance. 2008. *The 2008 Sourcebook for Long-Term Care Insurance Information*. Westlake Village, CA: AALTCI.

ADA. 1997a. *Becoming a Registered Dietitian*. American Dietetic Association. Retrieved November 2008 from http://www.eatright.org/ada/files/RD_Check_it_Out.pdf.

ADA. 1997b. *Becoming a Dietetic Technician, Registered*. American Dietetic Association. Retrieved November 2008 from http://www.eatright.org/ada/files/DTR_Check_it_Out(1).pdf.

BLS. 2007. *Occupational Outlook Handbook, 2008–09 Edition*. Bureau of Labor Statistics. Retrieved November 2008 from http://www.bls.gov.

CMS. 2005. *State Operations Manual: Appendix B—Guidance to Surveyors: Home Health Agencies*. Centers for Medicare and Medicaid Services. Retrieved November 2008 from http://cms.hhs.gov/manuals/Downloads/som107ap_b_hha.pdf.

CMS. 2006. *Intermediate Care Facilities for the Mentally Retarded*. Centers for Medicare and Medicaid Services. Retrieved October 2008 from http://www.cms.hhs.gov/Certificationand Complianc/09_ICFMRs.asp.

Cheek, P., et al. 2005. Aging well with smart technology. *Nursing Administration* 29, no. 4: 329–338.

Council on Social Work Education. 2008. *Commission on Accreditation, June 2008 Decisions*. Retrieved November 2008 from http://www.cswe.org/NR/rdonlyres/9F229762-8A02-4C3C-8E6C-FDC33B946F6B/0/Actions_2008_June.pdf.

Dieckmann, J.L. 2005. Home health administration: An overview. In M.D. Harris (ed.), *Handbook of Home Health Care Administration*, 4th ed. (pp. 3–15). Sudbury, MA: Jones and Bartlett Publishers.

Feldstein, M.J. 2008. Companies moving steadily in adult day care business. *St. Louis Post-Dispatch*. Retrieved October 2008 from http://www.stltoday.com/stltoday/business/stories.nsf/story/02D1846F93FE494F862573D4000E735E?OpenDocument.

Hawes, C. 2001. In S. Zimmerman et al., (eds.), *Assisted Living: Needs, Practices, and Policies in Residential Care for the Elderly*. Baltimore: The Johns Hopkins University Press.

Hughes, S.L., & Renehan, M. 2005. Home health. In C.J. Evashwick, (ed.), *The Continuum of Long-Term Care*, 3rd ed. (pp. 87–111). Clifton Park, NY: Thomson Delmar Learning.

IFAS. 2005. *The Long-Term Care Workforce: Can the Crises be Fixed?* Washington, DC: Institute for the Future of Aging Services.

Kramer, R.G. 2003. Financial benchmarks: Signs of struggle and hope. *Nursing Homes Long Term Care Management* 52, no. 9: 68–69.

Liu, K., et al. 1999. *Medicare's Post-Acute Care Benefit: Background, Trends, and Issues to be Faced*. Retrieved October 2008 from http://aspe.hhs.gov/daltcp/reports/mpacb.htm#secIII.

LTCPA. 2006. Mission. Long-Term Care Pharmacy Alliance. Retrieved February 2009 from http://www.ltcpa.org/mission/default.asp.

Mead, L.C. et al. 2005. Sociocultural aspects of transitions from assisted living for residents with dementia. *The Gerontologist* 45, special issue 1: 115–123.

MedPAC. 2004. *New Approaches in Medicare: Report to the Congress*. Washington, DC: Medicare Payment Advisory Commission.

MedPAC. 2008. *Long-Term Care Hospitals Payment System*. Washington, DC: Medicare Payment Advisory Commission.

MetLife. 2008. *The MetLife Market Survey of Nursing Home and Assisted Living Costs, October 2008*. New York: Metropolitan Life Insurance Company.

Mollica, R., et al. 2008. *Adult Foster Care: A Resource for Older Adults*. New Brunswick, NJ: Rutgers Center for State Health Policy.

NAB. 2007. *Residential Care–Assisted Living Administrators Licensing Examination: Information for Candidates*. National Association of Long-Term Care Administrator Boards. Retrieved October 2008 from http://www.nabweb.org/NABWEB/uploadedFiles/Examinations/2008 CandHand-RCAL.pdf.

NAHC. 2008. *Basic Statistics About Home Care*. National Association of Home Care and Hospice. Retrieved October 2008 from http://www.nahc.org/facts/08HC_Stats.pdf.

NADSA. 2008. *Adult Day Services: Overview and Facts*. National Adult Day Services Association. Retrieved October 2008 from http://www.nadsa.org/adsfacts/default.asp.

NASPAC. 2005. What is the definition of subacute care? Retrieved March 2009 from http://www.naspac.net/faq.asp.

National Center for Health Statistics. 2007. *Health, United States, 2007*. Hyattsville, MD: U.S. Department of Health and Human Services.

NHPCO. 2008. *NHPCO Facts and Figures: Hospice Care in America*. National Hospice and Palliative Care Organization. Retrieved October 2008 from http://www.nhpco.org/files/public/Statistics_Research/NHPCO_facts-and-figures_2008.pdf.

O'Keeffe, J., & Siebenaler, K. 2006. *Adult Day Services: A Key Community Service for Older Adults*. Washington, DC: U.S. Department of Health and Human Services.

PIC. 2003. *National Study of Adult Day Services: 2001–2002*. Winston-Salem, NC: Wake Forest University School of Medicine, Partners in Caregiving.

Prudential. 2008. *Research Report 2008: Long-Term Care Cost Study*. Newark, NJ: The Prudential Insurance Company of America.

Sanofi-Aventis. 2008a. *Managed Care Digest Series, 2008: Senior Care Digest*. Bridgewater, NJ: Sanofi-Aventis US, LLC.

Sanofi-Aventis. 2008b. *Managed Care Digest Series, 2008: Government Digest*. Bridgewater, NJ: Sanofi-Aventis US, LLC.

Shi, L., & Singh, D.A. 2008. *Delivering Health Care in America: A Systems Approach*, 4th ed. Boston: Jones and Bartlett Publishers.

Skaggs, R.L., & Hawkins, H.R. 1994. Architecture for long-term care facilities. In S.B. Goldsmith (ed.), *Essentials of Long-Term Care Administration* (pp. 254–284). Gaithersburg, MD: Aspen Publishers.

Stevenson, D.G., et al. 2007. *Medicare Part D, Nursing Homes, and Long-Term Care Pharmacies*. Retrieved February 2009 from http://www.medpac.gov/documents/Jun07_Part_D_contractor.pdf.

U.S. Census Bureau. 2008. *Statistical Abstract of the United States, 2008*. Washington, DC: U.S. Government Printing Office.

Wright, B. 2006. In brief: Training programs for certified nursing assistants. *AARP: Policy and Research for Professionals in Aging*. Retrieved November 2008 from http://www.aarp.org/research/longtermcare/nursinghomes/inb122_cna.html.

Chapter 8

Douglas A. Singh, PhD, MBA

Internal Environment and Culture Change

What You Will Learn

- Building codes, construction, and layout for a young and growing nursing home industry in the 1960s were adapted from hospitals. Competition during the 1980s prompted nursing homes to emphasize residential and aesthetic features. Contemporary models focus on person-centered care.

- The philosophy of long-term care greatly diverges from the sick-role model that governs hospital care. The long-term care model of person-centered care must integrate three major components: socio-residential, clinical, and overarching human factors.

- Nursing homes encounter four main challenges to a full integration of the three main components. The challenges include need for clinical care, economic constraints, patient-related constraints, and regulations.

- The clinical organization of a nursing home includes nursing units, and adequately staffed and well-equipped nursing stations.

- The socio-residential environment should emphasize both personal and public domains. These domains emphasize security of person and property, safety against potential hazards, wayfinding, autonomy and self-determination, personal privacy, compatible relationships, the dining experience, and opportunities for socializing.

- Modern architectural designs, such as cluster design and nested single rooms, emphasize many of the socio-residential factors.

- Aesthetics are an important element of homelike environments that also promote a sense of well-being. Choice of lighting, colors, and furnishings require special considerations in creating therapeutic environments for nursing home residents.

- Enriched environments are physically and psychologically support-ive environments. They incorporate the theories of biophilia and thriving. Creating an enriched environment first requires a philoso-phy of person-centered care in which clinical care, socio-residential elements, and human factors are integrated. The environment then incorporates elements that provide a moderate degree of positive stimulation and also opportunities for silent contemplation and in-ner reflection.

- A growing movement has been advocating culture change in nurs-ing homes. Culture change requires person-centered care, enriched environments, and staff empowerment based on adoption of new mindsets of managing people.

- The Eden Alternative and the Green House Project are two contem-porary models of culture change.

- Environments for dementia patients are based on the modern con-cepts of creating enriched environments.

The internal environment and organization of nursing homes have traditionally evolved as both a direct and indirect result of health pol-icy. It is only recently that enriched environ-ments and innovative designs have started to emerge through the influence of consumer ad-vocacy and market forces.

Evolution of Nursing Home Internal Environments

The poorhouses (discussed in Chapter 7) were the common ancestors of both hospitals and nursing homes. In the late 1800s and early 1900s, hospitals became separate insti-tutions mainly because medical discoveries—such as anesthesia, antiseptic surgery, and X-ray imaging—required an institutional setting where physicians could administer medical and surgical treatments and where

physicians could be trained. It was not until 1935, when the Old Age Assistance (OAA) program was created, that a private nursing home industry emerged. The OAA enabled many elderly to pay for services in homes for the aged and boarding homes. The new law had purposely prohibited payments to any-one living in poorhouses. Poorhouses closed down in large numbers, and private old age homes were in high demand. Private opera-tors acquired various types of buildings—old schools, hotels, and dormitories—and con-verted them into old-age homes. At this time, building standards and oversight for care de-livery were practically nonexistent. The old age homes provided basic nursing care and supervision, much as today's personal care homes do, and the very sick stayed in hospi-tals. Policies during the 1950s expanded the OAA program, and additional funding was made available for care in nursing homes. Legislation in 1958 and 1959 authorized the

Small Business Administration and the Federal Housing Administration to aid the construction of for-profit nursing homes, and there was a nursing home construction boom. The industry experienced explosive growth after the creation of Medicare and Medicaid in 1965.

By this time, hospitals were well established as institutions where the healing arts were practiced. For a young and growing nursing home industry, hospital layout and clinical arrangements became the obvious model. Building codes for nursing home construction were also adapted from hospitals. The result was hospital-like nursing homes characterized by long corridors, shared occupancy, and large cafeteria-style dining rooms. Licensing and certification rules further reinforced the hospital design because the nursing home was viewed as a place where convalescent treatment would continue following discharge from hospitals, as laid out in Medicare rules. Thus, by default, hospital design was adapted for nursing home construction. Clinical organization in nursing homes also followed the hospital-based medical model, with central nursing stations, buzzers, and call signals; noisy shower and bathing areas; lack of privacy; scheduled routines; and hallways cluttered with medication carts, soiled linen hampers, food carts, housekeeping carts, and similar items.

During the 1980s, construction of new nursing facilities and renovation of existing ones began emphasizing residential and aesthetic features. These changes were triggered mainly by market competition, which created the need to attract new patients to keep the beds filled. Competition also prompted efforts by nursing facilities to cater to the private-pay clientele. Competition came from newer nursing homes that adopted contemporary designs, the emergence of modern assisted living facilities, and expansion of substitute services such as home health care. Many private-pay patients have found the residential and social lifestyles in assisted living facilities to be much more appealing than skilled nursing facilities. In response, most nursing facilities operating today have taken at least some steps toward creating homelike and social environments that are more aesthetically pleasing than those found in older facilities.

New choices and alternatives to traditional nursing home care are molding people's expectations about long-term care (LTC). In response to the changing expectations, current trends suggest a gradual transformation from traditional hospital-inspired facilities to contemporary architectural features with a more residential look and feel. Other contemporary models are focusing on ***person-centered care***, a philosophy that integrates physical layout and design with empowerment of the residents, families, and staff. A cultural and social change is under way, with clients demanding that nursing home environments be made more appealing and less institutionalized. A gradual move away from the medical model and toward a more holistic socio-residential model that allows individuals to pursue their own lifestyles—rather than be governed by established routines and schedules—is where we are today in nursing home evolution.

Philosophy of Care Delivery

Traditionally, both the physical architecture and the philosophy of care delivery in nursing homes was influenced by hospitals. In a hospital, the ***sick-role model*** proposed by Parsons (1972) governs patients' social relationships. The patient is expected to relinquish individual control to medical personnel and comply with their directives. The sick role promotes an institutional orientation to patient care, which is manifested in four ways: (1) rigid daily routines; (2) social distance between staff members and the patient; (3) care practices that lend to depersonalization, such as loss of privacy; and (4) "blocking routines" that require patients to do certain things at prearranged times, mainly for the convenience of staff (Kruzich & Berg, 1985).

Unlike acute care hospitals, however, a nursing facility is both a clinical and a social establishment. It took some time for nursing home professionals and regulators to fully grasp this. Unlike hospitals, patients stay in nursing homes for extended periods of time. For some, the stay is permanent and, in a sense, the nursing home becomes their home. Although patients are admitted to skilled nursing facilities primarily to receive therapeutic interventions, these services must be delivered according to a philosophy that emphasizes personal preferences, independence, dignity, and self-esteem as overarching factors in the living environment and the delivery of care. Today, quality of life has become just as important as quality of care.

Creation of an environment of person-centered care (also called client-centered care) in modern nursing facilities is guided by three main factors (Figure 8–1):

- The socio-residential component creates the physical environment in which the resident receives room-and-board services and considers the nursing facility as his or her home. Amenities in the environment include personal and social spaces, aesthetic décor and designs, and various conveniences such as a barber/beauty salon. Accommodations must pro-

vide privacy, even though the most common type of living arrangement in nursing homes is a semi-private room. The environment must promote individual pursuits and leisure on the one hand and social interaction and engagement on the other. Meals must meet the nutritional and therapeutic needs, but must also be palatable and attractively served. Internal spaces must facilitate private visits with family and other visitors from the community. Social spaces must allow for a communal environment in which people can engage in meaningful social relationships.

- The elements of clinical care (listed in Figure 8–1) are highly individualized. They must be delivered by qualified professionals and paraprofessionals in accordance with accepted standards of clinical care.

- The overarching human factors—personal preferences, independence, dignity, and self-esteem—must blend into every aspect of the patient's life and the delivery of services. Such integration is not naturally achieved and requires staff training. Traditional nursing home care has been based on an expert approach to meeting the physical and medical needs of patients (Collopy, 1995). Well-meaning staff members are often ill-prepared to reconcile their technical training and priorities with the fact that residents are entitled to make their own choices. As a result, caregivers may experience difficulty relating to residents because of this conflict (Chapman et al., 2003).

When human factors are integrated into the other two components, it creates an

Figure 8-1 *Main Components of Client-centered Care*

Overarching Human Factors		
Personal preferences **Independence** **Dignity** **Self-esteem**		
Socio-Residential Component		**Clinical Component**
Room and Board	**Amenities**	**Clinical Care**
Accommodation • Privacy • Safety • Cleanliness • Comfort Meals • Nutrition • Choice • Adequacy • Attractiveness • Palatability	Private rooms Personal space Social space Dining rooms Layout Décor and aesthetics Barber/beauty salon Gift shop Library Chapel	Medical oversight Nursing care Rehabilitation Social services Dietary services Recreational activities End-of-life care

environment in which a person's physical, mental, social, and spiritual needs are met. Unlike the sick-role model, the person-centered model is characterized by shared control between the patient and the facility personnel. It promotes individual autonomy and decision making, even when a resident's decision-making capacity is limited. It embraces the idea that a LTC facility is not merely a clinical setting; it is also a place that many people call home.

Challenges to a Full Integration

Integration of the three components will continue to be a challenge for nursing home professionals, and there are four main reasons: primacy of clinical care, economic necessity, patient-related constraints, and regulatory burden. In spite of these constraints, nursing home professionals must strive to achieve a balance among the three factors just discussed.

Primacy of Clinical Care

The primary reason for admitting patients to a nursing facility is to meet their clinical needs. The fundamental purpose of a nursing home is defeated if it does not provide clinical care in accordance with accepted standards that require current medical and nursing knowledge and use of technology. As explained in Chapter 5, this is also a nursing facility's primary legal and moral duty. Hence, the sick-role model can be compromised but cannot be entirely dispensed with. For example, giving medications and other treatments in a patient population of any size requires certain routines based on medical directives. Medical examinations result in some loss of personal control by the patient. Necessary staff assistance with daily living activities does create some dependency.

Economic Constraints

Nursing facilities exist because of economic necessity. If it were feasible, almost every nursing home patient would choose to be cared for in a private residence by a private-duty nurse. The reality, however, is that unless an individual is very wealthy, neither the individual patient nor the society can afford to incur the expense that private-duty care would entail. Expensive as it is, delivery of care in a nursing facility is highly cost effective compared with private-duty nursing. From this perspective, the residential nature of a nursing facility should not be construed to mean that it is a private residence. It must, by necessity, provide services to a relatively large number of patients 24/7. In spite of suggestions to downplay or to criticize the institutional nature of nursing facilities, the fact remains that nursing facilities must function as efficient organizations.

Patient-Related Constraints

Nursing homes face constraints related to patient characteristics. Examples include behavioral problems, such as frequent combativeness or screaming episodes that can disrupt the environment. By its very nature, any group living arrangement, whether large or small, creates an environment in which small-scale conflicts of everyday life are likely to occur. First, respecting autonomy can be "vexatious because the conditions that bring elders into long-term care—confusion, dementia, wandering, and a host of chronic conditions associated with being old—are such that the very capacity for choice and rational decision making is seriously compromised, if not absent" (Agich, 1995, p. 113). In a relation of dependency, it may be quite natural for a caregiver to simply take over the care-delivery process. Yet, an effort must be made to return to the elder patient some of the responsibilities for his or her own health care in a caring and respectful way.

Regulatory Burden

Nursing home regulation and enforcement were discussed in Chapter 6. The nursing home industry particularly views the regulatory process to be onerous, adversarial, and punitive. As a result, the culture of nursing home administration has suffered from paranoia of the regulatory system. Inadequate financing under Medicaid, the largest payer for nursing home care, is also seen as a major constraint to procure needed resources. Collopy (1995, p. 149) argued that the nursing home industry is often slow to respond and is largely reactive in the way that it invokes moral values, mainly to protect itself against possible regulatory sanction. Such a highly risk-averse stance mutes the providers' own moral agency, so regulators and advocates for the elderly have seized the ethics agenda and have taken the initiative to prescribe minute regulatory details. Such a state of affairs will change only when the industry's leadership asserts the values that are most desired by its clients. The culture change, discussed later in this chapter, is an effort in this direction initiated by the industry's leadership, not by any regulatory requirements.

Need for Balance

A perfect integration of clinical, socioresidential, and human factors is almost impossible. Nevertheless, nursing home staff must strive for a balance in person-centered caregiving. There is, however, no standard rule that can be followed to help people adapt to change in their lives. People try to adapt in their own unique ways through various interpretive efforts. The nursing facility, however, can provide physical surroundings and a basic sense of personal space to help the process of adjustment. Familiarity and closeness in the caregiver–patient relationship that is built on the foundation of respect for the patient can also help patients maintain their sense of identity despite the ravages of impairment (Agich, 1995). In a nursing facility, each resident's desires, interests, and actions can directly affect the interests and legitimate expectations of other residents (Arras, 1995). For example, patients who wander into others' rooms, rummage through others' belongings, dip their hands into other diners' plates, make yelling noises, or display combativeness disrupt the quality of life of other residents. To deal with such conflicts in an institutional setting, the facility must achieve an appropriate balance among the needs of these groups. Arras (1995) suggested that a model

other than the one in which the patient's best interest becomes the overriding goal is necessary. This alternative model is based on the notions of fairness, accommodation, compromise, and negotiation. Again, each situation is going to be different, but in a social environment, no one patient's interests are legitimately outweighed by the competing interests of other patients. Also, modern architectural features and adoption of cultural change can facilitate the creation of a balanced environment.

Clinical Organization

The vast majority of nursing homes use a traditional clinical set-up, which is described in this section. Many newer facilities that are being built use innovative design concepts to downplay the clinical organization.

Nursing Units

A nursing unit or wing is a section of a facility that consists of a certain number of patient rooms served by a nursing station. Depending on its size, a facility may have clinically distinct nursing units, each providing a somewhat distinct level of care, such as rehabilitation, dementia care, or specialized care. Distinct nursing units can also be designated according to the type of certification. To achieve staff efficiency, most clinical units are self-contained, having their own bathing rooms, dining or feeding rooms and lounges for patients and visitors. An adequate number of clean linen closets should be located in the hallways of each nursing unit. An enclosed area or a hallway nook for depositing soiled linens is located in the unit, with marked containers to ease sorting and to separate lightly soiled linens from those that are heavily soiled. When utility closets are easily accessible to staff, hallways are kept free of clutter, and odors are kept to a minimum. An enclosed soiled utility area, rather than a nook in the hallway, is ideal because it can be equipped with a rinse tub to eliminate heavy wastes. Modern ventilation and waste-elimination systems are designed to keep odors to a minimum. Also, staff members should be trained in sanitation and odor control methods. Chemical deodorizers should not be used to mask odors.

A facility of 80 or more beds is likely to have more than one nursing unit. To the extent that it can do so, a facility should segregate patients on the basis of clinical criteria. Distinctly separate specialized care units are often provided for subacute care or Alzheimer's care. Such specialized units allow the facility to match staff skills to special patient needs. Rehabilitation aides (paraprofessionals who follow up on rehabilitation therapies), for instance, are most appropriately stationed in the SNF unit where most of the Medicare patients are located. A separate nursing unit, however, is not generally feasible for every type of specialization. Several clinically complex services such as ventilator care, head trauma care, care for spinal injuries, and treatment for pressure ulcers and wounds can be located on one unit that is served by the same nursing station. Also, neatly categorizing patients in terms of their needs for care is not always practical. Comorbidities often present a challenge to LTC clinicians about where a patient with given health conditions can be best accommodated. On the other hand, facilities must give due consideration to each patient's clinical needs as well as the patient's quality of life. For instance, every effort should be made to segregate patients with cognitive impairments or behavioral problems from those who do not have such disorders.

Some facilities focus on private-pay clients by furnishing a separate noncertified unit where the living environment is enhanced and amenities are upgraded. This type of segregation in a noncertified section allows a facility to provide upscale services to private-pay clients without discriminating against those on public assistance. It also shelters the noncertified section from certification surveys.

Nursing Station

The hub of clinical care is an appropriately located, adequately staffed, and well-furnished nursing station. This station can be regarded as a service center from where all nursing care is delivered to a certain number of patients, generally on an entire nursing unit.

Location of Nursing Stations

A nursing station should be centrally located to enable the nursing staff to observe and supervise a certain number of patient rooms and to respond effectively to patient needs. A facility may have more than one station, depending on its size, acuity level of patients, and complexity of care. On the other hand, having too many stations would be inefficient because each station must be individually staffed. As a general rule, a separate nursing station serves each clinical unit or wing in a facility. The maximum distance allowed from a nursing station to the farthest patient room is generally specified in state licensure regulations.

Other areas of a clinical unit that may be adjacent to the nursing station include rooms for bathing and showering, special dining areas to accommodate patients who need assistance with eating, and patient lounges, including any lounges designated for smokers.

Of course, not all patient dining rooms and lounges need to be in the vicinity of a nursing station—only those where supervision from staff is necessary.

Staffing of Nursing Stations

Staffing is one of the most important issues in nursing homes. State licensure regulations often specify minimum staff-to-patient ratios, and facility administrators may tend to believe that those minimum standards represent adequate staffing levels. State standards set a minimum requirement (which is, at best, arbitrary) because it does not take into account the level of patients' clinical acuity. Clinical load rather than state regulations should govern staff-to-patient ratios, and higher ratios are needed in specialized and heavy-care units.

Nursing Station Furnishings

The layout and furnishing of a nursing station should enhance staff effectiveness. The station itself is an enclosed area, with a counter behind which nurses and other staff members perform administrative tasks. No one but authorized staff members should have access to the area behind the counter. Among other things, a nursing station's furnishings must include three important components: a patient call signal system, medical records, and a pharmaceuticals room.

Patient Call Signals

A call system is a critical component of a nursing unit. The system connects devices at all patient bedsides and in toilets to the nursing station. It should also connect the station to the bathing-and-shower rooms, dining areas, and lounges located on a given nursing unit. The system enables the patients themselves and staff members working with patients to summon help when needed. Ideally, the system should have audio-visual as well as voice capabilities. A patient uses a sensory device—such as a call button—that sets off the audio-visual signal at the nursing station. This audio-visual signal consists of a light and a sound to alert the staff that a patient is calling for assistance and also to identify the patient who needs help. A voice or "talk-back" feature is useful when the staff member attending to a patient needs to communicate with staff members located at the station; this device saves time that otherwise will be spent walking back and forth from the nursing station. For communication among staff members, modern wireless communication devices such as portable pagers are increasingly being used. They reduce the need for frequent paging over the intercom, which makes the environment noisy and stressful.

Medical Records

Located at the nursing station, there must be a separate medical chart for every patient on the unit. The medical records must be readily accessible to all authorized staff members. Confidentiality, however, must be maintained at all times. Medical records are increasingly being automated by using computer-based information systems. Automation can greatly facilitate the tasks of keeping records up to date and retrieving them quickly. Privacy practices must comply with HIPAA standards.

Pharmaceuticals Room

The pharmaceuticals room, or medication room, as it is commonly called, should be quickly accessible from the nursing station.

This room is locked to safeguard all medications. The pharmaceuticals room is also commonly used to store nursing treatment supplies and a first-aid box. The room is furnished with a refrigerator for storing medications that require refrigeration.

Socio-Residential Environment

Although a nursing facility is considered a patient's home, it is also a community. The social and residential elements are closely intertwined, and the environment itself should promote the healing of the body, mind, and spirit. A healing environment relieves the clinical infrastructure of pressures that might otherwise be imposed on it from social conflict or individual ill-adjustment. As mentioned earlier, segregating patients with severe dementia and those with behavioral problems from other patients is particularly important. A disruptive environment creates commotion and confusion. It is mentally and emotionally upsetting for those who prefer quietude and wish to engage in productive social, mental, and spiritual pursuits. The facility's set-up should also make it easier for patients to explore their compatibilities with others and engage in social interactions in accordance with personal preferences. The socio-residential environment should emphasize both personal and public domains.

Personal Domain

At a personal level, the main concerns people have are security, safety, wayfinding, autonomy, and privacy. In coping with change, opportunities for introspection, a sense of personal space, and the support of others may be more important for the patient than the ability to socialize with others.

Security

Security is a basic human need. It entails physical safety and psychological peace of mind. It includes a variety of conditions that contribute to freedom from risk, danger, anxiety, or doubt (Schwarz, 1996). A nursing facility is responsible for its patients' personal security and the safekeeping of their belongings and private funds if the latter are deposited in a patient's trust account that the facility manages. Security considerations often vary from one patient to another. A patient may have a tendency to wander out unnoticed and compromise his or her safety. But if this same person can wander out into a protective environment, such as a fenced-in walkway, it can have a therapeutic effect. Another may insist on wearing expensive jewelry that someone could remove or that could get lost. Another may hallucinate and imagine that someone is assaulting her.

Not all nursing homes are located in safe neighborhoods. The administrator must evaluate external security concerns, which include protecting residents and their property from intruders. To the extent that patients can feel safe and secure, they can choose to spend time indoors and outdoors.

Safety

In building design, safety requirements are primarily governed by federal, state, and local codes and regulations. Among these, the *Life Safety Code* provides the most comprehensive set of rules. Other considerations are also important in creating a safe environment:

- The elderly are particularly vulnerable to falls. Great caution and vigilance needs to be exercised around wet floors, power cords, fallen objects, and throw rugs.

- Potential hazards should be eliminated or closely monitored. Access to products such as drugs, lotions, and ointments on medication and treatment carts should be adequately supervised. Patients could also gain access to other unattended toxic substances, such as cleaning chemicals left unattended on housekeeping carts, or sharp objects, such as certain maintenance tools.

- Access to areas such as the kitchen, mechanical rooms, and laundry are generally prohibited. However, kitchen and laundry areas can provide stimulating and meaningful engagement for some patients, including those with mild to moderate dementia. With some supervision, cooking or laundry activities can add to patients' quality of life, particularly when smaller household-style kitchens are included in the facility's design.

- All major safety concerns should be incorporated into the patient's plan of care, and they ought to be addressed by a multi-disciplinary team of professionals because the patient may require therapeutic intervention from trained staff. For example, a person's medications may need to be reviewed or behavior modification may be necessary.

Wayfinding

Wayfinding refers to features that can help people find their way through a large institution with relative ease. Residents in nursing homes are often susceptible to disorientation because of a decline of various senses. Sameness and repetition—similar layouts, regular pattern of doors, and similar furniture throughout a facility—are the common sources of disorientation (Drew, 1992). Orientation involves much more than use of signs. In addition to clear and readable signage, wayfinding can be facilitated by using a variety of means such as employing different color schemes and patterns in different sections of the facility; color-coded handrails; varying furniture styles; varying layout and arrangement; use of pictures, tapestry, hanging quilts, and window displays; and placement of public accessories such as telephones and water coolers in planned locations. On the other hand, doors leading to utility rooms and areas not meant for residents should be painted to blend with the adjacent walls.

Autonomy

Autonomy can be defined as "a cluster of notions including self-determination, freedom, independence, and liberty of choice and action. In its most general terms, autonomy signifies control of decision making and other activity by the individual. It refers to human agency free of outside intervention and interference" (Collopy, 1988). In any type of health care delivery, the patient assumes a dependent role in relation to the provider of care, as observed by Talcott Parsons (1972) in the sick-role model; the patient must concede some degree of autonomy. This dependence, however, does not mean that the patient should be made to give up all choice and decision making. To the contrary, because health care by its very nature creates dependency, providers have an obligation to ensure the maximum preservation of patient autonomy.

On the other hand, a patient's autonomy cannot be taken to an extent that it infringes on the rights of others.

Autonomy for patients also requires that they be allowed to personalize their living quarters with familiar things, and such personal items as radios, small television sets, family pictures, mementos, artifacts, plants, music, personal furniture, bed accessories, etc. Emotions and memories from past experiences and events often stimulate conversation and social interaction. Although space is almost always limited, a display shelf in each room can help people personalize their space by displaying memorabilia and other items. Certain personal belongings may also pose safety concerns. For instance, too many electrical gadgets may overload the circuits and create a fire hazard. Long extension cords and floor rugs pose a tripping hazard.

Autonomy also means that a patient must be able to make informed choices. Although the nursing facility must encourage informed choice, it also has the responsibility to do what is in the patient's best interest. Occasionally, conflicts may arise between a patient's autonomy and the facility's duty toward the patient. Such conflicts should be resolved by taking into consideration legal requirements, regulatory constraints, and ethics. Such situations are often not clear-cut. For instance, should a nursing facility use funds out of a patient's trust account to purchase new glasses or new hearing aids after the patient has already broken or lost two or three of them? Such decisions can be best addressed in a multi-disciplinary forum—such as an ethics committee—in which decision makers take into account the patient's wishes and past practices if the patient is unable to participate in decision making. But, if the patient can participate, his or her wishes must be carried out.

Privacy

Almost all individuals require some privacy in terms of space, time, and person.

Privacy of Space

In a health care facility, privacy of space is first determined by the type of accommodation: private or shared. Many facilities maintain a small number of private rooms for single accommodation. As a general rule, however, occupying a private room is considered a luxury for which someone has to pay more. Unless a medically determined need exists for private accommodation, public as well as private insurers do not cover it. So, in most instances, a patient must spend out-of-pocket funds if a private room is desired. Hence, for most patients, shared accommodation is the norm, which in most facilities constitutes double occupancy (rather than triple or quadruple accommodation). In these circumstances, privacy rests on how much physical space each individual has, including closet and storage space. Privacy also entails the need for intimacy (Westin, 1967). *Intimacy* refers to a person's privacy during visits with family, friends, and legal or spiritual counselors. Residents can also express their sexuality in a private environment if their intimacy is assured. Because privacy is generally compromised in a multiple-occupancy setting, the facility should provide secluded areas that may be used for intimate dining experiences with family and friends, for private visits, or for sexual intimacy.

Privacy of Time

Privacy of time is often compromised by clinical routines that are established for the sake of staff efficiency. However, such routines tend to make patients' lives regimented. In most nursing homes, wake-up and morning hygiene chores must be completed before breakfast. Because assigning staff members to every resident at the same time is not possible, certain residents must wake up before others, and there may be little provision for patients to sleep in late. Meal hours are also generally fixed. Bathing and shower routines are scheduled ahead of time. Yet, within the parameters of such scheduled routines, patients' individual preferences should be accommodated whenever possible. Privacy of time also includes the need for personal reclusion, that is, have time for oneself and be free from unwanted intrusion, to be alone for quiet reflection. For this purpose, quiet and secluded spaces such as small libraries and chapels are highly desirable.

Privacy of Person

A disregard of privacy of person is dehumanizing. Privacy of person can be equated with dignity. A basic rule for facilities to follow is to treat every person with dignity, regardless of whether he or she can perceive indignities (Kane, 2001). Knocking at the door before entering a patient's room, closing the door for a patient while that patient is using the toilet, drawing privacy curtains during treatment, providing appropriate personal covering for a trip to the common bathing-and-shower area, providing proper grooming during a trip to the therapy room or dining room, and giving lap robes to female patients in wheelchairs are examples of how personal privacy is respected to preserve individual dignity.

Public Domain

Loneliness and isolation are common concerns among the elderly. Unless a person chooses to remain alone, opportunities must be provided for wholesome social interaction. The range of opportunities depends on how well a nursing facility functions as a social community. The three most important experiences from this perspective are compatibility, the dining experience, and socializing.

Compatibility

Social interactions in the public domain are primarily driven by compatibility because compatible relationships are something people naturally seek. The issue of compatibility first arises when a new patient is admitted to the facility and has to share a room with another patient who is a complete stranger. Gender compatibility has been a long-established practice. Room sharing by two individuals of the opposite sex is permitted only in case of legitimate couples. Apart from such obvious types of compatibility, the main consideration in assigning a room to two people is how well the two individuals are likely to get along and engage in a meaningful social rapport. Compatibility is also an important consideration in other situations requiring social groupings, such as dining at the same table or participating in social and recreational events.

Relationship building and bonding can be facilitated in several ways. Some nursing home residents assist other residents with simple tasks, such as escorting a friend to the dining room or assisting someone in a wheelchair. People who have disabilities of their own can find meaning in being helpful to others; it builds their own self-esteem. Nursing home residents can also develop appropriate relationships with volunteers and staff members.

Dining

Dining goes beyond mere physical sustenance and good nutrition. It can provide opportunities for people to interact with others in a social setting. Seating arrangements should be such that they create opportunities for those who can socially interact. Of course, a patient's clinical condition will determine to what extent interaction is possible. For patients who require feeding assistance or who may have other special needs, dining may become a clinical event, but staff interaction can still help make it a social event. To the extent possible, clinical dining areas for those who cannot eat on their own should be separated from social dining areas so that those who are able to dine in a social setting can enjoy the dining experience without interruption or distraction.

The dining environment should be relaxed. Comfortable chairs, tablecloths or placemats, cloth napkins, table centerpieces, and soft music contribute to a relaxed and enjoyable experience. A facility should also have some special tables to accommodate wheelchairs, but ambulatory and wheelchair patients should be allowed to sit and dine together.

Socializing

Socializing often depends on an individual's capacity to interact with others. Well-planned facilities offer varied spaces where people can spend time in the company of others. The facility must schedule programs that offer numerous daily opportunities for patients to socialize according to their personal interests. Social events also enable patients with dementia and other limitations to receive sensory stimulation by just being present. Events should be held in both interior and exterior spaces.

Interior spaces include lounges, dining areas, craft and game rooms, and chapels. Some modern facilities also have spaces such as mini-malls, ice cream parlors, and barber and beauty shops where residents can enjoy some of the social activities they once pursued. Interior spaces should be comfortable and pleasing, with appropriate furniture, lighting, fixtures, and décor that allow people to associate with one another in pleasant surroundings.

Exterior spaces include courtyards, patios, balconies, terraces, vegetable and flower patches, gazebos, and the spaces around bird feeders and fountains. The building's design should permit all residents easy access to the exterior. The outdoor spaces should have appropriate seating arrangements so that the patients can spend time relaxing, socializing, and simply enjoying the surroundings.

Modern Architectural Designs

The average size of a nursing facility has increased by 44% from 75 beds in 1973 to 108 beds in 2006 (National Center for Health Statistics, 2007). Although the larger size creates operational efficiencies, it detracts from a residential environment. In response, some innovative architectural plans have emerged. Modern architectural designs try to incorporate a balance between the clinical and socio-residential factors. A homelike environment is achieved by a facility's structural design, furnishings, décor, and a proper emphasis on the socio-residential elements discussed earlier. Increasingly, in new constructions, private rather than shared rooms are in vogue, to give patients more personal space. In addition, current architectural designs no longer feature the traditional long corridors that are lined with rooms on both sides, which often get cluttered with all kinds of barrels and carts and create an institutional look and feel. High-pitched roofs, varied plan configurations, and the connection of indoor to outdoor spaces can make a building seem more like a condominium than a nursing home (Nursing home architecture, 1997). The medical character of the facility can be further deemphasized by eliminating the traditional nursing station and creating more shared spaces for social contact (Cohen & Day, 1993). In large institutions, some smaller self-contained units can be created, each with its own household-style kitchen and a common room that can serve as a multipurpose room for dining, activities, and socializing.

Cluster Design

The cluster design is gradually replacing the traditional corridor design in modern nursing home architecture. The design places decentralized self-contained clusters within the larger clinical units, creating relatively small residential groupings. Even though a nursing station is present, the design helps deemphasize it. The cluster concept is sometimes called "neighborhood living," and the clusters may be called "household clusters." Each cluster functions as a residential unit or neighborhood, with its own living room and a room for various activities and for dining, surrounded by resident rooms (Dunkelman, 1992). Seating configurations are designed to create intimate social spaces. The design allows for plenty of windows for natural lighting and a panoramic view of the exterior. Clusters also tend to offer better flexibility in segregating residents than traditional layouts do. For instance, patients requiring heavy care could be accommodated in the same cluster.

Clusters are typically designed for between 8 and 12 residents, and three or more clusters are grouped together for staffing efficiency (Browning, 2003). As an example,

Figure 8–2 illustrates three 9-bed clusters, totaling 27 beds. High construction costs for clusters present a major challenge to facilities, although better functional efficiencies are often gained. By decentralizing staff and services and giving associates quick access to utilities, a cluster layout can make associates more productive and the delivery of care can be improved. Small nurse aide stations—generally no more than a desk and chair—enable the staff to be in close proximity to residents, allowing for prompt attention to their needs. In Figure 8–2, each of the three clusters has its own nurse aide station. The self-contained clusters also have their own bathing rooms, linen closets, and soiled utility closets. Associates can function more efficiently because this arrangement shortens walking distances and saves time. Services are brought to each cluster instead of transporting residents to the nursing station, dining room, or therapy room (Dunkelman, 1992). A group of permanent caregivers assigned to each cluster can also provide opportunities for interaction and bonding between caregivers and residents.

Nested Single-Room Design

To counter the high construction costs of private rooms, the architectural firm of Engelbrecht & Griffin (now named EGA, PC) pioneered the design of nested single rooms. Cost is conserved by efficient use of space. Although nested rooms are much smaller than regular rooms, they are self-contained bedrooms with their own private half-bathrooms that have a toilet and a sink (Figure 8–3). Nested single rooms offer privacy, and when they are placed in a cluster setting, they can also provide opportunities for socializing through "neighborhood living" arrangements (Figure 8–4). Easy access to common lounge

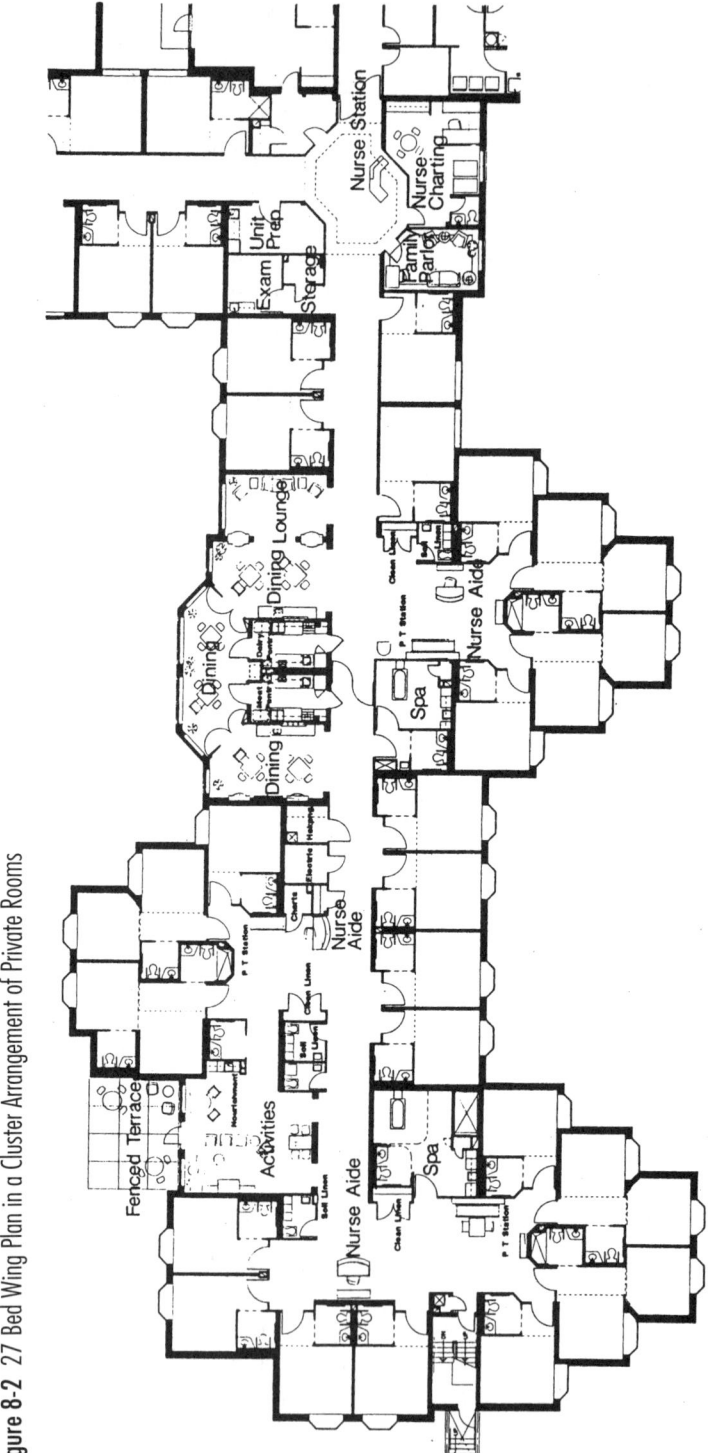

Figure 8-2 27 Bed Wing Plan in a Cluster Arrangement of Private Rooms

Source: PDT Architects/Planners, Cincinnati, Ohio. Designed by Mark B. Browning, AIA, for Cedar Village, Mason, Ohio. Reprinted with permission from Mark B. Browning.

Figure 8-3 Overhead One-Point Interior Perspective of Nested Rooms

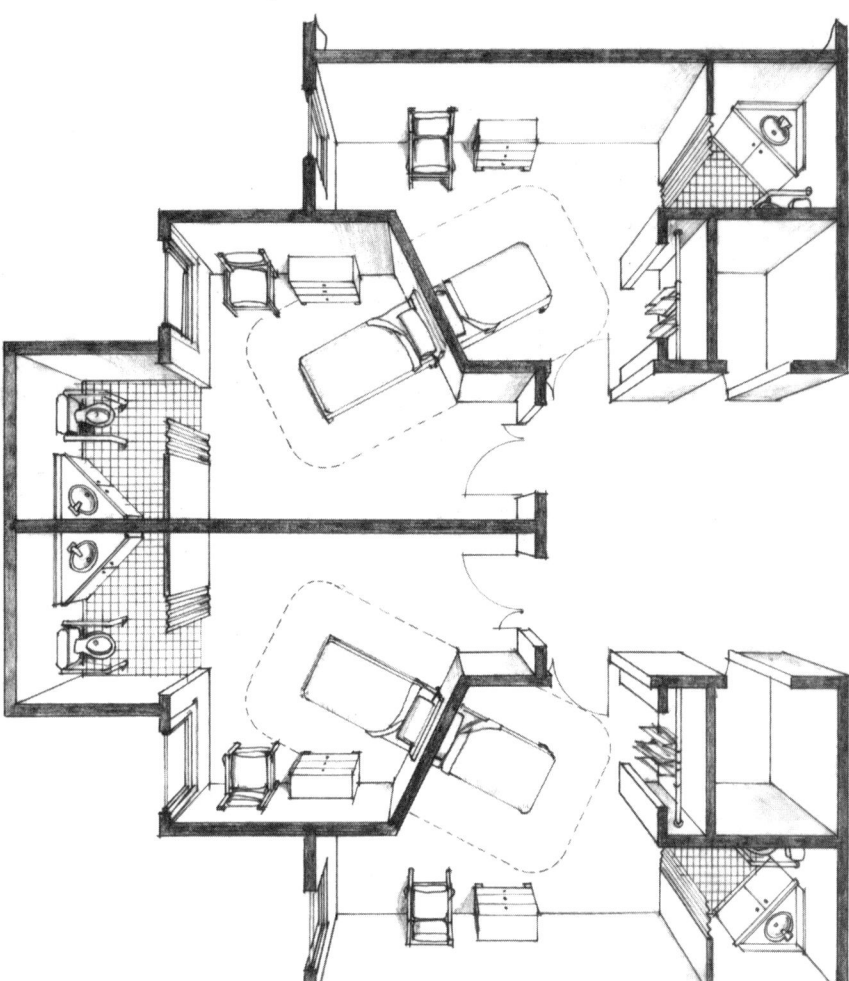

Source: EGA, P.C. "Designs for Living." Reprinted with permission from EGA, P.C.

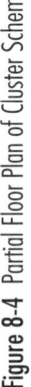

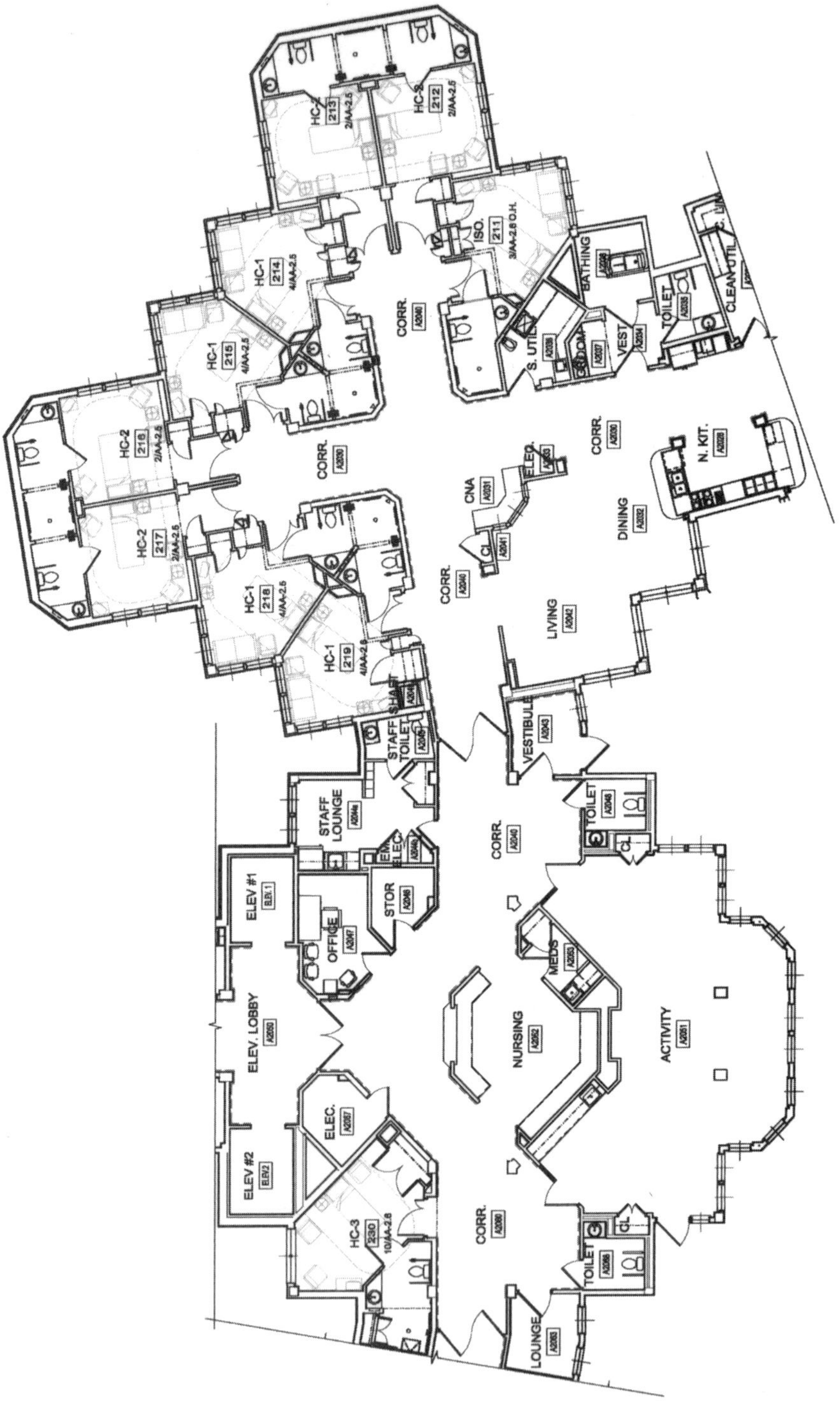

Figure 8-4 Partial Floor Plan of Cluster Scheme

Source: EGA, P.C. "Designs for Living." Reprinted with permission from EGA, P.C.

areas in the vicinity of the rooms encourages residents to get out of their rooms to meet and converse with familiar neighbors and provides a comfortable setting for visiting with family and friends.

Aesthetics

Aesthetics are necessary to promote a sense of well-being. Light and color, for example, influence patients' sleep, wakefulness, emotions, and health. Use of lighting, color, and furnishings create an environment that is both aesthetically appealing and comfortable. The physical environment can also affect social behavior and certain clinical outcomes.

Lighting

Vision impairment increases with age and it diminishes people's quality of life. Compared with community-dwelling elders, nursing home residents suffer from far greater visual impairment (West et al., 2003). Inadequate lighting affects sleep and depression and can cause falls that can otherwise be prevented. Lighting issues in LTC facilities should be addressed by (1) raising light levels substantially, (2) balancing natural light and electric light to achieve even light levels, and (3) eliminating direct as well as reflected glare (Brawley & Noell-Waggoner, Undated).

Natural sunlight is known to have positive effects on overall health. Facility design should incorporate as much natural lighting as possible, while also incorporating artificial light. Patios and porches enable residents to enjoy fresh air as well as direct sunlight. Windows, skylights, atriums, and greenhouse windows can be used to bring some of the natural daylight indoors. Low windows in patient rooms, lounges, and corridors allow residents to see the exterior grounds from their beds and wheelchairs. Window treatments should be used to regulate sunlight and minimize glare. Horizontal mini-blinds are generally preferable to vertical blinds, but light-filtering pleated shades are considered even better. Valances can be added to create a homelike look.

Lighting needs of the elderly are quite different from those of younger people. As their sight and visual acuity decline, the elderly require higher levels of illumination, but glare must be minimized. Glare can lead to agitation, confusion, anger, and falls. Most glare can be controlled either by shielding the light source from direct view or balancing the light in the room. A facility can ensure proper lighting for patients and also enhance the homelike feel by using chandeliers, wall sconces, recessed lighting, table lamps, floor lamps, and other light fixtures. In resident rooms, night lights are essential. Along with clear pathways to the toilet, night lights can facilitate safe trips to the bathroom and help prevent falls (Brawley, 1997).

Color

Colors used in health care settings have changed dramatically in recent years. Traditional colors such as white, bold yellow, beige, and green are no longer considered appropriate. More pleasing and stimulating colors have now become popular. Such colors include soft apricot, peach, salmon, coral, soft yellow-orange, and a variety of earth-colored tones. Patterns and colors in wall coverings and decorative borders can liven up some otherwise unexciting areas. Bedrooms, bathrooms, dining rooms, living rooms, and alcoves are all appropriate places where wall coverings can enhance residential quality. Coated wall coverings can be used in areas such as hallways, where soiling is a serious problem. Handrails are necessary in hallways and other areas, but with a natural wood finish, they help maintain the residential look.

Colors are also used to promote safety. Aging reduces a person's ability to distinguish colors. To compensate for this reduced visual function, high-contrast colors should be used. For example, the color of grab bars in the toilet should contrast sharply with the color of the wall, to ensure maximum visibility. Countertop colors should stand out strongly from those of floors. For many nursing home residents, being able to use the toilet may depend on being able to locate it. In a totally white bathroom, some patients will find it difficult to distinguish the toilet from the floor or the adjacent wall. Colored toilet seats create visible contrasts against the surroundings and can facilitate locating the toilet. Conversely, a colored wall can provide visual contrast against a white toilet.

Furnishings

Carpeting adds warmth and softens sounds. It also provides cushioning against falls and can prevent serious fractures of the hip or wrist. Today's high-performance carpets, which are resistant to stains and odors, are also cost effective. New carpets are treated with a vinyl moisture barrier and an antimicrobial coating (Yarme & Yarme, 2001). Proper installation and regular maintenance can make carpeting last for several years. Of course, carpeting is not appropriate for all areas in the building. Slip-resistant tile is by far the most widely used flooring material. Resilient flooring with low sheen can be used in certain high-use areas without creating an institutional appearance. For example, these hard-surface floorings also come in beautiful wood-grain patterns that add a homelike

touch. Also available are new soft-surface floorings that are made of easy-to-maintain sheet vinyl material with a dense, soft, carpet-like surface and a cushioned backing. These materials have been tested to ensure that they reduce injuries from falls (Yarme & Yarme, 2001). Highly polished and buffed surfaces are not recommended for the elderly because they produce glare, appear wet or slick, and can be a source of anxiety and confusion.

A variety of furniture is now available that is specifically designed for LTC facilities. Lounge chairs, sofas, and rocking chairs can add charm and variety as well as comfort. Use of upholstered furniture has actually become quite common. Some manufacturers are producing foam cushions that are soft enough to be comfortable and yet firm enough for residents to rise easily from chairs and sofas (Child, 1999). Brawley (1997) commented on several enhancements in high-tech finishing of upholstery fabrics. These include soil- and stain-resistant finishes, lamination with vinyl, fluid barriers, and antimicrobial finishes. For nursing home use, these fabrics must also be flame-retardant. "Super fabrics," such as Crypton, have built-in stain and moisture resistance and have been tested for fire and microbial resistance. These new fabrics have replaced vinyl coverings for chairs and sofas, and a range of colors, textures, and patterns are now available to enhance the residential environment in nursing facilities.

Enriched Environments

The environment is viewed as a "silent partner" in caregiving because it is a contributing factor to the healing process (Noell, 1995). *Enriched environments* (or enhanced environments) are physically and psychologically supportive environments that promote positive feelings, harmony, and thriving and reduce boredom and stress.

Theoretical Foundations

Creation of enriched environments finds support in two complementary theories: biophilia framework and theory of thriving.

Biophilia Framework

E.O. Wilson, a biologist, coined the term ***biophilia*** for the human propensity to affiliate with other life forms. In short, it describes the human tendency to pay attention to, affiliate with, and respond positively to nature (Wilson, 1984). People not only have an inborn biophiliac tendency to relate to animals and to natural settings, but people's relationship with nature is essential to their thriving. Plants, animals, water, and soil are the most common elements of the natural environment (Wohlwill, 1983). Based on an integrative review of the literature, Jones and Haight (2002) reported consistent findings that interactions with the natural environment, which can be experienced both indoors and outdoors, produce beneficial effects in human beings, such as positive mood and mental restoration. A recent study of hospitalized patients recovering from an appendectomy showed that patients with plants in their rooms had a significantly lower need for pain medication, had lower blood pressure and heart rates, and had less anxiety and fatigue than their counterparts in the control group with no plants in their rooms (Park & Mattson, 2008).

Theory of Thriving

Thriving means living life to the full. It is also a growth process that occurs as a result of humans interacting in a symbiotic relationship with their environments to enhance their physical, mental, social, and spiritual well-being. According to Haight et al. (2002), the integrative model of thriving includes three elements (1) the person; (2) the human environment comprising family, friends, caregivers, and others; and (3) the nonhuman environment comprising the physical and ecological surroundings of the person. Thriving occurs when the relationship among the three entities is mutually engaging, supportive, and harmonious. Conversely, a failure to thrive occurs when discordance exists among the person, the human environment, and the nonhuman environment. When thriving occurs, certain critical attributes are noticeable in the person: social connectedness, finding meaning in life, adaptation, and positive cognitive/affective function.

Principles of Enrichment

Enriched environments are created by incorporating three main principles:

- All three elements of person-centered care (clinical care, socioresidential elements of the physical environment, and overarching human factors) must be integrated, as discussed earlier. In a person-centered environment, care delivery is congruent with the values, needs, and preferences of care recipients (Eales et al., 2001). Health care professionals empower residents to assert their rights and preferences. This empowerment is achieved through a bonding between residents and caregivers who place supreme value on listening to the individual's preferences while offering professional advice and instruction on the risks and benefits of the choices the resident wants to make. The resident's autonomy and the freedom to take some risks are respected.

- The environment provides a moderate degree of positive stimulation and distraction. Prolonged exposure to low levels of environmental stimulation can lead to boredom, negative feelings, and depression. In the absence of positive distractions, patients begin to focus on their own problems and end up increasing their level of stress. Positive distractions elicit good feelings, hold attention, and generate interest. Happy faces, laughter, people passing by, pets, fish in aquariums, birds, flowers, trees, plants, water, pleasant aromas, and soothing music can all be positive distractions. Negative distractions, on the other hand, are stressors. They simply assert their unwanted presence because it is difficult to ignore them. Visual stimulation from pictures, artwork, and television watching can be positive for patients, but abstract art and uncontrolled loud noise from television are negative distractions.

- Thriving is not entirely a function of external stimulus. Thriving also requires solitude, reflection, introspection, spiritual contemplation, study, and a sense of one's individuality and self-worth. Contemplation and inner reflection often occur in a passive relationship with serene natural surroundings. On the other hand, thriving also requires active engagement in meaningful social relationships, caring for live plants or animals, lending a helping hand to a fellow patient, playing with children, or working on hobbies such as gardening or woodworking. In its ultimate sense, thriving is achieved when a person feels a deep sense of belonging to and connection with the physical environment comprised of people and things, and also feels closeness to a Supreme Being in accordance with one's own belief system.

Culture Change

The ideas presented in this chapter are at the heart of what has been loosely referred to as "culture change." The change is from the traditional nursing home environments and care processes driven by the sick-role model to the ones that promote client-centered care in enriched environments. Hence, *culture change* is the integration of the three elements of person-centered care along with enriching the environments in which people live. In addition, culture change requires empowerment of associates. Empowerment requires a change in management philosophy and practice. As a guiding principle, administrators and department managers start treating their associates as they would want the associates to treat the elders. There is no room for any practices that devalue workers, most of whom are women who typically earn just a little above the federal minimum wage. Empowerment also requires a decentralized management approach in which decision making is taken back to the elders and to the families and caregivers, and these stakeholders are given a voice in the elders' daily routine and life. For example, in the archetypal nursing home culture, the resident must comply with schedules and routines preset by the organization. Through culture change, residents and staff design schedules that reflect the residents' personal needs and desires. For instance, within reason, residents can decide whether they prefer a shower or a bath in the morning or in the evening (Andreoli et al., 2007). Culture change requires a new mindset on the part of management and associates.

The *Pioneer Network* played a critical role in advocating culture change in nursing homes. It began as a grassroots movement of caregivers, consumer advocates, and others who were concerned about the quality of life in even some of the finest conventional nursing homes. Beginning in 1997, nursing home professionals and advocates, referred to as "pioneers," began informal meetings to define common areas of endeavor and opportunities for bringing about a cultural change in nursing facilities. A few nursing home professionals, who had already experimented with some innovative approaches, were invited to share their experiences with various stakeholders, including regulators, nursing home administrators, directors of nursing, and social workers. Subsequently, regular meetings of these pioneers led to the formation in 2000 of a formal organization, named the Pioneer Network, an organization that had the aim of providing leadership to the grassroots movement. Since then, it has evolved into a growing national movement. The Network has continued to make some impact in the areas of education, in sharing information and ideas to form coalitions, and in advocacy to influence public policy.

The Centers for Medicare and Medicaid Services (CMS) has endorsed the principles of culture change. From 2004 to 2006, CMS sponsored a project in 21 states to teach nursing home operators the principles and practices of culture change. In 2006, the CMS funded and co-developed the Artifacts of Culture Change, a tool to help nursing homes measure concrete changes realized as a result of implementing the culture change philosophy (Appendix 8–I). Culture change

is also referenced in consumer guidelines issued by the CMS in choosing a nursing home.

There is no single model of culture change because of several variables involved. For example, leadership, ownership, and case-mix factors vary from facility to facility (Wiener et al., 2007). According to a 2007 national survey of nursing homes, 43% of the facilities were operating according to the traditional model, 31% had adopted the changes, and 25% were striving to adopt culture change. In general, nursing homes have been most successful in increasing resident autonomy and, to a certain extent, empowering caregivers. But, very few facilities have changed their physical environment to support culture change. For example, very few nursing homes have renovated their traditional facilities into "neighborhoods" or "households" with their own kitchens, dining areas, and living areas (Doty et al., 2008). The high cost of constructional modifications is one reason. Also, many of the older buildings present daunting challenges because of their layout and lack of available space that must be devoted to providing essential services such as nursing care and rehabilitation.

Doty et al. (2008) demonstrated that a greater degree of adoption of culture change results in greater benefits in terms of staff retention, higher occupancy rates, better competitive position, and improved operational costs. As these benefits become more widely known, a greater degree of adoption is likely to occur. It is also surmised that, compared with previous generations, baby boomers on the verge of retirement will be more inclined to search for LTC options that promote comfort and quality of life in an environment comparable to their own homes (Ragsdale & McDougall, 2008).

Contemporary Models of Culture Change

The Eden Alternative

Of all the various movements advocating enriched environments in LTC facilities, the Eden Alternative is perhaps the best known. In the early 1990s, Dr. William Thomas, while working as a physician in nursing homes, undertook a pilot project sponsored by the state of New York. Working with the staff in an 80-bed nursing home, which served mostly patients with dementia, Thomas developed some new ideas and a set of principles for creating a garden-like environment. As an advocate for change, Thomas explained:

> I want an alternative to the institution. The best alternative I can think of is a garden. I believe when we make a place that's worthy of our elders, we make a place that enriches all of our lives—caregivers, family members, and elders alike. So the Eden Alternative provides a reinterpretation of the environment elders live in, going from an institution to a garden . . . There are kids running around and playing. There are dogs and cats and birds, and there are gardens and plants. I want people to think that this can't be a nursing home. Which it isn't—it's an alternative to a nursing home . . . The future of caregiving belongs to people and organizations who can dream new dreams about how to care for our elders (McLeod, 2002, pp. 14–15).

The *Eden Alternative*, a trademark of its founding organization, entails viewing the surroundings in facilities as habitats for human beings rather than as facilities for the frail and elderly, as well as applying the lessons of nature in creating vibrant and vigorous settings. It is based on the belief that the companionship of pets, the opportunity to give meaningful care to other living creatures, and the spontaneity that marks an enlivened environment have therapeutic values (Eden Alternative, 2002). One of the main objectives of Eden Alternative is to banish from the lives of nursing home residents the loneliness, helplessness, and boredom that Thomas has called "the three plagues of nursing homes" (Bruck, 1997). To counteract these ills, residents need companionship, variety, and a chance to feel needed (Stermer, 1998).

According to the 10 principles on which the Eden Alternative is founded (Exhibit 8–1) the antidote to loneliness is meaningful contact with plants, animals, and children, as well as easy access to human and animal companionship; the remedy for helplessness is giving as well as receiving care; and the cure for boredom is unexpected and unpredictable interactions and happenings in surroundings that deliver variety and spontaneity (Eden Annual, 2003). Among methods to build relationships between staff members and residents, alternative means of healing such as massage therapy and aromatherapy are suggested, based on the belief that a back-rub or foot-rub may eliminate the need for sleep-inducing medications, and the belief that the smell of lavender or peppermint can have a calming effect.

Edenizing is the expression used for achieving culture change by implementing the Eden principles. For a long time, many nursing homes have, at least to some extent, involved their residents in nature-oriented activities such as pet therapy, gardening, and nature walks. Programs in collaboration with local schools and day care centers have also been developed to promote intergenerational companionship. Edenizing more fully incorporates the concepts of biophilia. It promotes surroundings rich in plants, animals, and children. Involving the residents in the care

Exhibit 8-1 The Eden Alternative Principles

1. The three plagues of loneliness, helplessness and boredom account for the bulk of suffering among our Elders.

2. An Elder-centered community commits to creating a Human Habitat where life revolves around close and continuing contact with plants, animals and children. It is these relationships that provide the young and old alike with a pathway to a life worth living.

3. Loving companionship is the antidote to loneliness. Elders deserve easy access to human and animal companionship.

4. An Elder-centered community creates opportunity to give as well as receive care. This is the antidote to helplessness.

5. An Elder-centered community imbues daily life with variety and spontaneity by creating an environment in which unexpected and unpredictable interactions and happenings can take place. This is the antidote to boredom.

6. Meaningless activity corrodes the human spirit. The opportunity to do things that we find meaningful is essential to human health.

7. Medical treatment should be the servant of genuine human caring, never its master.

8. An Elder-centered community honors its Elders by de-emphasizing top-down bureaucratic authority, seeking instead to place the maximum possible decision-making authority into the hands of the Elders or into the hands of those closest to them.

9. Creating an Elder-centered community is a never-ending process. Human growth must never be separated from human life.

10. Wise leadership is the lifeblood of any struggle against the three plagues. For it, there can be no substitute.

Source: Eden Alternative. Retrieved April 2009 from http://www.edenalt.org/about/our-10-principles.html. Used with permission of Eden Alternative®.

of plants and animals, and in interaction with children such as playing with them, helping them color, or reading them stories, enriches everyone's lives. A facility can have an on-site child day care center, providing opportunities to integrate child care with the care of the elderly. Children playing with toys in the facility's living room, or playing outdoors on a swing and slide set add to variety and spontaneity. But edenizing goes beyond these steps. It also incorporates other aspects of culture change, such as resident and caregiver empowerment.

Actions by a few states, such as North Carolina and South Carolina, to establish coalitions promoting the Eden Alternative have legitimized the concept by establishing partnerships with the respective state's regulatory and public health agencies. Voluntary regional coordinators have also been appointed in various locations across the country, under the auspices of the Eden organization, to promote education about the Eden Alternative and to create a registry program to recognize organizations that make a commitment to change. On the other hand, widespread adoption of the Eden principles by individual nursing homes has failed to materialize; only 300 to 400 facilities (2% or less) nationwide have edenized to date.

Published literature on the actual outcomes of edenizing is scant, but one unpublished study of five nursing homes in Texas concluded that adopting the Eden Alternative had decreased behavioral incidents by 60%, formation of pressure sores by 57%, prevalence of bed confinement by 25%, and use of restraints by 18%. Positive outcomes were also reported on increased occupancy (11%), reduced employee absenteeism (48%), and decreased worker injuries (11%) (Cerquone, 2001). A more recent study reported lower levels of boredom and helplessness, but not loneliness (Bergman-Evans, 2004). Some individual nursing homes have also reported decreases in staff turnover as a result of edenizing. On the other hand, a peer-reviewed published study that compared an edenized facility with a control (nonedenized) facility, using indicators of residents' well-being measured at baseline and a year later, reported that the Eden site had significantly greater proportions of residents who had fallen, residents who were experiencing nutritional problems, and those who required hypnotic drug prescriptions. However, because of a number of uncontrolled variables in the study, the authors concluded that quantitative measures suggested no major effects of the Eden intervention, but anecdotal qualitative information indicated that an extended period of implementation of edenizing may yield positive changes (Coleman et al., 2002). In short, at this time, scientific evidence in favor of the Eden Alternative remains inconclusive.

Edenizing may pose some risks in the form of allergies, injuries, and illnesses. *Zoonosis* is the transmittal of infections from vertebrate animals to humans. Examples of zoonotic diseases include dermatophytosis, psittacosis, bartonellosis, toxocariasis, pasturellosis, Q fever, and leptospirosis (Guay, 2001). However, potential problems can be managed with appropriate veterinary care and infection-control practices.

Proponents of the Eden Alternative explain that their approach is not a quick fix for serious problems. Not every facility should embark on making such changes. Acceptance of the Eden Alternative by staff members and their training are necessary prerequisites because, right off the bat, questions come up about the staff's extra responsibilities of caring for the pets and cleaning up after them. Particularly in unionized facilities where union–management contracts prescribe tasks and duties of staff members, edenizing can be challenging. Costs of training and implementation may be another deterrent: in 2000, the costs to implement the Eden Alternative were estimated to be $30,000 over two years (Reese, 2000). Also, the quality of life in long-term care facilities can be improved in ways other than edenizing.

Changing an organization's culture takes time, effort, and leadership skills. Implementing the Eden principles can take an estimated three to five years (Hannan & Schaeffer, 2003).

The Green House Project

The founder of the Eden Alternative had envisioned edenizing as a never-ending process. But, perhaps because of the inherent difficulties in initiating and maintaining the necessary changes in large institutional settings, the Eden model has not been widely adopted (Rabig, 2003). An outgrowth of the Eden Alternative, and also a brainchild of Dr. Thomas, the Green House Project takes edenizing a step further by revolutionizing the way in which nursing home services are organized and delivered in small-scale settings.

In the New York State pilot project described earlier, Thomas experimented with restructuring the caregiving staff into permanent care teams designed to serve a particular "neighborhood" of elders according to those elders' special needs. The teams—consisting of nurses, social workers, housekeepers, dietary employees, and members of the activities staff—tried to adapt the traditional large-scale caregiving approach for smaller groups of residents. Each team participated in extensive training in communication and problem solving, and some teams eventually became responsible for scheduling their own hours of work (Hannan & Schaeffer, 2003). In the Green House model, these organizational ideas are applied to physically distinct small-neighborhood architectural units. Also, unlike edenizing a large institutional structure, the Green House model relies more on natural outdoor activities, such as watching and feeding birds and squirrels, and less on indoor pets because the small design of the buildings allows ready access to the outdoors (Rabig, 2003).

The term **Green House** stands for architectural renderings of small freestanding cottages, each designed to house just 7 to 10 residents who live together in a homelike setting (Figure 8–5). The freestanding cottages are spread across a campus (Figure 8–6). The first Green House project in Tupelo, Mississippi, opened its doors in June 2003.

Each Green House has self-contained private rooms that include a commode, a sink, and a shower. To accommodate even the frailest elders, rooms are equipped with ceiling lifts for transferring. The lift operates on a ceiling track that runs from the bed to the bathroom sink and commode. In some instances, these lifts can be operated independently by the residents. Residents can bring their own furniture and they can choose their room's décor. The residential units are connected by short hallways to a central hearth room, open kitchen, and dining area. Other amenities include a spa room, laundry room, alcove, and storage space. The small size eliminates the need for nursing stations and

medication carts. The nurse-call system is wireless, using silent pagers that can be activated from pendants worn by the residents (Rabig & Thomas, 2003). In all aspects, the Green Houses fully comply with *Life Safety Code* and other building and safety standards described in Chapter 6.

Each Green House is staffed by cross-trained nursing assistants, who do cooking and cleaning in addition to delivering personal care. The Green Houses are supported by the traditional organization of a skilled nursing facility in which functions such as professional nursing, rehabilitation therapies, medical records, accounting, billing, purchasing, and plant maintenance are located (Rabig & Thomas, 2003). The cross-trained, self-managed worker teams create a decentralized organizational structure that eliminates the typical supervisor–subordinate relationships. Interdisciplinary clinical support teams that include physicians, nurses, therapists, social workers, dieticians, and others located in the support organization carry out individualized clinical assessment and care planning and visit the elders to meet their treatment needs. Clinical practice guidelines based on medical research and standards, as well as emergency protocols, are developed for use by caregivers (Rabig & Thomas, 2003).

The Green House Project proposes other cultural changes, such as referring to the cross-trained workers as "elder assistants" instead of "nursing assistants" or "nurse aides" and referring to patients as "elders" instead of "residents," who are "welcomed into" rather than "admitted to" the Green Houses. Physicians, nurses, and other clinical professionals who visit the patients are expected to assume a "visitor's role" and behave as guests, giving the elders the maximum control possible over clinical information

Figure 8-5 10-Bed Skilled Nursing Green House (Methodist Senior Services, Tupelo, Mississippi)

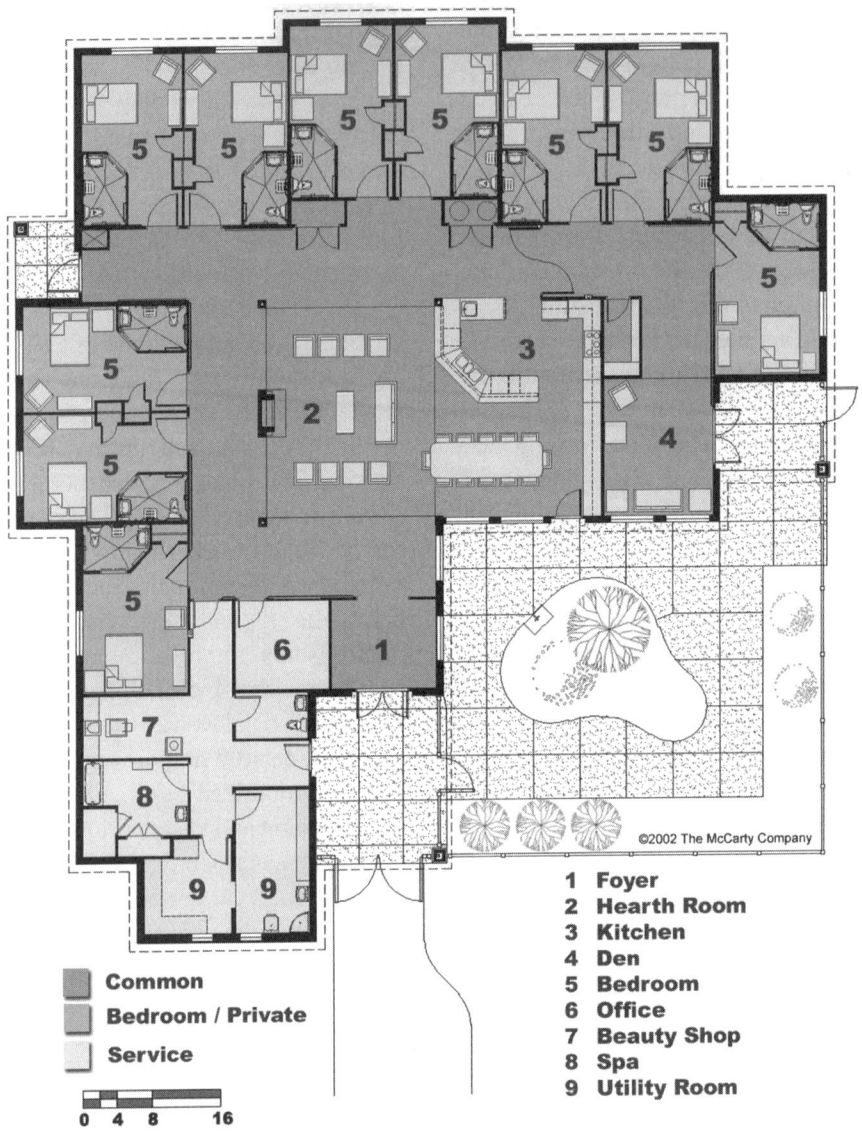

■ **Common**	1 **Foyer**
■ **Bedroom / Private**	2 **Hearth Room**
□ **Service**	3 **Kitchen**
	4 **Den**
	5 **Bedroom**
	6 **Office**
	7 **Beauty Shop**
	8 **Spa**
	9 **Utility Room**

0 4 8   16

©2002 The McCarty Company

Source: The McCarthy Company, Tupelo, Mississippi. Reprinted with permission from The McCarty Company (courtesy of Stephen Ladd).

and decisions. Individual choices and preferences are preserved by allowing the elders the maximum possible latitude in establishing their own daily routines for sleep, rest, meals, personal care, and activities. Elders are also encouraged to participate in meal preparation, gardening, cleaning, and laundry work. Weekly joint meetings or "house discussions" between elder assistants and elders provide feedback on quality of care, identify unmet

Figure 8-6 Overhead Perspective of Green Houses (small residential structures spread across a campus)

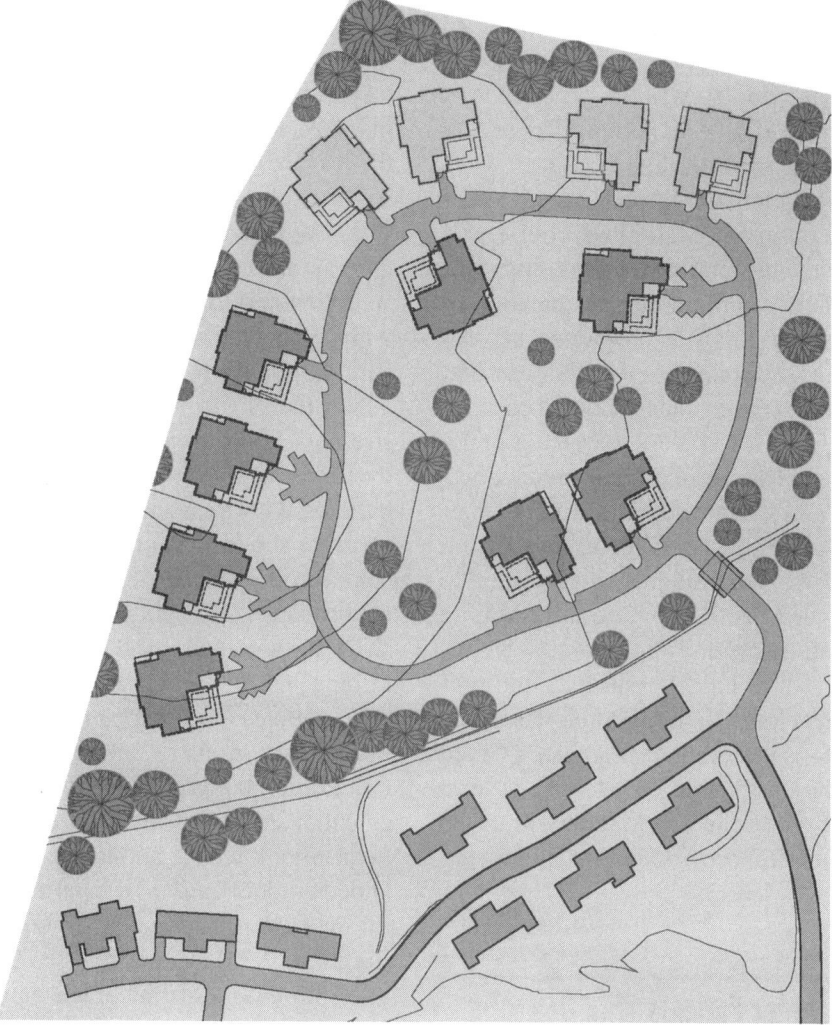

Source: The McCarty Company. Schematic Site Plan: Greenhouse Project, Methodist Senior Services, Tupelo, Mississippi. Reprinted with permission from the McCarty Company (courtesy of Stephen Ladd).

needs or concerns, and give input for household decisions (Rabig & Thomas, 2003).

The Green House philosophy requires close relationships between staff members and elders based on the concept of *intentional community*, the intrinsic need shared by elders and caregivers to "come together" to form a bond and "live together" for a common purpose. For example, the concept is applied when assistants and elders sit around a large common dining table and together enjoy a family-style meal. The assistant may help feed the patient sitting in the next chair. Even tube-fed patients may be brought to the dining table for sensory stimulation from the music, the chatter, and the aroma. The term *convivium* (from Latin, meaning "feast" or, more broadly, "living together") is used in Green Houses to describe the experience of a pleasurable dining experience in an enriched environment (Rabig, 2003).

To date, a number of positive outcomes have been observed: high satisfaction levels among residents, family members, and staff; few regulatory complaints; no unexpected weight loss and almost no nutritional supplement use; less decline in ADLs; staff turnover of less than 10%; no transfer-related back injuries to elders or staff; less prevalence of depression; and less use of anti-psychotic drugs (Robert Wood Johnson Foundation, 2005).

The Robert Wood Johnson Foundation has awarded a $10 million five-year grant to NCB Development Corp. to establish more Green Houses around the country. NCB's staff provides technical assistance and predevelopment loans to support long-term care organizations that want to establish a Green House. The objective is to establish at least one Green House in every state within the next 5 years (Robert Wood Johnson Foundation, 2005).

Environment for Patients With Dementia

For people with dementia, small groupings of residents in a setting that resembles a home—and not a large institution—provide a more effective therapeutic setting. The smaller scale of the living quarters reduces stress that such patients may experience from the overwhelming effect of being placed in complex, unfamiliar surroundings. This is because a link to the person's past home environments becomes essential for exercising his or her remaining capabilities. In dementia patients, long-term memory generally remains relatively intact until the later stages of the disease (Cohen & Day, 1993).

In a pilot study, Brush et al. (2002) found that improved lighting and table-setting contrast had a positive effect on food consumption and functional abilities of patients with dementia. Generally, a moderate level of stimulation from the environment is best. When the environment provides too many stressors and fewer opportunities to relax, dysfunctional behaviors are observed among patients with dementia (Rader, 1991). Unpleasant sounds, intense lighting, and bold colors produce a high level of stimulation that causes stress. For patients with Alzheimer's, sharp color contrasts and patterns can be disturbing. Pastel colors tend to work best for these patients (Kretschmann, 1995).

Patient safety is an important factor. Electronic guards to prevent wandering are essential. Protected pathways for wandering, residential kitchens and laundries, and contained outdoor gardens are particularly helpful in caring for patients with dementia (Regnier, 1998). Nature-related activities are often an essential but unused therapeutic resource in environments for people with dementia (Day & Cohen, 2000). Connection to nature extends to people's interaction with animals. There is some evidence that meaningful decreases in agitated behaviors and improvements in social interactions of dementia patients can occur as a result of pet therapy (Richeson, 2003).

For Further Thought

1. As a nursing home administrator who has just been appointed to manage a skilled nursing facility that was built in the 1970s, how would you go about delivering person-centered care?

2. Many nursing homes have limited financial resources. What can they do to enrich their environments?

3. The presence of dogs and cats does not appeal to everyone because of allergies or other health-related factors. As a nursing home administrator, how would you address such concerns?

For Further Learning

Eden Alternative: Official website

www.edenalt.com

The Green House Project. Access through the NCB Capital website

http://www.ncbcapitalimpact.org

The Pioneer Network: Official website

http://www.pioneernetwork.net

REFERENCES

Agich, G.J. 1995. Actual autonomy and long-term care decision making. In L.B. McCullough and N.L. Wilson (eds.). *Long-Term Care Decisions: Ethical and Conceptual Dimensions* (pp. 113–136). Baltimore: Johns Hopkins University Press.

Andreoli, N.A., et al. 2007. Serving culture change at mealtimes. *Nursing Homes: Long Term Care Management* 56, no. 9: 48–50.

Arras, J.D. 1995. Conflicting interests in long-term care decision making: Acknowledging, dissolving, and resolving conflicts. In L.B. McCullough and N.L. Wilson (eds.). *Long-Term Care Decisions: Ethical and Conceptual Dimensions* (pp. 197–217). Baltimore: Johns Hopkins University Press.

Bergman-Evans, B. 2004. Beyond the basics: Effects of the Eden Alternative Model on quality of life issues. *Journal of Gerontological Nursing* 30, no. 6: 27–34.

Brawley, E.C. 1997. *Designing for Alzheimer's Disease: Strategies for Creating Better Care Environments.* New York: John Wiley & Sons.

Brawley, E., & Noell-Waggoner, E. Undated. Lighting: Partner in Quality Care Environments. Retrieved April 2009 from http://www.pioneernetwork.net/Data/Documents/BrawleyNoell-WagonerLightingPaper.pdf.

Browning, M.B. 2003. Letter to the author dated August 18, 2003, on cluster design plan.

Bruck, L. 1997. Welcome to Eden. *Nursing Homes Long Term Care Management* 46, no. 1: 28–33.

Brush, J.A., et al. 2002. Using the environment to improve intake for people with dementia. *Alzheimer's Care Quarterly* 3, no. 4: 330–338.

Cerquone, J. 2001. Administrating Eden. *Balance* 5, no. 6: 4–6.

Chapman, S.A., et al. 2003. Client-centered, community-based care for frail seniors. *Health and Social Care in the Community* 11, no. 3: 253–261.

Child, M. 1999. Comfort is the key. *Nursing Homes Long Term Care Management* 48, no. 9: 61–62.

Cohen, U., & Day, K. 1993. *Contemporary Environments for People with Dementia*. Baltimore: Johns Hopkins University Press.

Coleman, M.T., et al. 2002. The Eden Alternative: Findings after 1 year of implementation. *Journal of Gerontology* 57A, no. 7: M422–M427.

Collopy, B.J. 1988. Autonomy in long-term care: some crucial distinctions. *The Gerontologist* 28, suppl.: 10–17.

Collopy, B.J. 1995. Safety and independence: Rethinking some basic concepts in long-term care. In L.B. McCullough and N.L. Wilson (eds.). *Long-term care decisions: Ethical and conceptual dimensions* (pp. 137–152). Baltimore: Johns Hopkins University Press.

Day, K., & Cohen, U. 2000. The role of culture in designing environments for people with dementia: A study of Russian Jewish immigrants. *Environment and Behavior* 32, no. 3: 361–399.

Doty, M.M., et al. 2008. *Culture Change in Nursing Homes: How Far Have We Come?* New York: The Commonwealth Fund.

Drew, S.G. 1992. Designing for special needs of the elderly. In A. Bush-Brown and D. Davis (eds.). *Hospitable Design for Healthcare and Senior Communities*. New York: Van Nostrand Reinhold.

Dunkelman, D.M. 1992. Individualized cluster. In A. Bush-Brown and D. Davis (eds.). *Hospitable Design for Healthcare and Senior Communities*. New York: Van Nostrand Reinhold.

Eales, J., et al. 2001. Seniors' experiences of client-centered residential care. *Aging and Society* 21: 279–296.

Eden Alternative, The. 2002. What is Eden? http://www.edenalt.com/about.htm.

Eden Annual 2003. 2003. *Come Grow with Us*. In J. Thomas (ed.). Norwich, NY: Chenango Union Printing.

Guay, D. 2001. Pet-assisted therapy in the nursing home setting: Potential for zoonosis. *American Journal of Infection Control* 29, no. 3: 178–186.

Haight, B.K., et al. 2002. Thriving: A life span theory. *Journal of Gerontological Nursing* 28, no. 3: 15–22.

Hannan, M., & Schaeffer, K. 2003. The Eden Alternative: More than just fuzzy props and potted plants. http://www.edenmidwest.com/about_eden.html.

Jones, M.M., & Haight, B.K. 2002. Environmental transformations: An integrative review. *Journal of Gerontological Nursing* 28, no. 3: 23–27.

Kane, R.A. 2001. Long-term care and a good quality of life: Bringing them closer together. *The Gerontologist* 41, no. 3: 293–304.

Kretschmann, A. 1995. Design touches to make the SCU a "home." *Nursing Homes Long Term Care Management* 44, no. 6: 31–34.

Kruzich, J.M. & Berg. W. 1985. Predictors of self-sufficiency for the mentally ill in long term care. *Community Mental Health Journal* 21, no. 3: 198–207.

McLeod, B.W. 2002. *And Thou Shalt Honor: A Caregiver's Companion*. Emmaus, PA: Rodale Press. www.rodalestore.com.

National Center for Health Statistics. 2007. *Health, United States 2007*. Hyattsville, MD: Department of Health and Human Services.

Noell, E. 1995. Design in nursing homes: Environment as a silent partner in caregiving. *Generations* 19, no. 4: 14–19.

Nursing home architecture. 1997. *Contemporary Long-term Care* 20, no. 8: 43–44.

Park, S. & Mattson, R.H. 2008. Effects of flowering and foliage plants in hospital rooms on patients recovering from abdominal surgery. *HortTechnology* 18: 549–745.

Parsons, T. 1972. Definitions of health and illness in the light of American values and social structure. In E.G. Jaco (ed). *Patients, Physicians and Illness: A Sourcebook in Behavioral Science and Health*, 2nd ed. New York: Free Press.

Rabig, J. 2003. Personal conversation, September 25, 2003.

Rabig, J., & Thomas, W. 2003. The Green House project: An alternative model of elder care. Unpublished manuscript.

Rader, J. 1991. Modifying the environment to decrease use of restraints. *Journal of Gerontological Nursing* 17, no. 2: 9–13.

Ragsdale, V., & McDougall, G.J. 2008. The changing face of long-term care: Looking at the past decade. *Issues in Mental Health Nursing* 29, no. 9: 992–1001.

Reese, D. 2000. Alternative lifestyle. *Contemporary Long-term Care* 23, no. 7: 38–42.

Regnier, V. 1998. Look homeward. *Contemporary Long-term Care* 21, no. 3: 92–94.

Richeson, N.E. 2003. Effects of animal-assisted therapy on agitated behaviors and social interactions of older adults with dementia. *American Journal of Alzheimer's Disease & Other Dementias* 18, no. 6: 353–358.

Robert Wood Johnson Foundation. 2005. Developing small community homes as alternatives to nursing homes. Retrieved January 2009 from http://www.rwjf.org/newsroom/newsreleases detail.jsp?productid=21757.

Schwarz, B. 1996. *Nursing Home Design: Consequences of Employing the Medical Model*. New York: Garland Publishing.

Stermer, M. 1998. Notes from an Eden alternative pioneer. *Nursing Homes Long Term Care Management* 47, no. 11: 35–36.

West, S.K., et al. 2003. A randomized trial of visual impairment interventions for nursing home residents: Study design, baseline characteristics and visual loss. *Ophthalmic Epidemiology* 10, no. 3: 193–209.

Westin, A. 1967. *Privacy and Freedom*. New York: Atheneum Press.

Wiener, J.M., et al. 2007. *Nursing Home Quality: Twenty Years After the Omnibus Budget Reconciliation Act of 1987*. Menlo Park, CA: Henry J. Kaiser Family Foundation.

Wilson, E.O. 1984. *Biophilia: The Human Bond with Other Species*. Cambridge, MA: Harvard University Press.

Wohlwill, J.F. 1983. The concept of nature: a psychologist's view. In I. Altman and J.F. Wohlwill (eds.). *Behavior and the Natural Environment* (pp. 5–37). New York: Plenum Press.

Yarme, J., & Yarme, H. 2001. Flooring and safety. *Nursing Homes Long Term Care Management* 50, no. 10: 82–83.

Appendix 8-1 Artifacts of Culture Change

Home Name _____ Date _____	
City _____ State _____ Current number of residents _____	
Ownership: _____ For Profit _____ Non-Profit _____ Government	

Care Practice Artifacts	
1. **Percentage of residents who offered any of the following styles of dining:** • **restaurant style where staff take resident orders;** • **buffet style where residents help themselves or tell staff what they want;** • **family style where food is served in bowls on dining tables where residents help themselves or staff assist them:** • **open dining where meal is available for at least 2 hour time period and residents can come when they choose; and** • **24 hour dining where residents can order food from the kitchen 24 hours a day.**	_____ 100 – 81% (5 points) _____ 80 – 61% (4 points) _____ 60 – 41% (3 points) _____ 40 – 21% (2 points) _____ 20 – 1% (1 point) _____ 0 (0 points)
2. **Snacks/drinks available at all times to all residents at no additional cost, i.e., in a stocked pantry, refrigerator, or snack bar.**	_____ All residents (5 points) _____ Some (3 points) _____ None (0 points)
3. **Baked goods are baked on resident living areas.**	_____ All days of the week (5 point) _____ 2–5 days/week (3 points) _____ < 2 days/week (0 points)
4. **Home celebrates residents' individual birthdays rather than, or in addition to, celebrating resident birthdays in a group each month.**	_____ Yes (5 points) _____ No (0 points)
5. **Home offers aromatherapy to residents by staff or volunteers.**	_____ Yes (5 points) _____ No (0 points)
6. **Home offers massage to residents by staff or volunteers.**	_____ Yes (5 points) _____ No (0 points)

(continues)

Appendix 8-1 Artifacts of Culture Change (Continued)

7. Home has dog(s) and/or cat(s).	_____ At least one dog or one cat lives on premises (5 points) _____ The only animals in the building are when staff bring them during work hours (3 points) _____ The only animals in the building are those brought in for special activities or by families (1 point) _____ None (0 points)
8. Home permits residents to bring own dog and/or cat to live with them in the home.	_____ Yes (5 points) _____ No (0 points)
9. Waking times/bedtimes chose by residents.	_____ All residents (5 points) _____ Some (3 points) _____ None (0 points)
10. _Bathing without a Battle_ **techniques are used with residents.**	_____ All residents (5 points) _____ Some (3 points) _____ None (0 points)
11. Residents can get a bath/shower as often as they would like.	_____ Yes (5 points) _____ No (0 points)
12. Home arranges for someone to be with a dying resident at all times (unless they prefer to be alone)—family, friends, volunteers, or staff.	_____ Yes (5 points) _____ No (0 points)
13. Memorials/remembrances are held for individual residents upon death.	_____ Yes (5 points) _____ No (0 points)
14. "I" format care plans, in the voice of the resident and in the first person, are used.	_____ All care plans (5 points) _____ Some (3 points) _____ None (0 points)
Care Practice Artifacts Subtotal: Out of a total 70 points, you scored _____.	

(continues)

Appendix 8-1 Artifacts of Culture Change (Continued)

Environmental Artifacts	
15. Percent of residents who live in households that are self-contained with full kitchen, living room, and dining room.	_____ 100 – 81% (100 points) _____ 80 – 61% (80 points) _____ 60 – 41% (60 points) _____ 40 – 21% (40 points) _____ 20 – 1% (20 point) _____ 0 (0 points)
16. Percent of residents in private rooms.	_____ 100 – 81% (50 points) _____ 80 – 61% (40 points) _____ 60 – 41% (30 points) _____ 40 – 21% (20 points) _____ 20 – 1% (10 point) _____ 0 (0 points)
17. Percent of residents in privacy enhanced shared rooms where residents can access their own space without trespassing through the other resident's space. This does not include the traditional privacy curtain.	_____ 100 – 81% (25 points) _____ 80 – 61% (20 points) _____ 60 – 41% (15 points) _____ 40 – 21% (10 points) _____ 20 – 1% (5 point) _____ 0 (0 points)
18. No traditional nurses' stations or traditional nurses' stations have been removed.	_____ No traditional nurses stations (25 points) _____ Some traditional nurses' stations have been removed (15 points) _____ Traditional nurses' stations remain in place (0 points)
19. Percent of residents who have a direct window view not past another resident's bed.	_____ 100 – 51% (5 points) _____ 50 – 0% (0 points)
20. Resident bathroom mirrors are wheelchair accessible and/or adjustable in order to be visible to a seated or standing resident.	_____ All resident bathroom mirrors (5 points) _____ Some (3 points) _____ None (0 points)

(continues)

Appendix 8-1 Artifacts of Culture Change (Continued)

21. **Sinks in resident bathrooms are wheelchair accessible with clearance below sink for wheelchair.**	_____ All resident bathroom sinks (5 points) _____ Some (3 points) _____ None (0 points)
22. **Sinks used by residents have adaptive/easy-to-use lever or paddle handles.**	_____ All sinks (5 points) _____ Some (3 points) _____ None (0 points)
23. **Adaptive handles, enhanced for easy use, for doors used by residents (rooms, bathrooms, and public areas).**	_____ All resident-used doors (5 points) _____ Some (3 points) _____ None (0 points)
24. **Closets have movable rods that can be set to different heights.**	_____ All closets (5 points) _____ Some (3 points) _____ None (0 points)
25. **Home has no rule prohibiting, and residents are welcome, to decorate their rooms any way they wish including using nails, tape, screws, etc.**	_____ Yes (5 points) _____ No (0 points)
26. **Home makes available extra lighting source in resident room if requested by resident such as floor lamps and reading lamps.**	_____ Yes (5 points) _____ No (0 points)
27. **Heat/air conditioning controls can be adjusted in resident rooms.**	_____ All resident rooms (5 points) _____ Some (3 points) _____ None (0 points)
28. **Home providers or invites residents to have their own refrigerators.**	_____ Yes (5 points) _____ No (0 points)
29. **Chairs and sofas in public areas have seat heights that vary to comfortably accommodate people of different heights.**	_____ Chair seat heights vary by 3" or more (5 points) _____ Chair seat heights vary by 1–3" (3 points) _____ Chair seat heights do not vary in height (0 points)
30. **Gliders that lock into place when person rises are available inside the home and/or outside.**	_____ Yes (5 points) _____ No (0 points)

(continues)

Appendix 8-1 Artifacts of Culture Change (Continued)

31. **Home has store/gift shop/cart available where residents and visitors can purchase gifts, toiletries, snacks, etc.**	_____ Yes (5 points) _____ No (0 points)
32. **Residents have regular access to computer/Internet and adaptations are available for independent computer use such as large keyboard or touch screen.**	_____ Both Internet access and adaptations (10 points) _____ Access without adaptations (5 points) _____ Neither (0 points)
33. **Workout room available to residents.**	_____ Yes (5 points) _____ No (0 points)
34. **Bathing rooms have functional and properly installed heat lamps, radiant heat panels, or equivalent.**	_____ All bathing rooms (5 points) _____ Some (3 points) _____ None (0 points)
35. **Home warms towels for resident bathing.**	_____ Yes (5 points) _____ No (0 points)
36. **Protected outdoor garden/patio accessible for independent use by residents.** Residents can go in and out independently, including those who use wheelchairs, e.g., residents do not need assistance from staff to open doors or overcome obstacles in traveling to patio.	_____ Yes (5 points) _____ No (0 points)
37. **Home has outdoor raised gardens available for resident use.**	_____ Yes (5 points) _____ No (0 points)
38. **Home has an outdoor walking/wheeling path that is not a city sidewalk or path.**	_____ Yes (5 points) _____ No (0 points)
39. **Pager/radio/telephone call system is used where resident calls register on staff's pagers/radios/telephones and staff can use it to communicate with fellow staff.**	_____ Yes (5 points) _____ No (0 points)
40. **Overhead paging system has been turned off or is only used in case of emergency.**	_____ Yes (5 points) _____ No (0 points)
41. **Personal clothing is laundered on resident household/neighborhood/unit instead of in an general all-home laundry, and residents/families have access to washer and dryer for own use.**	_____ Available to all residents (5 points) _____ Some (3 points) _____ None (0 points)
Environmental Artifacts: Out of a total 320 points, you scored _____.	

(continues)

Appendix 8-1 Artifacts of Culture Change (Continued)

Family and Community Artifacts	
42. Regularly scheduled intergenerational program in which children customarily interact with residents at least once a week.	_____ Yes (5 points) _____ No (0 points)
43. Home makes space available for community groups to meet in home with residents welcome to attend.	_____ Yes (5 points) _____ No (0 points)
44. Private guestroom available for visitors at no, or minimal, cost for overnight stays.	_____ Yes (5 points) _____ No (0 points)
45. Home has café/restaurant/tavern/canteen available to residents, families, and visitors at which residents and family can purchase food and drinks daily.	_____ Yes (5 points) _____ No (0 points)
46. Home has special dining room available for family use/ gatherings, which excludes regular dining areas.	_____ Yes (5 points) _____ No (0 points)
47. Kitchenette or kitchen area with at least a refrigerator and stove is available to families, residents, and staff where cooking and baking are welcomed.	_____ Yes (5 points) _____ No (0 points)
Family and Community Artifacts Subtotal: Out of a 30 possible points, you scored _____.	
Leadership Artifacts	
48. CNAs attend resident care conferences.	_____ All care conferences (5 points) _____ Some (3 points) _____ None (0 points)
49. Residents or family members serve on home quality assessment and assurance (QAA) (QI, CQI, QA) committee.	_____ Yes (5 points) _____ No (0 points)
50. Residents have an assigned staff member who serves as "buddy," case coordinator, Guardian Angel, etc. to check with the resident regularly and follow up on any concerns. This is in addition to any assigned social service staff.	_____ All New residents (5 points) _____ Some (3 points) _____ None (0 points)
51. Learning circles or equivalent are used regularly in staff and resident meetings in order to give each person the opportunity to share their opinion/ideas.	_____ Yes (5 points) _____ No (0 points)
52. Community Meetings are held on a regular basis bringing staff, residents, and families together as a community.	_____ Yes (5 points) _____ No (0 points)
Leadership Artifacts Subtotal: Out of a total 25 points, you scored _____.	

(continues)

Appendix 8-1 Artifacts of Culture Change (Continued)

Workplace Practice Artifacts	
53. RNs consistently work with the residents of the same neighborhood/household/unit (with no rotation).	_____ All RNs (5 points) _____ Some (3 points) _____ None (0 points)
54. LPNs consistently work with the residents of the same neighborhood/household/unit (with no rotations).	_____ All LPNs (5 points) _____ Some (3 points) _____ None (0 points)
55. CNAs consistently work with the residents of the same neighborhood/household/unit (with no rotation).	_____ All CNAs (5 points) _____ Some (3 points) _____ None (0 points)
56. Self-scheduling of work shifts. CNAs develop their own schedule and fill in for absent CNAs. CNAs independently handle the task of scheduling, trading shifts/days, and covering for each other instead of a staffing coordinator.	_____ All CNAs (5 points) _____ Some (3 points) _____ None (0 points)
57. Home pays expenses for nonmanagerial staff to attend outside conferences/workshops, e.g., CNAs, direct care nurses. Check yes if at least one nonmanagerial staff member attended an outside conference/workshop paid by home in past year.	_____ Yes (5 points) _____ No (0 points)
58. Staff is not required to wear uniforms or "scrubs."	_____ Yes (5 points) _____ No (0 points)
59. Percent of other staff cross-trained and certified as CNAs in addition to CNAs in the nursing department.	_____ 100 − 81% (5 points) _____ 80 − 61% (4 points) _____ 60 − 41% (3 points) _____ 40 − 21% (2 points) _____ 20 − 1% (1 point) _____ 0 (0 points)
60. Activities, informal or formal, are led by staff in other departments such as nursing and housekeeping or any departments.	_____ Yes (5 points) _____ No (0 points)
61. Awards given to staff to recognize commitment to person-directed care, e.g., Culture Change award, Champion of Change award. This does not include Employee of the Month.	_____ Yes (5 points) _____ No (0 points)
62. Career ladder positions for CNAs, e.g., CNA II, CNA III, team leader, etc. There is a career ladder for CNAs to hold a position higher than base level.	_____ Yes (5 points) _____ No (0 points)

(continues)

Appendix 8-1 Artifacts of Culture Change (Continued)

63. Job development program, e.g., CNA to LPN to RN to NP.	_____ Yes (5 points) _____ No (0 points)
64. Day care onsite available to staff.	_____ Yes (5 points) _____ No (0 points)
65. Home has on staff a paid volunteer coordinator in addition to activity director.	_____ Full time (30 hours/week or more) (5 points) _____ Part time (15–30 hours/week) (3 points) _____ No paid volunteer coordinator (0 pointss)
66. Employee evaluations include observable measures of employee support of individual resident choices, control and preferred routines in all aspects of daily living.	_____ All employee evaluations (5 points) _____ Some (3 points) _____ None (0 points)
Workplace Practice Artifacts Subtotal: Out of a total 70 points, you scored _____.	
Outcomes	
67. Average longevity of CNAs. Add length of employment in years of permanent CNAs and divide by number of staff.	_____ Your CNA average longevity Above 5 years (5 points) 3–5 years (3 points) Below 3 years (0 points)
68. Average longevity of LPNs (in any position). Add length of employment in years of permanent staff LPNs and divide by number of staff.	_____ Your LPN average longevity Above 5 years (5 points) 3–5 years (3 points) Below 3 years (0 points)
69. Average longevity of RN/GNs (in any position). Add length of employment in years of all permanent RN/GNs and divide by number of staff.	_____ Your RN/GN average longevity Above 5 years (5 points) 3–5 years (3 points) Below 3 years (0 points)
70. Longevity of the Director of Nursing (in any position).	_____ Longevity as DON _____ Longevity at home Above 5 years (5 points) 3–5 years (3 points) Below 3 years (0 points)

(continues)

Appendix 8-1 Artifacts of Culture Change (Continued)

71. Longevity of the Administrator (in any position).	_____ Longevity as NHA _____ Longevity at home Above 5 years (5 points) 3–5 years (3 points) Below 3 years (0 points)
72. Turnover rate for CNAs.	Number of CNAs who left, voluntary or involuntary, in previous 12 months divided by number of total CNAs employed = turnover rate Your home's figure _____ 0 percent (5 points) 20 – 39% (4 points) 40 – 59% (3 points) 60 – 79% (2 points) 80 – 99% (1 points) 100% and above (0 points)
73. Turnover rate for LPNs.	Number of LPNs who left, voluntary or involuntary, in previous 12 months divided by number of total LPNs employed = turnover rate Your home's figure _____ 0 – 12% (5 points) 13 – 25% (4 points) 26 – 38% (3 points) 39 – 51% (2 points) 52 – 65% (1 points) 66% and above (0 points)
74. Turnover rate for RNs.	Number of RNs who left, voluntary or involuntary, in previous 12 months divided by number of total RNs employed = turnover rate Your home's figure _____ 0 – 12% (5 points) 13 – 25% (4 points) 26 – 38% (3 points) 39 – 51% (2 points) 52 – 65% (1 points) 66% and above (0 points)

(continues)

Appendix 8-1 Artifacts of Culture Change (Continued)

75. Turnover rate for DONs.	_____ Number of DONs in the last 12 months 1 (5 points) 2 (3 points) 3 (0 points)
76. Turnover rate for Administrators.	_____ Number of NHAs in the last 12 months 1 (5 points) 2 (3 points) 3 (0 points)
77. Percent of CNA shifts covered by agency staff over the last month.	Total number of CNA shifts in a 24 hour period (all shifts no regardless of hours in a shift) _____ Multiplied by number of days in last the last full month _____ Of this number, number of shifts covered by an agency CNA _____ Your percentage (agency shifts/total number X days × 100) 0% (5 points) 1 − 5% (3 points) Over 5% (0 points)
79. Current occupancy rate.	_____ Your home figure Above 86% (5 points) At average 83 − 85% (3 points) Below 83% (0 points) (Using the national 2004 average of 84.2% form CMS)
Outcomes Subtotal: Out of a total 65 points, you scored _____.	

(*continues*)

Appendix 8-1 Artifacts of Culture Change (Continued)

Artifacts	Potential Points	Your Subtotal Scores
Care Practices	70	
Environment	320	
Family and Community	30	
Leadership	25	
Workplace Practice	70	
Outcomes	65	
Artifacts of Culture Change	**580**	**Grand Total**

Source: Developed by Centers for Medicare and Medicare Services and Edu-Catering, LLP. For more information contact Karen Schoeneman at karen.schoeneman@cms.hhs.gov or Carmen S. Bowman at carmen@edu-catering.com.

Chapter 9

John R. Pratt, MHA, FACHCA, LFACHE

Long-Term Care Reimbursement

What You Will Learn

- Understand how long-term care services are reimbursed.
- Identify and define key public sources of reimbursement, including Medicare and Medicaid.
- Identify and define private reimbursement sources, including private pay and private long-term care insurance.
- Understand how managed care works and its impact on long-term care.
- Understand the trends affecting long-term care reimbursement.

Introduction

The long-term care (LTC) system in the United States is reimbursement driven, meaning that the way care is provided is highly dependent on the way it is financed. Access to care, the availability of specific services, and even the quality of care provided are all dictated by the type and amount of reimbursement. It is unfortunate that such vital services are not universally and uniformly available, but the fact is they are not. Each of the provider segments along the continuum of care has its own unique mix of payment sources. Providers must understand what the various reimbursement agencies require of them. They have to understand the many different eligibility rules, the extent of coverage allowed, and the type and amount of documentation involved. It can be both bewildering and time-consuming.

The situation is even worse for consumers. As they move from one type or level of care to another, or even from one provider to another within the same provider category, they encounter a reimbursement system that must seem to them to be designed to be as confusing as possible. Long-term care reimbursement comes from a combination of public and private sources, but neither sector has satisfactory mechanisms for helping people anticipate and pay for their care (Weiner & Illston, 1993). This chapter presents an overview of current reimbursement options and methodologies, and it examines the trends and forces affecting the future of long-term care financing.

Origins and Development

The long-term care system has followed much the same pattern of development as the acute hospital system, although each stage seems to have developed somewhat later. Both systems began as charity-based care for all except the very wealthy. Most people needing health or custodial care received it at home, if there was someone available to provide it. As the need grew and families found themselves less able to care for the sick or disabled, private charitable organizations, often religious, took over some of the care in institutions operated and financed by them.

In time, state and federal governments began to get involved in protecting the welfare of the poor and needy. In 1935, following the Great Depression, Congress passed the Social Security Act, which included certain "categorical assistance" programs to help with care of the elderly, those who were blind, and families with dependent children (Goldsmith, 1994). This began serious government involvement in the financing of health care, including long-term care. During the next several decades, private coverage for hospital care became more available through formation of Blue Cross/Blue Shield plans and the growth of private health insurance. In the 1960s, with creation of the Medicare and Medicaid programs, government involvement in reimbursing health care was greatly expanded.

Yet with the exception of Medicaid, which requires individuals to become "medically indigent" to be eligible, little of this coverage applied to long-term care. Medicare reimbursement remained very limited. Private long-term care insurance was virtually nonexistent. Those with private financial resources had to use them to pay for their care. That situation remained pretty much the same up to the 1990s, when several factors forced the government, the long-term care industry, and society in general to reconsider how the system should be financed.

First, the number of elderly needing ever-larger amounts of long-term care was large and growing exponentially. In part because of this, the costs associated with providing long-term care were escalating. This made it more difficult for individuals to pay for their own long-term care, which, in turn, increased the burden on state governments funding Medicaid to the point where they were in desperate need of new financing sources, or at least new reimbursement methodologies.

These pressures have led to a considerable amount of examination of existing ways of reimbursing for long-term care services. They have also stimulated some reimbursement initiatives, which are discussed later in this chapter, but there has not been any significant improvement in either methods or results. The abortive Clinton healthcare financing reform effort in 1994, even had it passed, would have done little to change reimbursement of long-term care.

Current Reimbursement Options

An overview of the options that are currently available for financing of the long-term care system in general, and for reimbursing the individual segments, begins this discussion. These options can be broken into three categories for easier study: public sources, private sources, and public–private partnerships.

Public Reimbursement Sources

Medicare and Medicaid are by far the most prominent sources of public funding of long-term care and other types of health care. They were both created in 1965 as amendments to the Social Security Act. A centerpiece of

President Lyndon B. Johnson's Great Society, the two programs provided first-time healthcare coverage for millions of Americans. They have been amended many times in the past three decades, most often clarifying eligibility rules or tightening enforcement of provider regulations. Now, they are being reviewed with major change in mind. New payment methods are being tried, and the very structure of the programs is under review.

Medicare

The Medicare program was created as Title XVIII of the Social Security Act. Its primary purpose was to provide healthcare coverage for the elderly, who were defined at that time as anyone 65 years of age or older. In 1972 provisions were added to the act to include people who were permanently disabled and those with kidney disease.

The four main elements of the program are Part A, which provides hospital insurance, including some sections of long-term care (skilled care, home health care, hospice); Part B, which provides supplementary medical insurance that covers physician care; Part C, the so-called Medicare Advantage plans that deal with managed care organizations; and Part D, which covers medications. Parts A and B are the sections most closely related to long-term care, so we concentrate on them in our discussions in this chapter.

Part A is automatic for anyone meeting the eligibility criteria. Part B is purchased by beneficiaries with payment of a small premium. That separation pretty well defines the major thrust of the program. It is oriented to the acute care, medical model. Although some limited forms of long-term care coverage have been added over the years, this was not the original intent of the Medicare program.

Medicare is an entitlement program, meaning that anyone belonging to a particular population group is entitled to coverage. There is no requirement that recipients demonstrate financial need (as there is with Medicaid). The wealthiest retiree has the same rights to Medicare coverage as the poorest. This has become a major issue in recent years as the program struggles to provide coverage for a population that has grown many times faster than was predicted. In fact, the funding source for the program, the Medicare Trust Fund, is currently in considerable jeopardy. In their 2008 report, the trustees of the fund stated that the financial condition of the Social Security and Medicare programs remains problematic and that projected long-run program costs are not sustainable under current financing arrangements. Social Security' current annual surpluses of tax income over expenditures will begin to decline in 2011 and then turn into rapidly growing deficits as the baby boom generation retires. Medicare' financial status is even worse. In 2008, Medicare' Hospital Insurance (HI) Trust Fund would pay out more in hospital benefits and other expenditures than it received in taxes and other dedicated revenues, with the difference to made up from general revenues that pay for interest credits to the Trust Fund. Growing annual deficits are projected to exhaust HI reserves in 2019 and Social Security reserves in 2041 (CMS, 2008).

There is widespread disagreement about what should be done to solve the problem, but there is virtually complete agreement that there is a problem.

Why does this situation exist? When Medicare was developed in the 1960s, it adopted the retirement age built into the Social Security Act in 1935. At that time (1935) the average life expectancy was far shorter than today. However, from 1900 through 2004, life expectancy at birth increased from 46 to 75 years for men and from 48 to 80 years for women (NCHS, 2007). Sixty-five was chosen initially as a retirement age on the assumption that a relatively small number of people would take advantage of it and would not live for many years thereafter. Because the life span has increased steadily to where it is today, many more people now qualify for Medicare. What is more significant is the number of years each of them can expect to continue qualifying and continue to collect benefits.

Longer life is not the only factor not adequately anticipated by the framers of the Medicare program. They also failed to realize that increased availability of coverage would lead to increased usage. The frequency with which people visited their doctors or were admitted to hospitals was part of the equation used to predict the rate at which Medicare funds would be needed in the future. Although there was undoubtedly some consideration of inflation, there appears to have been no realization that many of the elderly were not availing themselves of medical services for the simple reason that they could not afford them. Once the Medicare program made those services available, the rush was on. Pent-up demand for needed, although postponable, care resulted in considerably more usage of health care than had been expected.

The politicians and others responsible for developing Medicare (probably innocently) contributed to the use, and even overuse, of Medicare when they touted it as being much more all-inclusive than it actually was. As they got caught up in the euphoria of having taken such a major step toward helping the elderly with their medical needs, they were not above implying that it would meet most, if not all, of those needs. In fact, it was never intended to do that. This erroneous public perception led many of the elderly, and their families, to expect much more from Medicare than it could provide.

During the more than 40 years of Medicare's life, medical technology has also developed and expanded at an unprecedented rate. That technology has created new treatments, the ability of which to save lives and improve the quality of life could hardly be denied by a public entitlement program. An example of the extent of the problem that introduction of such technological improvements has caused is treatment for end-stage renal disease. Patients who would have died can now live prolonged, useful lives through the wonders of renal dialysis. As beneficial as these treatments are, they are also ongoing and expensive. Finding it difficult to deny such life-saving treatment, and anticipating a relatively small volume of usage, the Medicare program added it to the list of categories of eligibility, regardless of the age of the patient. Kidney transplantation soon became a viable alternative to dialysis. Although very expensive initially, it eliminated the need for very costly, thrice-weekly treatments, although it did require life-long use of extremely expensive medications. It, too, was allowed as a Medicare-reimbursable procedure.

It is not hard to guess what happened next. The technology continued to improve, and large numbers of patients became medically eligible for dialysis, transplantation, or both. As with most medical technology, it became more expensive, not less so. Also, those receiving such treatments lived for years, and the cost to Medicare for this one category mushroomed; yet once it had been given as an entitlement, it could not easily be taken away.

This example represents much of what has happened to the overall Medicare program. It is, in many ways, suffering from its own success. It is worth noting here that, as other types of organ transplantation (e.g., heart, lung) became medically feasible, the Medicare program did not rush to include them, having learned from its experience with kidney transplants. Even in that, there has been criticism from those people needing such transplants because they feel discriminated against.

What does all of this have to do with long-term care? It is indicative of the systemic problems facing Medicare in the next few years. It is also why adding any new coverage is difficult. As noted earlier, long-term care was not intended to be a major component of Medicare. Attempts to find less costly alternatives to hospitalization and other institutionalization have led the program to add coverage for some types of long-term care, including subacute care, home health care, and hospice care. In many cases, however, experience is showing that the elderly using these services are not necessarily those who would otherwise be institutionalized. When this is the case, those services become added, rather than replacement, costs. Nevertheless, providing coverage of more forms of care does give Medicare a more prominent role in the reimbursement of long-term care than has been traditional. It is likely that it is a role that will continue to grow as the system experiences further pressures to reduce costs.

Medicare: What's Covered?

The Medicare coverage situation is changing so rapidly that it is not feasible to attempt to describe it in detail here, because any such description would soon be outdated. However, the following is a brief summary of the long-term care services Medicare does cover at this time.

Skilled Nursing Services

Medicare covers what it defines as "skilled nursing care" in nursing facilities or units in hospitals. Skilled nursing facilities (SNFs) may be freestanding, or they can be units in hospitals or nursing facilities. Skilled care is health care given when individuals need skilled nursing or rehabilitation staff to treat, manage, observe, and evaluate their care. Examples of skilled care include intravenous injections and physical therapy. Care that can be given by nonprofessional staff is not considered skilled care and is not covered by Medicare (CMS, 2007).

Skilled services must be certified as necessary by a physician, be related to a hospital admission (occur within 30 days of a hospital stay of at least 3 days for the same condition), and be needed on a daily basis. Coverage of SNF care by Medicare is limited to 100 days per benefit period, with the patient paying a portion of the cost from day 21 through day 100. A benefit period is defined as beginning when the Medicare beneficiary first enters the hospital until there has been a 60-day break in hospital or SNF services.

Medicare reimbursement for skilled nursing services has historically been retrospectively determined based on a combination of costs and per diem payments. However, payment by Medicare to provider organizations is in the middle of a drastic change of methodology. In 1997 Congress passed legislation creating a prospective payment system (PPS) for Medicare-funded postacute care. Similar to the payment system used to reimburse hospitals for acute services, it began on July 1, 1998, and was phased in completely over a three-year period. The basic premise is that providers be given an incentive to operate more efficiently. Instead of being paid for costs already incurred, they are given a set rate for certain services and must find ways to provide those services within that rate. If they are able to save more than that, they get to keep the remainder. If they fail to do so, they must absorb the difference between their costs and the PPS rate.

The PPS is designed to reduce cost inflation to Medicare. There had been a steady increase in skilled nursing care payments by Medicare for years. At the beginning of the new system, average Medicare payments to nursing facilities were reduced by 17 percent, an amount that Congress determined to be the inefficiency rate. This change created a great deal of concern among providers, as might be expected. It also resulted in as much confusion for nursing facilities as the original PPS did for hospitals when it began. Routine, ancillary, and capital costs were all included in one payment instead of separately as in the past. Payment was and is based on a formula that takes into consideration the mix of residents, their acuity levels, and the amount and type of care those residents receive—similar to the resource utilization groups used in an earlier PPS demonstration project. The new system required facilities to develop new resident management and cost-tracking systems, in many cases meaning acquiring and learning to use new technology. Hospital-based SNFs would appear to have somewhat of an advantage, given the head start their parent organizations had with PPS.

Recognizing the magnitude of the change for nursing facilities, the Centers for Medicare & Medicaid Services (CMS), formerly the Health Care Financing Administration (HCFA), developed a phase-in period for some of them—namely, those that were receiving Medicare payments prior to 1995. That phase-in process gradually changed the balance from a facility-specific rate to a federally set rate.

As is usually the case with any major change in payment methodology, the regulations governing PPS are still, several years later, undergoing some revision and refinement, including some changes based on challenges by providers. It cannot be stressed strongly enough here that readers wanting detailed and current information about PPS should seek other sources. It is simply not possible for a text, which takes months to prepare, to include all of the changes that have taken place since its publication process began.

Subacute Care

Subacute care is not a separate category under Medicare. It is covered under the category "postacute care," is generally provided in Medicare-certified SNFs or units, and is reimbursed through the SNF mechanism. However, subacute care may be provided in other settings. When this is the case, the reimbursement mechanism of that licensure category governs the reimbursement. For example, Medicare allows some hospitals to participate in a swing-bed program under which small rural hospitals may use certain beds interchangeably at a hospital, SNF, or nursing facility level of care as needed. The reimbursement for those beds is based on the type of care provided in the bed.

Home Health Care

Medicare embraced home health care as an alternative to institutionalization early on and is the primary provider of reimbursement for home healthcare services. To receive that reimbursement, these services must be provided by agencies certified by the Medicare program. As was the case with Medicare skilled nursing coverage, the former retrospective payment system was changed to a PPS as the result of the Balanced Budget Act of 1997. It was phased in over three years, during which home health providers were reimbursed on the basis of an interim payment system. With the PPS, Medicare pays for each 60-day "episode of care." The amount paid for that 60-day period is a set amount based on a standard rate adjusted for the type and intensity of care provided in what is known as a case-mix formula.

The original intent of Medicare was that it would cover home health care only after discharge from a hospital. This has been broadened to allow consumers to choose home health care as another option, including as an alternative to hospital care. Medicare beneficiaries must (1) be confined to home; (2) be under the care of a physician; (3) be in need of skilled services; (4) be under a plan of care; and (5) receive the services from, or under arrangements made by, a participating home health agency.

Hospice

Medicare covers hospice care for people who are certified to be terminally ill, with six months or less to live. The care must be palliative rather than curative and, as with other types of Medicare coverage, must be delivered by a provider organization that is certified by that program. The care may be provided in a healthcare facility or in the patient's home. It generally includes services such as pain management, nursing services, and some therapies.

Other Long-Term Care Services

Medicare does not regularly provide coverage in settings such as assisted living or adult day care. However, under some Medicaid waiver programs (discussed later in this chapter), these services may be included.

Medicaid

At the same time that the Medicare program was developed to provide health care for the elderly, Congress also created Medicaid as a program to provide health care for the poor. Enacted as Title XIX of the Social Security Act, Medicaid is different from Medicare in several very specific ways. First, it has no age limitations but covers people of all ages. Second, it does have income restrictions, covering only those who are "medically indigent" and who cannot pay for their own health care or do not have insurance. Third, Medicare is funded and operated by the federal government, but Medicaid is jointly funded by the federal and state governments and is run by the states under federal guidelines. In theory, Medicaid is funded half-and-half by the state and federal governments, but in practice some states receive as much as 75 percent of their Medicaid funding from the federal government. Finally, whereas Medicare coverage is limited in terms of the

types of services covered and the length of time they are covered, Medicaid essentially covers most services needed by its beneficiaries. This is not to say that it covers everything. In fact, the states have considerable flexibility in determining which healthcare services are covered by their state programs. They must cover certain basic services but may choose not to cover services beyond that. However, in most states, Medicaid coverage is extensive, particularly in long-term care. This makes it a major source of funding for long-term care consumers and providers. According to a report by the Henry J. Kaiser Family Foundation, Medicaid pays for more than 40 percent of long-term care (Kaiser Family Foundation, 2008). Medicaid also serves as a backup to Medicare, paying for services for low-income elders beyond those covered by Medicare.

Because Medicaid is a welfare-type program, it is not intended as a reimbursement source for anyone with other resources. This means that consumers must not be eligible for other forms of health insurance, public or private. They must also use up all of their available resources before becoming eligible for Medicaid.

Medicaid: What's Covered?

Like Medicare, Medicaid coverage for long-term care services ranges from none at all for some providers to being the primary funding source for others. Also, like Medicare, there are several changes, some experimental, in the works. Several of these changes are tied to the Medicaid waiver program. This program, included in the 1987 Omnibus Budget Reconciliation Act (OBRA), allows states to apply for a waiver from Medicaid rules to allow them flexibility in operating their Medicaid programs. The waiver programs give CMS authority to:

- Approve projects that test policy innovations likely to further the objectives of the Medicaid program.

- Grant waivers that allow states to implement managed care delivery systems, or otherwise limit individuals' choice of provider under Medicaid.

- Allow long-term care services to be delivered in community settings. (CMS, 2005)

Since passage of that act, which has been expanded twice, many states have been granted waivers. Working within those waivers, they have found ways to fund services other than the traditional medical-related services found in nursing facilities. The waivers permit them to selectively purchase nonmedical services (e.g., case management, respite care, personal care services, homemaker services, and transportation) if they can do so without raising expenses above the level of care received in nursing facilities (Meiners, 1996). They can also use waivers to change their focus from care in nursing facilities to home- or community-based care. This has had some effect on the funding of those services to date, and those services will probably expand.

Nursing Care Facilities

Medicaid accounts for more than 40 percent of all funding for most nursing facilities (Kaiser Family Foundation, 2008). There are a couple of reasons for this. To begin with, other sources of reimbursement for these facilities are very limited. As we noted earlier, Medicare coverage for nursing care is limited to skilled nursing care and does not include residents whose care needs fall below that level. Private sources of reimbursement are also very limited, although that seems to be changing. Given the lack of other payment sources, Medicaid is often left to fill the resultant coverage gaps.

A second, closely related, reason for the prominence of Medicaid as a reimbursement source for nursing facilities is its role as a safety net. Nursing care facility residents are often institutionalized for years, usually the last years of their lives. By that time, they have generally incurred heavy expenses, including hospitalization. They have used up any insurance coverage they may have had, as well as their personal savings.

Assisted Living

Medicaid is also a provider of reimbursement for assisted living facilities and programs (called "residential care facilities" in some states). That coverage is far from universal, varying from state to state, but it is growing. Much of the Medicaid coverage of assisted living has resulted from waiver programs. One of the primary goals of many of these states is to reduce the number of beds in nursing facilities. They see shifting payment to assisted living and residential care as one way of doing that.

Home Health Care

Medicaid is the second largest source of funding for home healthcare agencies, although it falls behind Medicare. That proportion has grown as states seek cost savings through waivers and try to move more of their Medicaid recipients from institutions to home-based care. In 2006, Medicare accounted for 38 percent of home healthcare expenditures, with Medicaid at 34 percent (Kaiser Family Foundation, 2008). Medicaid is often used to supplement Medicare coverage for low-income seniors. Medicaid spending for home and community-based care increased from $22 billion in 2000 to $45 billion in 2006 (Kaiser Family Foundation, 2008).

Other Long-Term Care Providers

Other forms of long-term care—such as subacute care, hospice, and adult day care—are generally not covered by Medicaid, but may be covered as a supplement to Medicare or under some of the waiver innovations.

State Efforts to Reduce Medicaid Expenses

In the past several years, both federal and state governments have found their Medicaid budgets rising to levels that threaten their ability to fund them. In 2006, total spending for Medicaid was $311 billion, with more than one-third of that amount being spent on long-term care (Kaiser Family Foundation, 2008). The portion funded by the states has grown just as fast.

Total Medicaid outlays in fiscal year (FY) 2007 had grown to $333.2 billion: $190.6 billion (or 57 percent) represented federal spending and $142.6 billion (or 43 percent) represented state spending (Truffer, Klemm, Hoffman, & Wolfe, 2008).

Many states have seen their portion of Medicaid grow to being one of the top two or three most expensive items in their budgets. This has led to a number of efforts to lower expenses.

One of the most common ways of doing so is by reducing the amount of care received by Medicaid recipients in nursing facilities. A method used by some states to accomplish this is raising the eligibility requirements. One of the primary criteria for admission to a nursing facility is the number of activities of daily living (ADLs) with which a person needs help. After increasing the minimum requirement from two to three ADLs, a significant portion of the Medicaid long-term care population was no longer eligible for admission. Several states have also reduced the allowed number of licensed beds in nursing facilities, arguing that they are excessive and expensive to operate. A third method of reducing state Medicaid expenses is through managed care, a topic that is discussed further later in this chapter.

Medicaid "Spend Down" Requirements

There has been a great deal of concern recently about one of Medicaid's most basic rules—or at least about reactions to it. That rule specifies that no one can qualify for Medicaid benefits who has other resources available, such as money in the bank, real estate, or other property. Before consumers can become eligible, they must use up all such resources, hence the term "spend down."

The rule is logical in and of itself. After all, Medicaid is a welfare-type program intended for those who have no other funds. However, enforcement of this restriction (and efforts to circumvent it) has generated much controversy. The situation has caused battle lines to be drawn, creating opposing camps. First are the consumers and their families. In another camp are the state and federal agencies charged with funding Medicaid. They identify Medicaid as a safety net for those who need help and find it unfair for taxpayers to provide healthcare coverage for people who have resources of their own that could be spent. Both sides have valid arguments, and it is a dispute that will not be solved easily.

Add to these two groups a couple of other not-so-innocent bystanders—providers and estate planners, both of whom have stakes in this argument and have something to gain or lose, depending on its outcome. The providers want to get paid for their services and fear that the Medicaid program will become insolvent, or at least cut reimbursement rates to below where they are already. Estate planners and tax lawyers have found a profitable business advising their clients on ways of avoiding the spend-down rule. They show how to create trusts and other financial mechanisms that protect funds from being taken.

A note of caution here: as much as picking on lawyers has become somewhat of a national pastime, we should not assume that all tax lawyers and estate planners seek to circumvent the Medicaid rules. Most do not. Even those that do so, do it within the letter of the law, so they cannot be criticized for illegal acts. Perhaps the saddest part of this situation is that the really wealthy are usually able to find a way to avoid spending down, while those in the lower- and middle-income categories are far less likely to know how to do that. The latter groups are the ones caught in the middle.

Both sides, providers and estate planners, have taken steps to solidify their positions, with neither clearly winning; however, there have been some interesting results. For example, in 1996 Congress made it a criminal act to willfully dispose of assets for the purpose of gaining eligibility for Medicaid. This was the first time there had been any legal sanction for such acts. Suddenly, anyone caught transferring or otherwise disposing of personal assets to avoid having to spend down would be subject to fines and possible imprisonment. It seemed like a good idea at the time, but Congress failed to anticipate the degree of concern and opposition it would generate. Amid a great deal of publicity claiming that the legislation would result in "jailing Granny," Congress did an about-face and, as part of the 1997 budget act, repealed that provision. In its place was put a new section that provided for criminal actions against those who advise consumers—attorneys and estate planners. Early interpretations of the change tended to deem it only slightly more enforceable.

Other suggested remedies for the spend-down problem range from tighter enforcement of existing laws and regulations to providing incentives for consumers to provide their own coverage. The enforcement advocates have had a weapon in place since 1982. It is the Tax Equity and Fiscal Responsibility Act, parts of which allow states to (1) restrict asset transfer within two years of Medicaid nursing home eligibility, (2) place liens on the property of living recipients, and (3) recover from the estates of deceased recipients. Despite the time that has elapsed since the act was passed, it appears that states have either had little success implementing these provisions or have not really tried. The 1993 OBRA did go a step further by actually requiring states to recover the costs of nursing facility and other long-term care services from the estates of Medicaid beneficiaries. OBRA does not appear to have made a significant difference in the states' success, at least to date.

Among the incentives that have been tried or proposed to reduce spend-down avoidance are several forms of public–private partnership demonstration projects, which are discussed in more detail later in this chapter.

Other Public Funding Sources

Medicare and Medicaid are by far the largest public reimbursers of long-term care. There are several other smaller sources of public funding for long-term care services. They include the Supplemental Security Income (SSI) program, the Veterans Administration, and the Older Americans Act. These programs serve limited populations, and, although they are very important to their recipients, their impact on the overall long-term care system is not great.

Private Reimbursement Sources

In addition to public payment for long-term care services, there are several private (meaning nongovernment) methods of reimbursing providers for those services. In 2002, private payments (including private insurance, out-of-pocket contributions, and other private sources) accounted for 34 percent of all spending on long-term care (Georgetown University, 2004).

Managed care, which includes a variety of prepayment options, is becoming a major force in health care, primarily as a private reimbursement source. However, because it is also increasingly being applied to public sources such as Medicare and Medicaid, and because of its large current and potential impact, it is discussed separately.

Out-of-Pocket Payments

Historically, the largest private reimbursement source for long-term care has been out-of-pocket payments by individuals and their families. As recently as 1993, this represented slightly more than one-third of all long-term care payments, public or private (Meiners, 1996). However, neither of the other primary sources, private long-term care insurance and managed care, had begun to have much impact at that time. The recent growth of these two sources is at least partly responsible for the fact that out-of-pocket payments dropped to less than one-quarter of the total at the beginning of the millennium (Georgetown University, 2004).

Private Long-Term Care Insurance

Private long-term care insurance has grown very slowly as an option until the past several years, when its availability and popularity increased considerably. Currently, about 10 percent of Americans over the age of 55 have private insurance protection for LTC costs (AHIP, 2007a). A report released by the American Association for Long-Term Care Insurance (AALTCI) showed that some 180,000 Americans with long-term care insurance policies were paid $3.5 billion in benefits in 2007 (AALTCI, 2008b). By definition, "long-term care insurance" is insurance sold by insurance companies specifically to pay for long-term care services. Some long-term care insurance is purchased through group plans, including employers and organizations, but most such insurance is sold to individuals.

Although most Americans get their health insurance through group plans offered at their places of work, until quite recently few employers offered long-term care insurance to their employees. This seems to be changing. According to AALTCI, there are now nearly 10,000 employer groups offering a form of employer-sponsored long-term care insurance with just over 2 million Americans insured by these plans (AALTCI, 2008a). However, during the latter part of 2008, the severe economic downturn experienced across the country most likely caused many firms to forgo adding this benefit. Hopefully, that will change as the economy rebounds.

There have been a number of reasons given for the reluctance of businesses to add long-term care insurance to their employee benefits. Some have said it is not well developed enough yet and that they are waiting for it to be improved more—an argument that is probably no longer valid. Most are concerned that it is too expensive and that the costs to them will be overwhelming when added to already high health insurance premiums. They find themselves caught in a dilemma. If they provide employer-funded long-term care insurance for all employees, their total premiums may well be prohibitive. However, if they make it optional, they run the risk of adverse selection—only those most likely to use it will take advantage of the option, and the company's premiums will escalate accordingly. If it is offered as part of a company plan but paid for by individual employees, the likelihood of adverse selection becomes even greater, raising premium rates beyond the ability of most employees to pay.

Perhaps the biggest reason companies are not offering long-term care insurance more regularly is that their employees have not demanded it, at least not in large enough numbers to convince them. Interest in long-term care insurance is still not high among people of working age. They have enough to worry about financially without thinking about something that may (or may not) occur several decades in the future. They have also been conditioned to believe that the government will provide for them when they get

old. They, like many of the elderly of today, believe that Medicare will cover the bulk of their healthcare needs when they reach the age of 65. The result is that younger people, those of working age, are not convinced of the necessity for purchasing long-term care insurance, yet it is for this group that long-term care insurance is most cost-effective. Jesse Slome, executive director of AALTCI, says,

> The risk of needing long-term care is higher than the risk of a serious car accident or house fire, but few people are aware of how many individuals and families already benefit from having purchased long-term care insurance. As more individuals become aware of, and understand the importance of, planning for long-term care needs, the number of individuals and families deriving benefit from this coverage will only increase. (AALTCI, 2008)

There is, however, a countering force that is prodding some younger people to look seriously at buying long-term care insurance, and that is their experience as members of what has come to be known as the "sandwich generation." They are caught between taking care of their own children and also taking care of their parents when those parents become elderly and dependent. As these young and middle-age adults struggle to make sure that their parents receive long-term care services, they learn just how difficult it can be to get reimbursement for them. They are now much more likely to seek ways to avoid putting their own children through the same hassle in future years. Long-term care insurance is one solution that has begun to catch on. In 2007, the average age of buyers was

58, dropping below 60 for the first time, after falling steadily for the past decade (Villagran, 2007).

One of the complaints from the elderly and their advocates, such as AARP (formerly the American Association of Retired Persons), is that long-term care insurance is too expensive. It is—for anyone who anticipates using it relatively soon. As might be expected, most individuals receiving benefits from their long-term care insurance policies are older. Nearly a third (32.3 percent) of new claims in 2007 began for individuals between 70 and 79. More than half (55.2 percent) began for those age 80 or over. However, 11.5 percent were for those between 50 and 69 (AALTCI, 2008). One of the basic precepts of any type of insurance program is that the longer a person pays premiums before collecting benefits, the lower those premiums will be per annum. According to a 2008 national price index, a 65-year-old considering long-term care insurance protection can expect to pay $1,342 a year, if married, or $1,999, if single, while a 55-year-old purchasing comparable coverage will pay $709 a year, if they are married, or $1,095, if they are single, depending on the type and amount of coverage (Senior Journal, 2008). This is clearly too expensive for many seniors. However, younger workers can find good coverage for as low as around $400 per year. For many of them, this is the equivalent of one month's payment on a car loan or a fraction of a monthly home mortgage payment.

Long-term care insurance, when first offered, was quite restrictive and gave individuals few options from which to choose. As it has developed, insurance companies have added benefit choices that allow purchasers to tailor their benefits to correspond to the amount they are willing to pay for premiums.

Long-term care insurance policies are nearly always indemnity-based, meaning that they pay a certain dollar amount of covered services per day. Buyers usually have several dollar amounts on which to base their policies. They may also choose to have their insurance cover nursing facility care, home care, other selected services, or any combination of these services, and they can select the amount of coverage for each. While most people associate long-term care insurance with nursing home care, quite the opposite is true. Most benefits paid today cover care at home or in an assisted living community. More than 97 percent of long-term care insurance policies sold today provide some form of home care benefit. That compares with 86 percent in 2000 and 67 percent in 1995 (AALTCI, 2008).

They also may have the option of determining the length of coverage, generally defined in years. Policies most commonly offer choices ranging from one to five years in nursing facilities and/or home care. Another option is an inflation provision that is designed to anticipate increases in service costs, keeping the same proportional coverage for the insured.

Long-term care insurance is destined to play a much larger role in the reimbursement of long-term care services in the future. There are too few other alternatives for that not to happen. It will not be effective, however, unless the public accepts both its necessity and its value. One factor that will help in gaining that acceptance is the increasing concern over the future viability of Medicare and Medicaid. The possible insolvency of these programs and some of the options suggested for saving them (e.g., raising the eligibility age for Medicare, converting it to a means-based program, and reducing benefits for both Medicare and Medicaid) are beginning to scare the public and shake their complacency. They are starting to realize that they have some responsibility to provide for their own future care needs to the extent they can, and they see long-term care insurance as one alternative.

The willingness of the public to invest in long-term care insurance would be greatly enhanced if there were some tax incentives to do so. One survey showed that the single most important step government could take to encourage the purchase of LTC coverage is to offer tax incentives. According to that survey, more than 80 percent of those who currently forgo purchase of LTC insurance would be more interested in buying a policy if they could deduct premiums from their taxes (AHIP, 2007b). Several states already allow credits or deductions for the premiums of long-term care insurance, but to date there has been nothing done at the national level. There has been some discussion of national tax incentives, and there will need to be more if private long-term care insurance is to be a significant factor in the near future. (See "Significant Trends and Their Impact" later in this chapter for a more detailed discussion.)

Public–Private Partnerships

One of the most promising initiatives to come along in long-term care reimbursement in recent years attempts to take advantage of the willingness of many people to accept social responsibility and to facilitate fulfillment of that willingness. It is the concept of developing public–private partnerships. Public–private partnership programs seek ways to provide incentives for individuals to purchase long-term care insurance. The primary incentive is asset protection in return for meeting some of the cost of long-term care.

Public–private partnerships began with a program sponsored by the Robert Wood Johnson Foundation. That program, titled "Partnership for Long-Term Care," provided financial support for innovative state initiatives that would encourage the purchase of private long-term care insurance by individuals, thus reducing the drain on their Medicaid budgets. Several states participated in the program, using different methods to make the purchase of long-term care insurance more attractive to consumers.

The program was so successful, the government endorsed it. In February 2006, Congress approved legislation clearing the way for expanded, nationwide public–private long-term care (LTC) insurance partnerships. The law authorizes changes in state law to allow individuals to purchase private LTC insurance that coordinates with Medicaid. Specifically, in states adopting the partnership approach, individuals can purchase private LTC insurance policies with the assurance that Medicaid will cover LTC costs incurred beyond the terms of the private coverage. In these states, under the terms of the partnership, people with private insurance are not required to "spend down" their remaining assets to qualify for Medicaid (AHIP, 2007a).

Public–private partnerships hold benefits for consumers and for state and federal Medicaid programs. Nationwide adoption of the concept, together with effective education and clear financial incentives to purchase private LTC coverage, would create a more robust market for private LTC insurance. This change would benefit consumers, whose assets would be protected even if they needed extended long-term care services and required assistance from Medicaid. It also would be good for U.S. fiscal policy, helping to limit growth in Medicaid spending and thus reducing pressure on federal and state budgets (AHIP, 2007a).

Managed Care

Few innovations, movements, or trends have affected health care in the United States as much as managed care has in the past several decades, yet we have to search hard to find a reasonably concise, descriptive definition of "managed care." Even the experts seem to have difficulty confining it to a single agreed-upon definition. For example, Peter Kongstvedt, who has written several texts dealing with managed care, calls managed health care:

> A regrettably nebulous term. At the very least, it is a system of health care delivery that tries to manage the cost of health care, the quality of that health care, and access to that care. Common denominators include a panel of contracted providers that is less than the entire universe of available providers, some type of limitations on benefits to subscribers who use non-contracted providers (unless authorized to do so), and some type of authorization system. (Kongstvedt, 2007)

He goes on to urge his readers to formulate definitions of their own.

Another author also describes managed care.

> The term managed care has two distinct meanings. Though sometimes used to refer to discrete initiatives that seek to combine financial and medical decisions (e.g., utilization management), managed care is most often used to refer to the continually adapting and developing alternative health care plans that, in varying degrees, integrate the financing and delivery of medical care. Despite the variations, all managed care plans "manage" physician and patient behavior through a host of financial and administrative mechanisms, reverse the economic incentives of traditional fee-for-service practice, and require physicians to assume some of the financial risk of their decisions. (Priester, 1997)

These two definitions eloquently describe the vagueness inherent in any discussion of managed care. It is truly many things to many people and includes a broad range of programs and arrangements. The definitions do, however, identify several basic components of managed care plans. First, managed care integrates, in some fashion, the financing and delivery of health care. Second, its purpose is to manage cost, quality, and access for a defined group of consumers. Third, it "manages" the behavior of both consumers and providers through financial and administrative mechanisms. Fourth, providers, and sometimes consumers, share the financial risk.

There are many variations of managed care plans or organizations. Some of the more familiar include health maintenance organizations (HMOs), preferred provider organizations (PPOs), physician-hospital organizations (PHOs), and exclusive provider organizations (EPOs). It is not the purpose of this book to present a comprehensive discussion of managed care, nor would it be feasible to do so in this chapter. The intent is to discuss managed care as it affects long-term care organizations. With that limitation, there are some points for the reader to keep in mind.

One is that it is recognized that managed care is more than just a reimbursement mechanism. It is a combination of reimbursement and delivery. Yet, to keep the discussion in proper perspective, managed care is approached here as a reimbursement source for long-term care. Also, managed care is still primarily oriented to physicians and hospitals, and its impact is being felt by long-term care organizations to differing degrees. Rather than attempt to describe all aspects of this very extensive topic, that impact is the focus here.

Managed Care: How It Works

What is now called managed care began with HMOs, a type of provider/reimbursement organization that delivered health care to a specified group of members on a fixed-rate basis, regardless of how much service they required. Enrollment was generally in groups, by employers or other distinct membership organizations. They prepaid the HMO an amount per member per month or per year; thus these were also known as prepaid health plans. It was a direct reversal of the traditional fee-for-service payment mechanism. The HMO employed physicians directly or contracted with groups of physicians. These physicians either received a salary or were paid on a capitation basis, meaning that they received a rate based on the number of enrollees for whom they were responsible, not on the amount of service rendered.

These early HMOs evolved over time, and several new variations have emerged. The changes include expanding the ways they charge their enrollee organizations, their financial relationships with their providers, and how they control costs. Actually, managed care represents a continuum of its own, with several types of plans offering an array of features that vary in their ability to balance access to care, cost, quality control, benefit design, and flexibility (Wagner & Kongstvedt, 2007). Today, they range from managing care for an insurance company or employer on an indemnity basis to constituting a fully integrated health system.

Managed Care and Long-Term Care

Managed care has taken hold much more in some parts of the country than in others. This is particularly true when it comes to long-term care. One early study found that more than 75 percent of long-term care facilities involved with managed care were in a few states: Arizona, California, Florida, Massachusetts, Minnesota, Oregon, Pennsylvania, and Washington (Fisher, 1997). That has certainly changed some, but the distribution is still uneven. It does not mean that managed care will not affect long-term care in other states, but merely that it may take longer to happen.

A relatively recent development in managed care is its use by public agencies. Several states, attempting to lower their costs through waiver programs, are contracting with managed care organizations (MCOs) to manage care for their Medicare and Medicaid beneficiaries. They find it to be a good way to reduce their costs or to minimize ongoing growth in those costs. They also see contracting care out to some external organization as a way to control or ration the distribution of care while separating themselves from the responsibility of making difficult political decisions (Kane, 1997). Managing care for public programs has already increased the involvement of long-term care organizations beyond the level it occupied when managed care was primarily private.

Institutionalized long-term care, including facilities that provide skilled nursing care, subacute care, nonskilled care, and/or assisted living services, are on the verge of having to become heavily involved with MCOs if they are not already involved. As the long-term care provider closest to acute hospitals, subacute care is leading the pack. The MCOs, in seeking less costly alternatives for hospital care, find nonhospital subacute care attractive. Being able to add that level of care to their comprehensive service packages makes them more competitive. As Medicare makes more use of managed care, this will only increase.

Facilities that do not provide subacute or skilled care are more likely to be influenced by the increasing desire of state Medicaid agencies to contract for management of their caseloads. As the largest source of reimbursement for nursing care and assisted living, the incursion of Medicaid into managed care will force those facilities to join as well.

Home healthcare organizations have also found themselves attractive to MCOs. Where they had relied mostly on Medicare for funding in the past, they are now finding MCOs, both public and private, becoming more important as buyers of their services. These MCOs need to offer a full spectrum of care, including community-based services. They generally do not have the capability to offer those services directly within their own organizations, so they must acquire the services on a contract basis.

Hospice care would seem to be a natural choice for managed care involvement. It already relies heavily on Medicare for reimbursement and has proven itself a less costly alternative during the final months of life. However, the rate of utilization of hospice by MCOs is still relatively low. This may be caused by several factors, including the complexity of MCO transfer rules. However, some hospice providers blame a lack of understanding of the benefits of hospice care on the part of MCO staff and blame themselves for not educating MCOs adequately. They note that hospice care is cost-effective, in addition to providing terminally ill patients and their families more freedom and support.

Types of Managed Care: Provider Arrangements

The possible forms of interaction between an MCO and a long-term care provider are almost endless. However, there are several general categories into which most tend to fall. Kathleen Griffin, a managed care consultant, has identified the following possibilities: per diem contract, case rate contract, preferred placement, bed-lease, and joint venture (Peck, 1996). The simplest and most common is the per diem contract, in which the provider agrees to accept referrals from the MCO. A case rate contract involves the provider in a bit more risk, because the payment is the same for all cases with a given diagnosis or all cases that require a particular type of treatment.

The last three arrangements identified by Griffin are forms of partnership between the MCO and the provider. Preferred placement gives the referring MCO or hospital priority placement in return for a per diem rate based on volume. A bed-lease arrangement has the MCO actually leasing a number of beds with separate rates for those that are occupied and those that are not. The last category, a joint venture, involves the two parties creating a new, separate entity to own and operate the service. These arrangements, and the endless number of possible permutations, give the long-term care provider seeking a relationship with an MCO lots of opportunities to find one that meets its needs.

Managed Care: Making the Transition

In looking at the need for long-term care organizations to embrace managed care, or at least become an active participant in it, there are several questions that should be asked.

1. How big a step is it for a long-term care provider to become involved in managed care?
2. What capabilities must they have in their operations to be successful?
3. How ready are they?

The short answers to those questions are:

1. It's a big step.
2. Many specific capabilities are needed.
3. They are generally not very ready.

These questions and answers are now explored in a bit more depth.

Taking the Big Step

Getting involved with managed care is a significant undertaking for most long-term care organizations. Granted, there are many who have already taken the step—and have done so successfully—but all indications are that the vast majority have not. Changing from traditional fee-for-service reimbursement to capitation or other managed care payment method means giving up some of its own control over its residents or clients. The MCO will have its own cost and quality control mechanisms, often different from those of the long-term care provider both in format and in focus. Given the traditional retrospective payment to which most long-term care providers have been accustomed, many were and are not nearly as cost-conscious as are MCOs. The PPS has changed that, making most long-term care organizations quite cost-conscious. MCOs are interested in quality of care but make their purchasing decisions based on price.

Even with the most at-arms-length arrangements, the MCO becomes another organization with which to work. This requires the provider to understand how the MCO works and what it is looking for in a relationship. Depending on how deeply involved the provider becomes with the MCO, the arrangement may interfere with, or even replace, relationships with other payers or acute care providers.

Capabilities Needed

MCOs look for providers that can meet their needs completely and efficiently. They choose providers able to demonstrate their experience in providing high-quality care and that are able and willing to adapt as necessary. There are also certain financial and administrative capabilities that a long-term care provider needs to have to interact successfully with an MCO. Perhaps the most important is a working case management function. This is also the area in which many of them fall short. Their existing utilization review programs, while meeting current needs, may not be stringent or detailed enough to satisfy the MCO.

A second major capability that providers must have is a highly sophisticated information system. To begin with, that system must make it possible for the provider to identify and manage costs. MCOs expect their contractors to have a sound grasp of where and how they are spending their money. That information system also prepares the provider for future negotiations with the MCO. The information system must also be capable of providing the data needed for measuring clinical outcomes. MCOs will look for outcomes-measurement capability on the part of contracting providers. They want measurement of utilization, length of stay, and use of quantitative outcome measurement tools.

State of Readiness

Most observers agree that much of the long-term care field is not adequately prepared for managed care. On the whole, the degree of involvement of long-term care organizations in managed care runs the gamut from highly involved to not interested. Some recognize the value of participation; others are not yet convinced. Some are in areas of the country where MCOs have made few inroads. Others are working on developing the capabilities needed.

Managed Care: A Tarnished Image

It is assumed here that managed care is here to stay and that long-term care organizations cannot afford to ignore it. There would appear to be plenty of justification for that assumption. However, all is not sweetness and light with managed care. From its inception, it has taken hits from all sides because of the perception that MCOs put cost control ahead of quality of care or the interests of consumers. The news media have been full of stories of MCOs denying tests and procedures to save money. Individual physicians and physician groups have complained of having their medical decisions overturned by nonmedical MCO staff. Public and teaching hospitals fear that they will be left to care for only the sickest and poorest patients while, through selective enrollment, MCOs skim off those patients who are less expensive to handle. Consumers who are enrolled, often by their employers, in managed care plans tell of losing their ability to choose their physicians and other providers.

These and other similar complaints have generated a great deal of consumer and political backlash against MCOs. Consumer advocacy groups such as AARP and Families USA work hard to protect the rights of their constituents, including providing them with the information needed to judge the care they are getting. This concern from healthcare professionals and the public has led to creation of a presidential commission. The President's Advisory Commission on Consumer Protection and Quality in the Health Care Industry eventually developed a Consumer Bill of Rights and Responsibilities. Although it addresses the entire healthcare system, it was clearly stimulated by worry about the direction that the system seemed to be taking as managed care became ever more influential.

This bill of rights addresses a number of consumer rights, focusing directly on the complaints heard about managed care. These rights include the rights of consumers to receive accurate, understandable information; to choose their healthcare providers; to have emergency care reimbursed; to participate in treatment decisions; to be treated respectfully and in a nondiscriminatory manner; and to appeal differences with providers and health plans (President's Advisory Commission, 1997). At the same time, several states have also been developing their own managed care consumer assistance legislation. Several states have considered bills aimed at helping people more easily navigate the often confusing world of managed care. These bills, strongly supported by AARP, are designed to support the national bill of rights and fill perceived gaps in the national bill.

The backlash against MCOs by both consumers and physicians caused some long-term care providers to question whether they want to become involved. It gave others an excuse to remain distant from a part of the system that they saw as changing their operations too radically. Managed care will weather this storm, will make some changes as a result of it, and will emerge as an even more important mechanism for providing and reimbursing health care. For that reason, long-term care organizations will continue to become more involved with it, although some will do so reluctantly.

Significant Trends and Their Impact on Long-Term Care Reimbursement

There are several changes taking place in long-term care reimbursement that will continue to have impact on providers and consumers alike. They include (1) the growing influence of private MCOs; (2) the degree to which public reimbursers, such as Medicare and Medicaid, use managed care; (3) the ongoing impact of the change from retrospective payment to a PPS; (4) an emphasis on noninstitutional forms of care; (5) the provision of incentives for consumers to purchase private long-term care insurance; and (6) efforts to reduce the cost of liability insurance through tort reform. These developments are,

not surprisingly, closely interrelated. They share a common goal of containing the rising cost of providing care.

These changes have been initiated primarily by public and private organizations responsible for paying for care. However, the stimulus actually comes from their customers, who are seeking financial relief. For private MCOs, the customers are the companies and others who contract for healthcare coverage for the members of their groups. They are looking for ways to reduce the expenses associated with providing that coverage. For the public agencies administering Medicare and Medicaid programs, the ultimate customers are taxpayers, who are also feeling the need for relief.

Private Managed Care

Managed care, in spite of the questions that have been raised about it, will continue to be a major player in the area of long-term care reimbursement for the foreseeable future. It experienced some growing pains, as happens with just about any new business concept. These growing pains are shaping it into a more stable entity. Trying to predict what shape that entity will ultimately take is risky, but it is likely to be somewhat less extreme than some of the earlier versions. The competing forces of cost containment and consumer choice are working to eliminate some of the provisions and characteristics most objectionable to each, which will result in a product both can live with. Government, acting in its regulatory mode, has already responded to some of these forces and has established some parameters within which managed care can operate.

Long-term care organizations are, and will be, faced with the reality of private managed care as a serious source of reimbursement. The percentage of their funding received from that source has grown slowly in most cases and, with some exceptions, will not exceed public reimbursement. However, the relationships between long-term care providers and other segments of the continuum may well hinge on how willing and able those providers are to embrace managed care. The influence of an organization's other stakeholders, particularly referring hospitals, will be significant. The importance of managed care is much greater for those hospitals than for most long-term care organizations. They are looking for long-term care partners who can help them as they compete for the business of the MCOs.

Public Managed Care

As was noted earlier, both the Medicare and Medicaid programs have actively increased their use of managed care. Like the private sector, they see it as a way of managing their costs. Because of their much larger role in long-term care reimbursement, their managed care involvement is affecting long-term care providers significantly.

The Centers for Medicare & Medicaid Services (CMS), which administers the Medicare program, has experimented with a number of managed care formats. The agency has contracted with private MCOs to develop and pilot a variety of different plans and options. These projects generally focus on acute care for Medicare recipients, but most include some long-term care elements as well. State Medicaid agencies are also trying managed care as an option for reducing, or at least containing, their growing costs. As trials or demonstration projects, the formats have varied considerably in structure and coverage and continue to do so. In most cases, Medicaid agencies also contract with private MCOs to develop and administer their plans, rather than attempting to create their own MCOs.

The long-range impact of these efforts on long-term care organizations is not yet clear. In areas in which demonstration projects have taken place, the impact has been significant, particularly with Medicaid projects. In others, it has not been felt yet. However, the necessity of finding solutions to the financial problems of Medicare and Medicaid make managed care look very attractive to those agencies. Add in the unknown factor of possible reform of both programs, and the potential impact on long-term care organizations could be much greater than anyone would have guessed.

Although changes in Medicare eligibility rules tend to get most of the spotlight, it is a safe bet that there will also be a continued and expanding search for ways to reduce expenses for coverage of those who are eligible. It is these actions, many of which are already under way, that will most significantly affect providers of long-term care services. CMS has stepped up its efforts to reduce fraud in Medicare billing. Many state Medicaid agencies, with assistance from CMS, have done the same. Case-mix payment programs, where providers (primarily nursing facilities) are paid according to the proportion of their residents needing certain levels of care, have been tried. And, finally, the various managed care experiments mentioned here will have the most impact in the long run.

Prospective Payment

As Medicare completes the change from a retrospective payment system to one that is prospective for providers of long-term care services, many of these providers have had to make significant changes in their record-keeping and operating practices. They have had to develop case management systems, if they did not already have them in place. There has been, and will continue to be, pressure on them to reduce their costs even further. For those providers whose primary service is subacute or skilled care, these changes have already been made or are at least under way. For others, such as the large and growing number of nursing facilities with small skilled care components, it is much more difficult. They must adopt a highly complicated billing and recordkeeping system for a small part of their facilities, one that is very different from what they use for the rest of their residents.

When long-term care providers were awaiting, and trying to prepare for, the new PPS for postacute care, Nursing Homes magazine interviewed a group of leaders in the field to get their reactions (Peck, 1997). Most accepted the fact of the coming changes but expressed a number of concerns. Some expressed concerns about how the new program would be implemented, fearing delays and confusion about reporting requirements. Opinions were mixed concerning how it would affect their competitive position with hospital-based subacute care units. On one thing, however, there seemed to be consensus: The intent of the PPS was to lower costs; therefore, providers could expect to receive less. In general, their concerns were realized, but most likely not to the degree they had anticipated.

Emphasis on Community-Based Care

As reimbursers of long-term care services, both public and private, begin to look for ways to ensure that their constituents receive appropriate care at the lowest possible prices, there has been a very clear and well-documented shift of reimbursement resources from institution-based care to that which is home or community based. This has obviously been a boon for home health and hospice organizations and a concern for nursing care, assisted living, and residential care providers. The shift is likely to continue, although some of the policy makers most enamored of the idea have come to realize that it does not work in all situations. Studies have shown that the population of consumers, particularly the elderly (who are the majority), who can best make use of home-based services are not necessarily the same ones who reside in nursing care or other residential facilities. Therefore, to some degree, the effect of shifting resources from institutional care to home-based care has been to create additional demand. This is good for those consumers who benefit from the added coverage and for the organizations providing the care. It has also forced institutional providers to be more cost conscious and competitive. However, it has not had the overall effect on the reimbursement system anticipated by some.

Incentives for Purchasing Private Long-Term Care Insurance

Because of the historic lack of interest of many consumers in purchasing private long-term care insurance, there needs to be, and will be, continued pressure for better incentives for them to do so. There have been some efforts in the past couple of years, and several bills have been filed in Congress to provide tax incentives for consumers paying premiums for long-term care insurance. Bills filed in the 108th Congress included two that are very similar, one in the House of Representatives and one in the Senate. They would have amended the Internal Revenue Code of 1986 to allow individuals a deduction for qualified long-term care insurance premiums, use of such insurance under cafeteria plans and flexible spending arrangements, and a credit for individuals with long-term care needs. (AHCA/NCAL, 2003) This action was hailed by providers and consumers alike as an excellent first step but one that must be carried to fruition. Hopefully, by the time this text is being read, it will have.

One question that stirs a lot of controversy today—and will in the future no matter what financing system we develop—is who should be the gatekeeper? Someone has to make healthcare decisions for each individual. Who should it be? In an ideal system, it should be the consumers, but they are often not well-enough informed. The players in this game do not trust each other. Providers and payers suspect that the consumers will want too much if they have control. If the providers are the gatekeepers, the payers are afraid they will prescribe too much expensive care. Yet, if the payers are the gatekeepers, both the consumers and providers accuse them of putting cost ahead of quality. There is no easy answer, and this question will only continue to get in the way as new systems develop.

Liability Costs and Tort Reform

In the past few years, all of health care, including long-term care, has been beset by increasing numbers of multimillion-dollar lawsuits. Without attempting to judge the validity of such lawsuits, it is easy to see that the effect on both providers and reimbursement organizations (including Medicare and Medicaid) has been nearly devastating. Although most of the costs have been borne directly by liability insurance companies, they pass that cost on to providers in the form of higher premiums. They, in turn, pass the cost on to their sources of reimbursement and, eventually, to the consumers. In several states, physicians have had to retire from practice or move to other states because they could not afford to pay their liability insurance premiums. Although the costs associated with this phenomenon are often higher in acute care, a recent study of the impact on long-term care revealed the following information:

- Countrywide, the number of claims incurred per 1,000 occupied beds doubled from 5.6 in 1995 to 11.1 in 2006.

- The average amount spent to defend a GL/PL claim has almost quadrupled in the past seven years from approximately $13,600 to $52,800.

- Currently, more than half of the total amount of claims costs paid for GL/PL claims in the long-term care industry is going directly to attorneys. This means that less than half of the dollars spent on liability is actually going to the patient and their families. (Bourdon & Coleianne, 2007)

That same report showed that there has been significant improvement in states that have enacted tort reform in the past several years as follows:

- As a group, the average loss cost of Florida, Georgia, Louisiana, Mississippi, Ohio, Texas, and West Virginia dropped from $5,110 in 1998 to $1,240 in 2006.

- For the providers represented in this study, tort reform has produced approximately $200,000,000 in annual savings in the cost of care.

- Both frequency and severity are down in states that have passed tort reform. The number of claims per 1,000 occupied beds for this group peaked at 18.7 in 2001 and dropped to 12.3 in 2006. The average size of a claim plummeted from $358,000 in 1998 to $101,000 in 2006. (Bourdon & Dubin, 2003)

It is perhaps the fact that so much of the money is going to lawyers that is most disturbing. Few would deny injured consumers fair compensation. However, much of the liability settlements is paid to their attorneys. Even CMS has expressed concern over the effect on providers, consumers, and the ability of CMS and state Medicaid agencies to keep up with the costs. In a healthcare industry market update, CMS took note of the increasing number of bankruptcies among long-term care providers; of the likelihood that providers, particularly multi-facility corporate chains, will move out of states where the crisis is particularly acute; and of the effect on access to services (Van Der Walde & Choi, 2003).

There has been a call for reform of current tort laws to address this problem. As with most such issues, this one is hotly contested in the political arena. The U.S. House of Representatives passed a reform act in July 2003, but opponents in the Senate succeeded in delaying, or possibly preventing, action by that body. Medical organizations, other provider groups, and insurance companies are lined up on one side of the issue, and trial lawyers and some consumer advocacy groups are on the other. Unless action is taken, this problem will continue to get worse and will have a major impact on the entire healthcare system.

Financing Reform

There has also been much talk about reforming the overall U.S. healthcare system, which really means reforming the healthcare financing system. The debate, which ebbs and flows, generally centers on providing coverage for people needing acute and preventive care. Throughout, there has been little attention given to providing more coverage for long-term care. There seem to be several reasons for this.

First, long-term care financing does not have the urgency of acute care. The public sees it as something that can be put off—unless they are already involved with it. Acute care, on the other hand, affects them now and in dramatic fashion. Lack of access to it can be immediately and permanently devastating. People unable to pay for emergency or preventive care, especially children, evoke a great deal of concern. They should—and they should receive the highest priority. However, the gap in public interest between that top priority and the somewhat lower priority of long-term care is far too great. Efforts by the elderly and their advocates have begun to raise public consciousness and close that gap, but it still exists.

A second reason long-term care financing is given low priority in reform talks is that it is so hard to get a handle on it. As has been demonstrated throughout this text, long-term care takes many forms; is constantly evolving into new forms; and is subject to many separate, uncoordinated methods of reimbursement. Politicians and other policy makers—those who must make reform happen—are having a hard enough time reforming the less complex acute care financing system. They find it exceedingly difficult to grasp a system that is not purely health care but is inextricably interwoven with other social systems. They are reluctant to attempt reforming the way long-term care is financed when that may require also reforming other social systems such as welfare, housing, and transportation.

The third, and probably most important, factor preventing meaningful reform of how long-term care is reimbursed is the cost. Most discussions of financing reform begin with an assumption that it means significantly greater government involvement, which means a level of public spending that would be unpalatable to most taxpayers. Even the most conservative estimates show that increased public spending on long-term care would mean a major increase in the burden on taxpayers. Given our history of underestimating such things, the actual result would be much higher.

Still, in spite of these barriers, reform is happening. It is not happening all at once or in dramatic fashion but incrementally. Changes are taking place. New ideas are being tried. The evolution of managed care, in both the public and private sectors, is one example. Another is the testing of public–private partnership innovations. Those tried so far have demonstrated that it is an appropriate approach to follow. Further experimentation should provide additional evidence of this and a refinement in methodology. One element that will contribute greatly to the success or failure of any public–private partnership attempt is consumer education. It will require an intensive, ongoing effort—one that may not pay off for many years—but one that is absolutely essential.

The growth of private long-term care insurance, although slow, can also have some impact. It is unlikely to become a major source of reimbursement, but it can be significant. What is needed to make that happen are more incentives for individuals and/or employers to invest in it. These incentives might take the form of tax credits or even subsidies. Tax incentives are already in place to a limited degree and show promise. The idea of the government subsidizing the purchase of private insurance premiums has been floated. It is attractive to those advocating more choice by consumers, but it is looked on with skepticism by others concerned about losing control.

Other reform discussions, particularly as they affect public programs, are taking place. Again, however, the direct involvement of long-term care is very limited. The discussions address the Medicare and Medicaid programs primarily, aimed at preserving the programs and the services they cover. The impact on long-term care reimbursement and on long-term care providers may be significant, but it is usually secondary to concerns for the programs themselves.

Summary

This chapter attempted to present a broad overview of how long-term care is reimbursed. It is far too complex a topic to do justice to in a single chapter, and there are some excellent books available that cover it in more appropriate detail. It is a topic that is, and probably always will be, in a state of constant evolution, meaning that even the best text on the subject is quickly out of date.

That complexity and dynamism are among the factors contributing to the increased importance given to the role of specialists in long-term care reimbursement. It is difficult for many administrators to keep up with the details of reimbursement and manage their organizations as well. A secondary, but directly related, result is the incentive for long-term care providers to become involved in integrated networks or systems where such specialists are more likely to be available. However, all administrators of long-term care organizations and anyone seeking an understanding of the continuum of care must understand, at least, the essentials of reimbursement.

Test Your Understanding

Terminology

beneficiary
case management
Consumer Bill of Rights and
 Responsibilities (managed care)
entitlement program
health maintenance organization
 (HMO)
 managed care
Medicaid
medically indigent
Medicare

Medicare Trust Fund
Part A
Part B
private long-term care insurance
private payment
prospective payment system
public–private partnerships
reimbursement driven
Robert Wood Johnson Foundation
spend down
waiver programs

Review Questions

The following questions are presented to assist you in understanding the material covered in this chapter. They tend to be general but lend themselves to detailed answers, which can be found in the chapter.

1. What do we mean when we say that the long-term care system is reimbursement driven?
2. Who is covered by Medicare? Medicaid?
3. What long-term care services does Medicare cover? What restrictions are placed on them?
4. What long-term care services does Medicaid cover? What restrictions are placed on them?
5. What is the "spend-down" provision of Medicaid, and why is it controversial?
6. What is the purpose of waiver programs?

7. What are public–private partnerships?
8. Why has managed care taken hold more slowly in long-term care than in other segments of health care?
9. What are the most common forms of managed care organizations?
10. What is the managed care consumer bill of rights, and why is it needed?

REFERENCES

AALTCI. (2008a, February 8). *Group LTC Insurance Sales & Claims Paid Up.* Retrieved September 17, 2008, from http://www.aaltci.org/subpages/media_room/story_pages/media020808.html

AALTCI. (2008b, August 6). *180,000 Americans Receive Long-Term Care Insurance Benefits.* Retrieved October 6, 2008, from EmaxHealth: http://www.emaxhealth.com/105/23764.html

AHCA/NCAL. (2003). *Grassley Long-Term Care Insurance Bill on Leading Edge of Nation's Debate on Seniors' Retirement Needs.* Retrieved October 22, 2008, from American Health Care Association/National Center for Assisted Living: http://www.ahca.org/news/nr030708.htm

AHIP. (2007a). *Long-Term Care Insurance Partnerships: New Choices for Consumers—Potential Savings for.* Washington, DC: America's Health Insurance Plans.

AHIP. (2007b). *Who Buys Long-Term Care Insurance?* Washington, DC: America's Health Insurance Plans.

Bourdon, T., & Coleianne, C. (2007). *Long Term Care 2006 General Liability and Professional Liability 2006 General Liability and Professional Liability.* Washington, DC: American Health Care Association.

Bourdon, T., & Dubin, S. (2003, June). *Long-Term Care General Liability and Professional Liability Actuarial Analysis.* Retrieved 2003, from American Health Care Association.

CMS. (2005, December 14). *Medicaid State Waiver Program Demonstration Projects—General Information, Overview.* Retrieved October 9, 2008, from Centers for Medicare & Medicaid Services: http://www.cms.hhs.gov/MedicaidStWaivProgDemoPGI

CMS. (2007). *Medicare Coverage of Skilled Nursing Facility Care.* Baltimore, MD: Centers for Medicare & Medicaid Services.

CMS. (2008, April 22). *Status of the Social Security and Medicare Trust Funds: A Summary of the Reports of the 2008 Annual Reports.* Retrieved October 7, 2008, from Social Security Online: http://www.ssa.gov/OACT/TRSUM/index.html

Fisher, C. (1997, October). Unprepared for Managed Care? *Provider,* pp. 9–10.

Georgetown University. (2004, July). *Who pays for long-term care?* Retrieved September 22, 2008, from Georgetown University Long-Term Care Project: http://ltc.georgetown.edu/pdfs/whopays2004.pdf

Goldsmith, S. (1994). *Essentials of Long-Term Care Administration.* Gaithersburg, MD: Aspen Publishers.

Kaiser Family Foundation. (2008, May 19). *Medicaid Today.* Retrieved October 8, 2008, from Kaiser Fast Facts: http://facts.kff.org/chart.aspx?ch=463

Kane, R. (1997). The Evolution of the American Nursing Home. In R. Binstock, L. Cluff, & O. Von Mering, *The Future of Long-Term Care: Social and Policy Issues* (pp. 145–168). Baltimore: Johns Hopkins University Press.

Kongstvedt, P. (2007). *Essentials of Managed Health Care*, 5th. ed. Sudbury, MA: Jones & Bartlett.

Meiners, M. (1996). The Financing and Organization of Long-Term Care. In R. Binstock, L. Cluff, & O. Von Mering, *The Future of Long-Term Care: Social and Policy Issues* (pp. 191–214). Baltimore: Johns Hopkins University Press.

NCHS. (2007). *Health, United States, 2007 with Chartbook on Trends in the Health of Americans (2007)*. Hyattsville, MD: National Center for Health Statistics.

Peck, R. (1996, June). Linking Subacute Care Services with Managed Care. *Nursing Homes*, pp. 33–35.

Peck, R. (1997). Medicare PPS: Here at Last. *Nursing Homes*, pp. 16–20.

President's Advisory Commission. (1997). *President's Advisory Commission Releases Consumer Bill of Rights and Responsibilities*. Washington, DC: President's Advisory Commission on Consumer Protection and Quality in the Health Care Industry.

Priester, R. (1997). Does Managed Care Offer Value to Society? In M. Brown, *Managed Care: Strategies, Networks, and Management* (p. 3). Gaithersburg, MD: Aspen Publishers.

Senior Journal. (2008, June 13). *Long-Term Care Insurance Cost Nears $2,000 a Year for a Senior Citizen*. Retrieved October 8, 2008, from Senior Journal: Today's News and Information for Senior Citizens & Baby Boomers: http://seniorjournal.com/NEWS/Money/2008/20080613-3-LongTermCare.htm

Truffer, C., Klemm, C., Hoffman, E., & Wolfe, C. (2008). *Medicaid Actuarial Report on the Financial Outlook for Medicaid*. Washington, DC: Centers for Medicare and Medicaid Services.

Van Der Walde, L., & Choi, K. (2003). *Health Care Market Industry: Nursing Facilities*. Retrieved October 21, 2008, from Centers for Medicare and Medicaid Services: http://www.achca.org/news/nr030522.pdf

Villagran, L. (2007, October 3). *Boomers Buying Long-Term Care Coverage*. Retrieved June 12, 2008, from BusinessWeek: http://businessweek.com/ap/financialnews/D8SJ3KQ01.htm

Wagner, E., & Kongstvedt, P. (2007). Types of Managed Care Plans and Integrated Healthcare Delivery Systems. In P. Kongstvedt, *Essentials of Managed Care*, 5th ed. (pp. 19–40). Sudbury, MA: Jones & Bartlett.

Weiner, J., & Illston, L. (1993). Options for LTC Financing Reform: Public and Private Strategies. *Journal of Long-Term Care Administration*, pp. 46–57.

Chapter 10

John R. Pratt, MHA, FACHCA, LFACHE

Long-Term Care Quality

What You Will Learn

- Understand the concept of quality improvement and how it applies to long-term care.
- Identify the similarities and differences between quality assurance and continuous quality improvement.
- Discuss and compare outcomes-based measures and process-based measures and the advantages of each.
- Discuss the value of a systemwide approach to management of quality.
- Identify government and private resources available to assist providers in developing and maintaining quality improvement programs.

Introduction

Long-term care managers must be dedicated to providing care that is of the highest possible quality. This means constantly striving not only to maintain quality, but to improve it. Today there is much emphasis on quality in all of health care, particularly in long-term care. Some is the result of a public that is concerned about the quality of long-term care services; some is the result of elected and regulatory officials expressing that concern. Politicians and advocacy groups such as AARP are demanding that the federal government exercise more oversight over the long-term care field. Lawyers are openly advertising in some states with ads that read something like, "Have you or a loved one been mistreated or harmed in a nursing home?"

The concern over quality in long-term care has resulted in several major studies by the National Institute of Medicine (IOM). First was the report of the IOM Committee on Nursing Home Regulations, *Improving the Quality of Care in Nursing Homes*. It was the basis for the Nursing Home Reform Act, passed as part of the 1987 Omnibus Budget Reconciliation Act (OBRA), which imposed significant new regulations on long-term care providers. More recently (2001), the IOM released two additional reports concerning quality. One, entitled *Crossing the Quality Chasm: A New Health System for the 21st Century*, reported on the findings of the IOM Committee on Quality of Health Care in America. It addressed the topic of quality in all of health care, including long-term care.

The other report focused directly on long-term care. It covered the work of the IOM Committee on Improving Quality in Long-Term Care. Entitled *Improving the Quality of Long-Term Care* (Wunderlich &

Kohler, 2001), it contained significant conclusions about the level of quality found in long-term care services, along with recommendations for improvement. The committee found that since implementation of OBRA, the quality of care has generally improved, even though nursing homes are serving a more seriously ill population, and that quality of life for nursing home residents has also shown some improvement, but to a lesser extent (Wunderlich & Kohler, 2001). The committee noted that information about the quality of care for long-term care other than nursing homes is scarce and inconsistent, making it difficult to evaluate.

There have been a number of quality initiatives aimed at long-term care and other segments of the healthcare field. In part, it is because of this kind of pressure. However, it is also because quality is important to providers. Organizations tend to embark on quality improvement for a variety of reasons, including accreditation requirements, cost control, competition for customers, and pressure from employers and payers (McLaughlin & Kaluzny, 2006). They recognize the benefits of establishing a comprehensive quality agenda that becomes part and parcel of daily operations—high-quality resident care, improved workforce retention, increased organizational effectiveness, better use of available resources, and a positive impact on the success of the operation (Schiverick, 2008). We discuss both government and private quality measurement a bit later in this chapter, but first, let us look at how quality is defined.

Defining Quality

Just about anyone involved with any form of quality assurance (QA) or quality measurement agrees that the first step to accomplishing anything is determining what is meant by quality. It is also the most difficult step. *Quality* means different things to different people and different things in different situations. There are many definitions, but as a 2001 IOM study noted, "no single or simple formula is available to guide those attempting to evaluate the quality of long-term care" (Wunderlich & Kohler, 2001).

The most commonly cited, perhaps easiest to use, definition comes from Dr. Avedis Donabedian of the University of Michigan, one of the earliest to teach and write about quality assessment in health care. He defines healthcare quality as "a judgment about the goodness of both technical care and the management of the interpersonal exchanges between client and practitioner" (Donabedian, 1991). This definition, while covering all of health care, has excellent application to long-term care. It is also brilliant in its simplicity. He describes the definition as "rather broad, but not so broad as to be crippling." Let us examine some of the key words and phrases in that definition:

1. Quality is a matter of judgment. There is no absolute measure of quality. It depends on many inconstant factors, as well as the perception of the person making the judgment.

2. Quality measures something Donabedian calls "goodness." Although that term seems to be pretty subjective and difficult to quantify, most of us have our own understanding of what goodness is.

3. Quality involves both technical care and interpersonal exchanges between the recipient of care and those providing it. This includes quality of life.

It has been suggested that there are five interrelated domains that should be measured to establish an evidence-based, actionable quality agenda:

- Consumer satisfaction.
- Employee satisfaction.
- Workforce stability.
- Clinical outcomes.
- Regulatory performance. (Schiverick, 2008)

These domains cover both clinical and nonclinical measurement areas and address an organization's primary stakeholders: residents (and their families), staff, and outside forces such as regulators.

These factors are even more important in long-term care than in acute settings because of the very nature of the relationship between consumer and provider. That relationship is ongoing and long-standing. It involves very personal, day-to-day interactions. Long-term care consumers are being cared for, not cured. Care for them means more than treatment of a disease or alleviation of a temporary medical condition. They rely on their caregivers for the quality of every aspect of their lives.

Quality of life is particularly difficult to measure. Most consider it to include at least physical health, cognitive status, and functional status, as well as psychological, social, spiritual, and economic well-being (Wunderlich & Kohler, 2001).

Yet, although all of these elements have a bearing on quality of life, each individual places different degrees of importance on each of them. It is hard for "outsiders"—that is, anyone other than the person directly involved—to measure the quality of life of that person. For this reason, measurement of quality in long-term care has moved toward including more input from consumers.

Where it had historically been based largely on empirical data (number of falls, infections, etc.), recent efforts have begun to add an element of consumer satisfaction. Although often overshadowed by measures of clinical process and outcomes, consumer satisfaction is emerging as an important indicator of quality (Bernard & Savitz, 2006). Long-term care consumers are now asked what is important to them and whether they are satisfied with the care they get.

Consumer satisfaction is only one element of quality measurement, and as important as it is, it is not always easy to measure. Many long-term care consumers have limited cognitive ability or are unable to communicate their thoughts clearly, making their input either impossible to get or of questionable validity.

There is still one more definition of quality that perhaps says it even better, although the quality it defines may not be as easy to measure or regulate. Someone once told a group of administrators that "Your customers may not know what quality is, but they know when they don't get it." On a practical basis, this says it well.

Whatever means are chosen to measure (and therefore ensure) quality, it probably involves one or more of three generally accepted measurement types: structure, process, and outcomes (Donabedian, 1966). *Structure measurement* deals with the makeup of the organization where the care is provided, including organizational structure, resources provided, and so on. *Process measurement* refers to how the care is delivered. *Outcomes measurement* focuses on the end result—the effect the care has on the individual.

Historically, most quality measures have focused more on structure and process than on outcomes, in large part because structure and process are easier to measure than outcomes. It is easier to document what was done and how it was done than what the resultant effect on the consumer was. Measurement of outcomes is more difficult in long-term care than in acute care settings. In acute care, successful outcomes often mean restoring patients to their level of functioning before the onset of illness. In long-term care, successful outcomes are usually aimed at maximizing quality of life and physical function in the presence of permanent, and sometimes worsening, impairment. They often focus on such things as overall health status, presence or absence of specific conditions (e.g., pressure sores), social and psychological well-being, and satisfaction with care (Wunderlich & Kohler, 2001). More recently, there has been an increased emphasis on achieving such outcomes, difficult though they may be to measure. One author calls outcome measures the "gold standard" for measuring the quality of care (DesHarnais & McLaughlin, 2006).

Yet outcomes depend in large part on both process and structure, and the three are invariably linked. Process (how care is delivered) depends on the structure of the delivery organization (staffing, equipment). As important as outcomes are, it is also necessary to measure process and structure as indicators of the reasons the outcomes may be less than optimal.

For example, a high rate of nosocomial infections (those contracted while in the facility) is definitely an undesirable outcome, yet the only way to deal with it is to examine the structure and processes involved in care of residents. Did poor infection control techniques cause the high rate? If so, that is a process issue. Did lack of resources resulting in overcrowding of residents or understaffing (structure issues) contribute to the high infection rate? As you can see, the outcomes are important in measuring results, but it is likely structure or process (usually process) that causes these outcomes, and only by focusing on the structure or processes can the outcomes be improved.

Total Quality Management/ Continuous Quality Improvement

Although sometimes called by other names, continuous quality improvement (CQI) is the most common name for what is essentially total quality management (TQM) as applied to health care. TQM was created by Dr. W. Edwards Deming. It has been used extensively in business and industry for years, but its acceptance by long-term care and other healthcare organizations has been quite recent. As they have adapted its principles to their organizations, they have generally chosen to call it continuous quality improvement. This slight difference in terminology is important because it better defines what they seek to accomplish.

The basis of CQI is that quality is not separate from other aspects of the organization's operations. It is a holistic approach that is based on a desire by the staff and administration to achieve excellence in what they do—provide care to the residents who rely on them. Deming based his approach to quality improvement on a set of principles known as his "Fourteen Points." They are not covered in depth here, nor are they all identified. Instead, the overall aspects of CQI and how they apply to long-term care is discussed. It is worth noting, however, that these principles recognize the inherent goodness of individuals and their desire to work, as well as the contributions they can make to-

ward improving quality and reducing costs. As a result, CQI encourages their active involvement. Another definition of CQI (or TQM) is that it is "a structured organizational process for involving personnel in planning and executing a continuous flow of improvements to provide quality health care that meets or exceeds expectations" (McLaughlin & Kaluzny, 2006).

Quality Initiatives

As noted at the beginning of this chapter, there are many initiatives and/or efforts aimed at measuring and improving quality in long-term care. Some of these are internal in nature in that they are administered by the provider organization primarily for the benefit of that organization and its consumers. Others are developed and administered by some entity external to any individual provider organization and are meant to ensure quality for the overall system or at least for major segments of the system. Although these separate types of quality initiative are generally quite well defined, the distinction is not always clear because some of the systemwide quality initiatives involve grouping several of the programs used by providers. These situations are pointed out as the discussion continues.

Systemwide Quality Programs

In addition to the internal quality improvement efforts of providers, there are several external initiatives in place that attempt to improve the overall quality of the long-term care system. Some of them are managed by government agencies, and others are operated by private organizations.

Government Programs

Much of what we have seen in the way of standardizing quality measurement and assurance has been dictated by government regulation. The government has, when paying for care through programs such as Medicare and Medicaid, a responsibility to ensure both the quality and cost-effectiveness of the care for which they pay. Unfortunately, the two aspects often become confused. In some cases, the idea of quality has taken on more of a focus on medical necessity—is the care provided medically necessary? Ideally, medical necessity should mean neither more nor less than is appropriate. In the past, the pressures to achieve cost-effectiveness seem to have tilted that equation toward ensuring that the government does not pay for more than it must. To be fair, it may only seem that such is the focus, but the evidence has been pretty strong and consistent. The requirement for utilization review was focused more on cost saving than on quality. You should not assume that government agencies are unconcerned with quality. They certainly are. It is just much harder to measure and ensure. Government concern with quality is shown by requirements that providers create and maintain quality assurance (QA) programs and, more recently, quality improvement programs.

There is a major difference in emphasis in externally mandated quality requirements and in internal, provider-administered, quality improvement. Typically, externally mandated requirements do not focus on improving the average performance of providers over time. They are aimed at weeding out poor performers and ensuring that providers meet minimal standards. Internal quality improvement, on the other hand, is designed to sustain and improve quality within the organizations.

Federal and state governments are concerned with quality of care, particularly for consumers covered by government-run eligibility plans such as Medicare and Medicaid. Government attempts at ensuring quality fall into three distinct approaches: regulation of quality, public information initiatives, and quality-related research.

Regulation of Quality

Government regulation of long-term care covers both regulation of quality and regulation of cost. Regulation of quality takes the form of measuring providers against minimally acceptable levels and punishing those providers who fall below those levels. It mostly involves setting standards, designing survey processes to monitor compliance, and determining sanctions for noncompliance. Because of the dominant role of Medicare and Medicaid in reimbursement of nursing facilities, subacute care, home health care, and hospice care, the federal government is the major source of quality regulations for these providers. For others not generally covered by Medicare and Medicaid (most notably assisted living/residential care), the states determine the quality regulations. This is changing somewhat as states increasingly use Medicaid waivers to cover some residential care consumers.

History of Government Quality Regulations

While government entities, particularly the federal government, have long regulated quality in long-term care, that regulation has evolved through several different formats and initiatives.

Quality Assurance

Quality assurance was one of the early forms of quality regulation required by the Medicare and Medicaid system. It was a method of quality management that identified quality issues, set minimum standards to be met for the issue, and then ceased to work on the issue once the minimum standards were met (Lighter & Fair, 2004). Because it was required for several decades, it was long seen as the primary method of measuring and ensuring quality in long-term care organizations. It is regulation driven, and, as with many regulations, much of the focus was on documentation of compliance rather than on the actual quality itself. Many long-term care managers and staff saw it as a requirement, not something they do by choice, which limited its effectiveness. QA involved eliminating defects (Kelly, 2003) and relied on reviews of reports of infections, accidents, transfer of residents (utilization review), and administration of medications to identify any real or potential problem areas. It was focused as much on cost savings as it was on quality. As such, it was only partially successful and had little effect on the mounting cost to the government of the Medicare and Medicaid programs (Shaw, Elliott, Isaacson, & Murphy, 2003).

"Quality assurance" also became a somewhat generic term referring to any such quality measurement and improvement methods—so much so that many feel as did one author who stated, "One of the most critical tasks for the health care industry is the conversion from a quality assurance framework to one of QI (quality improvement)" (Lighter, 2004).

Minimum Data Set for Long-Term Care

In 1998, the federal government mandated use of a Minimum Data Set (MDS) as a means of structuring the assessment of long-term care (nursing home) residents. The MDS, includes assessment of:

- Cognitive patterns.
- Communication and hearing patterns.
- Vision patterns.
- Physical functioning and structural problems.
- Continence.
- Psychosocial well-being.
- Mood and behavior patterns.
- Activity-pursuit patterns.
- Disease diagnoses.
- Other health conditions.
- Oral/nutritional status.
- Skin condition.
- Medication use.
- Treatments and procedures. (Shaw et al., 2003)

Using information collected from these assessments, the government provides the facility with a list of identified deficiencies when compared with the standards.

OASIS

The Centers for Medicare & Medicaid Services (CMS) uses a similar assessment tool for home health care, called the Outcomes and Assessment Information Set (OASIS).

Quality Improvement Organizations

CMS now contracts with one organization in each state, as well as the District of Columbia, Puerto Rico, and the U.S. Virgin Islands, to serve as that state/jurisdiction's quality improvement organization (QIO) contractor. QIOs are private, mostly not-for-profit organizations staffed by professionals, mostly doctors and other healthcare professionals, who are trained to review medical care and help beneficiaries with complaints about the quality of care and to implement improvements in the quality of care available throughout the spectrum of care (CMS, 2008b). The QIO's purpose is not to identify situations in which enforcement is necessary but rather to assist nursing homes to improve quality using quality improvement principles and techniques (CMS, 2002).

Pay-for-Performance

As part of its overall quality initiative, CMS also began several pay-for-performance programs, with a goal of improving quality and lowering costs. The pay-for-performance (also known as "P4P") programs involve identifying procedures for which providers will not be reimbursed, as CMS identifies them as not necessary or resulting from poor quality. For example, any procedures resulting from facility-acquired infections would not be reimbursed (Sultz & Young, 2009). Other "preventable" conditions might include falls, catheter-based urinary infections, and pressure ulcers. While the concept sounds good, not all agree with its effectiveness. Some have suggested that it is more effective as a cost-control measure, but dispute the relationship between payment and quality. For example, one study that compared P4P-participating hospitals and similar ones (both in a large multi-hospital system) showed no significantly different rates of improvement in the quality of care provided by the P4P-participating facilities (Grossbart, 2008).

Providers object to the implication that they will improve quality—or decrease provision of poor quality—if they are paid more.

Public Information Quality Initiatives

In recent years, government agencies have increasingly attempted to provide the public with information about healthcare quality with the intent of creating more knowledgeable consumers capable of judging quality for themselves. The most ambitious such project occurred in late 2002, when the CMS announced a nationwide quality initiative for nursing care facilities.

Nursing Home Compare

Under the initiative, the CMS released comparative data for all nursing facilities serving residents covered by Medicare and/or Medicaid. The approach was to identify certain quality measures and to show how individual facilities compared with the preset standard and with each other. Among the first quality measures chosen were the number of residents with loss of ability in daily tasks, residents with pressure sores, residents with pain and infections, and residents in physical restraints.

The CMS makes information about these measures and how providers rate available on its website in a section titled "Nursing Home Compare." On this site, consumers can get information about individual nursing homes, including number of beds and type of ownership; data on the selected quality measures; results of state surveys; and information about staffing. Although this initiative is quite different in nature from internal quality improvement programs, there is a relationship. The CMS initiative relies on reports submitted by the facilities through the MDS information that all must file with the government agency. The initiative uses numerical data in much the same way as was described earlier in the "Quality Assurance" section. CMS does not attempt to improve quality but strives to pressure the facilities to do so.

Similar initiatives concerning hospitals and home health providers are also in place. While there is at this writing no "compare" program for assisted living (not covered by Medicare), the government and assisted living stakeholders are collaborating on an initiative to develop a tool that helps consumers compare and select assisted living communities across the nation (NCAL, 2008).

"Five-Star" Ratings

In June 2008, CMS announced the launch of a ranking system of America's nursing homes, giving each a "star" rating. According to CMS, the new "five-star" rating system "will provide a composite view of the quality and safety information currently on Nursing Home Compare to help beneficiaries, their families, and caregivers compare nursing homes more easily" (CMS, 2008a). There have also been numerous efforts by state governments to publish report card–type information about providers in their state jurisdictions.

Quality-Related Research

There are several government agencies involved in quality-related research. They fund research studies and disseminate the results. They also serve as a valuable source for quality improvement guidelines, measurement tools, quality indicators, and other data.

AHRQ

Foremost among these resources is the Agency for Healthcare Research and Quality (AHRQ). Formerly known as the Agency for Health Care Policy and Research, this organization is a source of many studies concerning healthcare quality. It regularly produces reports documenting research studies it has funded. It has developed quality indicators (quality improvements) that serve as valuable measures used both by researchers and by individual provider organizations. The AHRQ also maintains the National Guideline Clearinghouse, a centralized source of information about clinical practice guidelines that provides recommendations for how care should be given.

National Library of Medicine

The National Library of Medicine (NLM), on the campus of the National Institutes of Health in Bethesda, Maryland, is the world's largest medical library (NLM, 2007). It collects materials and provides information and research services in all areas of biomedicine and health care and works closely with AHRQ to produce and disseminate data, guidelines, and other information for researchers and practitioners.

Private Quality Programs

Not all systemwide quality improvement efforts come from the government. Several private organizations and coalitions of organizations have produced their own quality programs. In fact, there has been such a proliferation of quality programs it is difficult to list them without omitting some. A good effort is made to do so, but apologies are in order in advance for any that were in-advertently missed.

Quality First

In 2002, several leading long-term care professional organizations created a voluntary five-year initiative designed to improve the quality of nursing home care and other long-term care services. That initiative, called "Quality First: a Covenant for Healthy, Affordable, and Ethical Long-Term Care," was developed by the American Association of Homes and Services for the Aging (AAH-SA), the American Health Care Association (AHCA), and the Alliance for Quality Nursing Home Care. These organizations signed a covenant that reads as follows:

> Through Quality First we are collectively and individually committed to healthy, affordable, and ethical long-term care. We commit to achieving excellence in the quality of care and services for older persons and strengthening public trust. We recognize that confidence on the part of consumers and policy makers is lacking and must be restored. We are committed to taking bold and deliberate steps, embedded in the principles of this Covenant to ensure quality. We believe that by doing so, there will be measurable improvements in defined outcomes as well as in ethical, compassionate, and resident-centered practices in the provision of care for those who are frail, elderly, or disabled. (AHCA, 2007b)

The covenant is rooted in the following seven principles, designed to "cultivate and nourish an environment of continuous quality improvement, openness and leadership":

1. Continuous quality assurance and quality improvement.
2. Public disclosure and accountability.
3. Patient/resident and family rights.
4. Workforce excellence.
5. Public input and community involvement.
6. Ethical practices.
7. Financial stewardship. (AHCA, 2007b)

Quality First represents a major commitment by long-term care providers to assure consumers, consumer advocacy organizations, and government that they will provide high-quality care. It is the most significant such initiative to date, in part because of the many providers represented by these organizations and because they are committing to going beyond what may be required by government regulation. In doing this, they are accepting their individual and collective responsibility to gain the trust and confidence of the public. The Quality First organizations originally outlined several specific outcomes to be achieved:

1. There will be continued improvement in compliance with federal regulations.
2. There will be demonstrable progress in promoting financial integrity and preventing occurrences of fraud.
3. There will be demonstrable progress in the quality of clinical outcomes and prevention of confirmed abuse and neglect.

4. There will be measurable improvements in all Centers for Medicare and Medicaid Services continuous quality improvement measures.

5. High rates on consumer satisfaction surveys will indicate improved consumer satisfaction with services.

6. There will be demonstrable improvement in employee retention and turnover rates. (AHCA, 2007b)

Although Quality First is a private initiative, the participating organizations have pledged to work with the government, particularly CMS. They use the quality improvement measures adopted by CMS and report on their progress to government officials on an annual basis. They also point out that Quality First and CMS share several common goals:

- Achieve excellence in the quality of care and services.
- Emphasize continuous quality improvement.
- Publicly report results to strengthen public confidence and trust. (AHCA/NCAL, 2004)

AAHSA

The American Association of Homes and Services for the Aging represents 5,600 mission-driven, not-for-profit nursing homes, continuing care retirement communities, assisted living and senior housing facilities, and home- and community-based service providers. The organization has state association partners that represent AAHSA members in most states. As one of the organizations signing the Quality First covenant, AAHSA developed a 10-point plan to involve all of its members in Quality First. The AAHSA 10-point plan focuses on

1. Commitment.
2. Governance accountability.
3. Leading-edge care and services.
4. Community involvement.
5. Continuous quality improvement.
6. Human resources development.
7. Consumer-friendly information.
8. Consumer participation.
9. Research findings and education.
10. Public trust and consumer confidence. (AAHSA, 2008)

AHCA/NCAL

The American Health Care Association/National Center for Assisted Living is a nonprofit federation of affiliated state health organizations, together representing more than 10,000 nonprofit and for-profit assisted living, nursing facility, and subacute care providers, as well as providers of services to the developmentally disabled. Together, these organizations care for more than 1.5 million elderly and disabled individuals nationally.

To assist its members in achieving the goals of Quality First, AHCA developed the AHCA/NCAL Quality Award: a criteria-based program that recognizes a commitment to performance excellence by member facilities. Quality Award recipients demonstrate their commitment to deliver ever-improving value to residents and other customers, to improve overall organizational effectiveness and capabilities, and to champion organizational and personal learning. Facilities may apply for recognition and awards at three levels, each of which requires a more detailed and comprehensive demonstration of systematic quality. Facilities must receive a quality award at each level to progress to the next level (AHCA/NCAL, 2008).

Alliance for Quality Nursing Home Care

The Alliance for Quality Nursing Home Care was the third major organization involved in the creation of Quality First to sign on to the Quality First covenant. The Alliance is a coalition of 14 national provider organizations that care for 650,000 elderly and disabled patients annually. As with the AAHSA and the AHCA, the Alliance has developed a more in-depth plan for achieving the goals of the Quality First covenant.

Although there is undoubtedly some cross-membership among these three organizations that created Quality First, it is clear that they represent the vast majority of providers of institutional long-term care. Their commitment to actively work toward the goals of the covenant and to work with government and other long-term care stakeholders is a major step toward achieving a high level of confidence in the quality of long-term care received by consumers.

Advancing Excellence in America's Nursing Homes

Advancing Excellence in America's Nursing Homes is an ongoing, coalition-based campaign concerned with how we care for the elderly, chronically ill, and disabled, as well as those recuperating in a nursing home environment. This voluntary campaign:

- Monitors key indicators of nursing home care quality—both clinical quality and organizational improvement goals.

- Promotes excellence in caregiving.

- Acknowledges the critical role nursing home staff have in providing care.

- Recognizes the important role of consumers to the success of the campaign by contributing ideas and suggestions.

The campaign builds on the success of other quality initiatives like Quality First and the CMS Nursing Home Quality Initiative (NHQI). It is made up of groups representing:

- Long-term care providers.

- Consumers and advocates.

- Nurses, healthcare professionals, medical directors, and healthcare administrators.

- Caregiver/support staff.

- Government agencies, foundations, and other quality-focused organizations. (Advancing Excellence Campaign, 2007)

In its first two-years, the Advancing Excellence Campaign developed the following measurable goals:

Clinical Goals:

Goal #1: Reducing high-risk pressure ulcers;

Goal #2: Reducing the use of daily physical restraints;

Goal #3: Improving pain management for longer-term nursing home residents;

Goal #4: Improving pain management for short stay, post-acute nursing home residents;

Operational/Process Goals:

Goal #5: Establishing individual targets for improving quality;

Goal #6: Assessing resident and family satisfaction with the quality of care;

Goal #7: Increasing staff retention; and

Goal #8: Improving consistent assignment of nursing home staff, so that residents regularly receive care from the same caregivers.

Participating providers will commit to focus on at least three of the eight measurable goals, with at least one clinical goal and one operational/process goal. (AHCA, 2007a)

The Advancing Excellence campaign has had dramatic success in its first two years. One sign of such success is the number of organizations that have become involved. Those participants include:

- Nearly 7,000 long-term care facilities—more than 43 percent of the nation's skilled nursing facilities.
- Thirty organizations, including the Centers for Medicare & Medicaid Services.
- More than 1,500 consumers. (Wagner, 2008)

Another sign of success is the degree to which participating facilities showed tangible improvement. They made clinical improvements at a faster rate than nonparticipants. For example, restraint use dropped by nearly 23 percent among Advancing Excellence facilities that set goals for this objective (Wagner, 2008).

American Health Quality Association

The American Health Quality Association (AHQA) is a charitable, educational, not-for-profit national membership association dedicated to healthcare quality through community-based, independent quality evaluation and improvement programs. It represents quality improvement organizations and professionals working to improve healthcare quality and patient safety. AHQA members:

- Develop and manage projects in healthcare quality improvement and evaluation for Medicare, Medicaid, and private payers and purchasers.
- Provide expertise in clinical care, quality improvement, health information management, statistical analysis, and communications to healthcare purchasers and providers.
- Collaborate with medical practices, hospitals, health plans, long-term care facilities, home health agencies, and employers to evaluate systems of healthcare delivery and to share best practices.
- Work to improve care in rural settings, as well as urban areas, and improve care for disadvantaged groups and ethnic minorities. (AHQA, 2008)

AHQA member organizations assist federal and state agencies and provider organizations by providing technical support. They work with long-term care providers such as nursing facilities and home healthcare agencies, providing them with guidelines, procedures, and hands-on assistance as needed.

National Quality Forum

The National Quality Forum (NQF) is a private, not-for-profit membership organization created to develop and implement a national strategy for healthcare quality measurement and reporting. The mission of the National Quality Forum is to improve the quality of American health care by setting national priorities and goals for performance improvement, endorsing national consensus standards for measuring and publicly reporting on performance, and promoting the attainment of national goals through education and outreach programs (NQF, 2008). The NQF develops and implements quality measures, working with government and private agencies.

Accreditation Organizations

There are several private accreditation organizations involved with long-term care, including the Joint Commission on Accreditation of Healthcare Organizations (JCAHO), the Commission on Accreditation of Rehabilitation Facilities (CARF), the Continuing Care Accreditation Commission (CCAC), and the Community Health Accreditation Program (CHAP). It is important to note that all organizations require a strong emphasis on quality improvement in the provider organizations they accredit.

Private Foundations

Numerous private foundations provide funding for quality-related research and project implementation. Among the largest and best known is the Robert Wood Johnson Foundation, which has a mission to improve the health and health care of all Americans. The core strategy of the Foundation's long-standing commitment to improve the quality of health care that Americans receive is *Aligning Forces for Quality*, working to lift the overall quality of health and health care in targeted communities across the country (RWJ Foundation, 2008). Because the

Robert Wood Johnson Foundation has long had an interest in chronic care, it is a very valuable source of information for long-term care providers.

The Robert Wood Johnson Foundation is not the only private foundation supporting this type of research. There are too many others to list all of them here.

College and University Research Institutes

Many colleges and universities maintain research institutes or other organizational divisions addressing quality of care. They generally rely on private and/or government grant funds to conduct research and disseminate the results. They are valuable sources of needed information.

A Combination of Efforts

These quality resources, both private and government sponsored, serve several purposes. First, they bring a great deal of emphasis to the topic of quality care, giving it the prominence it deserves. As noted by both CMS and the signatories to Quality First, consumers of long-term care have a right to expect high-quality care and to have access to enough information to adequately judge whether the care they receive meets those expectations.

Second, these initiatives make it easier for individual providers to develop and maintain quality improvement programs. It can be difficult for small provider organizations to allocate the staff and other resources needed for a good quality improvement program. By taking advantage of the processes, guidelines, standards, and quality indicators available from these sources, they can avoid the necessity of creating their own.

Finally, they help bring a high degree of uniformity and commonality to quality programs across the continuum. As providers become better at quality improvement in their own organizations, the level of quality in the long-term care system becomes better—and consumers are able to have a higher level of confidence in that system.

Other Organizations

There are many other organizations, associations, and coalitions working to improve long-term care—too many to list here. All strive for the same goals: the best possible care for consumers.

Provider-Administered Quality Improvement Programs

There are several programs used by long-term and other healthcare providers to ensure quality of care within their organizations. The term "quality improvement" is used here to cover them in general terms.

Quality improvement began in the acute care sector of health care and has more recently been adapted to long-term care. This has something to do with the fact that the OBRA now requires providers to implement and maintain quality improvement programs, but to be fair to those providers, many had embraced the concept well before that happened. Another impetus for development of quality improvement programs, both in acute care and in long-term care, has come from accrediting agencies such as JCAHO. Healthcare organizations seeking accreditation must have such programs in place. Even though these programs may be in place primarily because of regulations or encouragement from external entities, they fit the definition of internal because they are facility based or organization based and are implemented by staff of the organization.

Although several different types of quality improvement in long-term care are discussed, there are two that are most prominent: quality assurance (QA) and continuous quality improvement (CQI).

Developing a Quality Improvement Program

Creating an effective quality improvement program for a long-term care facility is not simply a matter of copying one developed for an acute care hospital. The focus is different, and the quality improvement plan must reflect that difference. In acute care, quality improvement focuses on episodes of care and ensuring the quality of care during those episodes. In long-term care facilities, the focus must be more on quality of life and must include ongoing monitoring and evaluation of physical, functional, and psychological indicators over a longer period of time (Cohan, 1997). The time period may include several acute episodes, but the overall objective of the quality improvement program is focused on the quality of life of the individual. What follows is a brief description of some of the important elements of a quality improvement program.

Top-Level Support

To begin with, a quality improvement program must have support from the very top levels of administration. In long-term care facilities, this includes the chief executive officer (CEO) of the facility and, if part of a larger corporation, the corporate officers. Studies have shown a correlation between involvement of senior management and successful quality improvement. One such study found five significant roles and/or activities of senior management that are of most importance:

1. *Personal engagement*, characterized by advocacy for quality improvement efforts, participation in quality improvement teams, and dissemination of quality improvement data.

2. *Relationship with clinical staff*, characterized by perceived understanding of clinical/professional staff activities and skill at negotiating with clinical/professional staff.

3. *Promotion of a quality improvement organizational culture*, characterized by goal setting consistent with quality improvement, and consensus-driven interdepartmental and/or multidisciplinary norms.

4. *Support of quality improvement with organizational structures*, characterized by the existence of quality improvement teams and linkages of quality improvement teams to central decision makers.

5. *Procurement of organizational resources*, characterized by procuring and allocating adequate staffing and information technology (IT) capability. (Larson, 2003)

This does not necessarily mean that the CEO must be involved in day-to-day quality improvement activities, but he or she must stay on top of the program. In most facilities, the program director will be someone who has other clinical duties, because many cannot afford to designate a full-time position for quality improvement. In multi-facility organizations, a full-time quality director may be designated by the corporate offices and shared among facilities. In either case, there should be a quality steering committee or council that oversees the work of other committees and individuals. That committee or council should include the top clinical and administrative staff, including the CEO, the director of nursing services, the medical director, and any others who are in charge of major divisions or service areas.

Mission-Based

Ideally, the quality improvement program should be an integral part of the mission of the organization. Most organizational mission statements include some, usually vague, reference to providing quality of care. If an organization has such a statement and really means it, then it can develop a quality improvement program based on the intent of the mission statement.

Defining the Customers

To improve quality, the organization must define who its customers are—those residents or other individuals served by the organization. If it already has a good strategic planning process in place, such data are probably available. However, a special effort should be made to be sure the data are up-to-date because such information can easily become obsolete.

Standards

Having defined its customers, the organization then needs to identify what it wants for them in terms of quality. Although there are many ways of defining that quality, there are some good benchmarking tools available to use, including predetermined quality standards. Standards represent levels of quality against which the care given in an organization can be measured. Some organizations may develop their own, but there are many good quality standards that have been set by various regulatory, accrediting, and professional organizations. These standards may represent an optimal level of quality, but more often they are set at the acceptable level, recognizing that the optimum may not be achievable, at least not at first. As such, standards become dynamic, continuously moving higher toward an optimal level as each standard is achieved (Larson, 1997). When standards developed by someone else are used, they should be evaluated carefully to see how closely they match the outcomes desired for the organization's own customers. If needed, the standards can be adapted to better serve their needs. However, in most cases, that will not be necessary until the quality improvement program becomes more mature.

Measurement

Once an organization has determined the standards against which its quality will be measured, it is time to move on to the measurement itself. Much of the measurement of quality is accomplished by monitoring certain key indicators, such as the number of residents with physical restraints, number of medication errors, or infection rates. Determining which indicators to use takes some effort, but once they have been chosen, the actual measurement is relatively uncomplicated. However, it can be time-consuming. Staff may need to organize into teams to measure the key indicators against the standards that have been chosen. Most likely, structure, process, and outcomes measures will all be used.

Evaluation

When measurement has taken place, producing a volume of data sufficient to draw conclusions, it is up to the quality improvement steering committee to evaluate how well the organization is doing. Initially, this probably involves comparing its performance in key indicator areas against standards set by outside agencies. As the program grows, the committee will increasingly want to compare current results with earlier results to determine how much progress has been made.

Improvement

Because the ultimate purpose of a quality improvement program is to improve quality in specific areas, the next step is to identify appropriate corrective steps to take to improve the quality level in a particular area. This may include changing procedures, reassigning resources such as staff or equipment, education and/or training of staff, restructuring of organizational responsibilities, or other similar steps. In some cases, the solutions may be difficult and expensive. For example, excessive use of physical restraints might indicate that there are not enough staff available, leading to a need to increase the staffing complement. On the other hand, it may simply involve retraining of staff, at little expense. Each quality area will have its own method of improvement, often a combination of several.

Ongoing Measurement and Evaluation

Once corrective steps have been taken, measurement against the standards must be ongoing. If measurement over a period of time indicates that significant progress has been made, the quality improvement team may determine that further steps are not needed. However, they may instead decide to raise the standard and attempt to reach it. Quality improvement is an ongoing program that continues to move on to new areas while keeping track of previously studied areas to make sure there has not been slippage back to an unacceptable level.

Quality Teams

Quality improvement borrows another philosophy from Deming's total quality management—namely, that the people involved in doing a job are usually best suited to solving problems related to that job. Instead of an individual or small committee doing all of the measurement and improvement, quality improvement usually involves teams consisting of staff closely involved with the area being evaluated. They do report to a steering committee, but the individual teams deal directly with identifying and solving the problem. For instance, staying with the example used earlier of a high nosocomial infection rate, the team would include at least representatives from the medical staff, nursing, others involved in hands-on care, and possibly outside consultants with expertise in infection control. A facility may have several quality teams at work at any given time, with some overlap in the personnel assigned to them. For that reason, the number of teams should not be too high.

Technology

Omission of a discussion about how valuable technology can be to a quality improvement

plan would be remiss. Much of the work of the quality teams, the designated quality director, and the steering committee relies on getting access to data that are current and accurate. Although much of that record-keeping was handled manually in the past, it can now be computerized. The result is not only less to do, but much more accurate and usable information. There are some excellent commercial software packages available that do much of the work, although the quality improvement team will still need to interpret it and act on it.

Summary

Quality in long-term care is of highest importance to everyone involved. There has been much improvement in quality in recent years, but there is more to be done. A report by the National Committee for Quality Assurance (NCQA) showed that the quality of health care for millions of Americans improved in 2007, but significant variations in performance continue. While quality improved for most people in private health insurance plans, there was little improvement in the care delivered to those enrolled in Medicare and Medicaid, the nation's two largest public healthcare programs (MarketWatch, 2008).

It is vital that any long-term care administrator understand that and understand how quality improvement is accomplished. Although the techniques of quality improvement are still being developed in many areas, particularly in long-term care, there is already enough information and technical support available for any long-term care organization to develop and implement an effective quality improvement program.

Test Your Understanding

Terminology

*continuous quality improvement
(CQI)*
outcomes measures
process measures
quality
quality assurance (QA)
Quality First
quality improvement

quality indicators
quality steering committee
quality teams
standards
structure measures
total quality management (TQM)
utilization review
W. Edwards Deming

Review Questions

The following questions are presented to assist you in understanding the material covered in this chapter. They tend to be general but lend themselves to detailed answers, which can be found in the chapter.

1. Why is quality difficult to define?
2. Why is quality of life of particular importance in long-term care?
3. What are the purpose and functions of a quality assurance (QA) committee?
4. How do process, structure, and outcomes measures differ?
5. What are the differences between QA and continuous quality improvement (CQI)? The similarities?
6. What are quality indicators?
7. What incentives are there, if any, for individual long-term care providers or groups of providers to think in terms of the overall system when focusing on quality?
8. What disincentives exist in the payment system when it comes to improving quality? How can they be overcome?

REFERENCES

AAHSA. (2008). *10 Elements of Quality: the Framework for Quality First.* Retrieved September 12, 2008, from American Association of Homes and Services for the Aging: http://www.aahsa.org/article.aspx?id=828

Advancing Excellence Campaign. (2007). *About the Campaign.* Retrieved April 2008, from Advancing Excellence in Long-Term Care Campaign: http://www.nhqualitycampaign.org/star_index.aspx?controls=about

AHCA. (2007a). *Advancing Excellence: AHCA's Quality First Focus for 2006–2008.* Retrieved July 21, 2008, from American Health Care Association: http://www.qualityfirstnursinghomes.com

AHCA. (2007b). *Quality First: The Covenant.* Retrieved January 17, 2008, from American Health Care Association: http://www.ahca.org/quality/qf_covenant.htm

AHCA/NCAL. (2004). *The Quality Connection: Bridging Quality First and the CMS.* Retrieved May 2, 2008, from American Health Care Association/National Center for Assisted Living: http://www.qualityfirstnursinghomes.com

AHCA/NCAL. (2008). *The AHCA/NCAL Quality Award: A Benchmark of Performance Excellence.* Retrieved September 12, 2008, from American Health Care Association/National Center for Assisted Living: http://www.ahcancal.org/quality_improvement/quality_award/Documents/2008_QualityAward_brochure.pdf

AHQA. (2008). *About AHQA.* Retrieved September 13, 2008, from American Health Quality Association: http://www.ahqa.org/pub/inside/158_670_2426.cfm

Bernard, S., & Savitz, L. (2006). Measuring Consumer Satisfaction. In C. A. McLaughlin, *Continuous Quality Improvement in Health Care: Theory, Implementations, and Applications*, 3rd ed. (pp. 131–153). Sudbury, MA: Jones & Bartlett.

CMS. (2002, May 22). *Nursing Home Quality Initiative.* Retrieved September 9, 2008, from www.cms.hhs.gov:http://www.cms.hhs.gov/NursingHomeQualityInits/Downloads/NHQIssaqiomergedoc200512.pdf

CMS. (2008a, June 18). *CMS to Rate Nursing Home Quality: New Five-Star System to Be Added to Nursing Home Compare Site.* Retrieved September 13, 2008, from Centers for Medicare & Medicaid Services: http://www.cms.hhs.gov/apps/media/press/release.asp?Counter=3163&intNumPerPage=10&checkDate=&checkKey=2&srchType=2&numDays=0&srchOpt=0&srchData=star&keywordType=All&chkNewsType=1%2C+2%2C+3%2C+4%2C+5&intPage=&showAll=1&pYear=&year=0&desc=&cboOrder=date

CMS. (2008b, August 15). *Quality Improvement Organizations: Overview.* Retrieved September 9, 2008, from Centers for Medicare & Medicaid Services: http://www.cms.hhs.gov/QualityImprovementOrgs/01_Overview.asp

Cohan, M. A. (1997). Improving Quality in Long-Term Care. In C. Meisenheimer, *Improving Quality: A Guide to Effective Programs*, 2nd ed. (pp. 507–520). Gaithersburg, MD: Aspen Publishers.

DesHarnais, S., & McLaughlin, C. (2006). The Outcome Model of Quality. In C. A. McLaughlin, *Continuous Quality Improvement in Health Care: Theory, Implementations, and Applications*, 3rd ed. (pp. 67–94). Sudbury, MA: Jones & Bartlett.

Donabedian, A. (1966). Evaluating the Quality of Medical Care. *Milbank Memorial Fund Quarterly*, pp. 194–196.

Donabedian, A. (1991). Reflections on the Effectiveness of Quality Assurance. In H. D. Palmer, *Striving for Quality in Health Care: An Inquiry into Policy and Practice* (p. 61). Ann Arbor, MI: Health Administration Press.

Grossbart, S. (2008, Spring). Effectiveness of Pay for Performance as a Quality Improvement Strategy. *Prescriptions for Excellence in Health Care*, pp. 2–4.

Kelly, D. (2003). *Applying Quality Management in Healthcare.* Chicago: Health Administration Press.

Larson, S. (1997). Standards: The Basis of a Quality Improvement Program. In C. Meisenheimer, *Improving Quality: A Guide to Effective Programs*, 2nd ed. (pp. 33–41). Gaithersburg, MD: Aspen Publishers.

Larson, S. (2003). The Roles of Senior Management in Quality Improvement Efforts: What Are the Key Components? *Journal of Healthcare Management*, p. 20.

Lighter, D. (2004). Strategies for Implementing Quality Improvement. In D. Lighter & D. Fair, *Quality Management in Health Care: Principles and Methods* (pp. 321–364). Sudbury, MA: Jones & Bartlett.

Lighter, D., & Fair, D. (2004). *Quality Management in Health Care: Principles and Methods.* Sudbury, MA: Jones & Bartlett.

MarketWatch. (2008, October 2). *Report: Health Care Quality Improves but Varies across Different Regions of the Country.* Retrieved October 2, 2008, from MarketWatch: News and Commentary: http://www.marketwatch.com/news/story/report-health-care-quality-improves/story.aspx?guid=%7B1B96F411-C7F4-4939-AD60-B4B86B82CDB3%7D&dist=hppr

McLaughlin, C., & Kaluzny, A. (2006). Defining Quality Improvement. In C. A. McLaughlin, *Continuous Quality Improvement in Health Care: Theory, Implementations, and Applications*, 3rd ed. (pp. 3–40). Sudbury, MA: Jones & Bartlett.

NCAL. (2008, September). Federal Effort Begins for Developing National Assisted Living Comparison Tool. *NCAL Focus*, pp. 1–2.

NLM. (2007, January 23). *Fact Sheet: The National Library of Medicine.* Retrieved September 9, 2008, from National Library of Medicine: http://www.nlm.nih.gov/pubs/factsheets/nlm.html

NQF. (2008). *About Us: Mission.* Retrieved September 12, 2008, from National Quality Forum: http://www.qualityforum.org/about/mission.asp

RWJ Foundation. (2008, June). *Quality/Equality: Our Strategy.* Retrieved September 13, 2008, from Robert Wood Johnson Foundation: http://www.rwjf.org/qualityequality/strategy.jsp

Schiverick, B. (2008, October). An Evidence-Based Quality Agenda Should Be Part of the Everyday Game Plan. *Provider*, pp. 2–7.

Shaw, P., Elliott, C., Isaacson, P., & Murphy, E. (2003). *Quality Performance Improvement in Healthcare: A Tool for Programmed Learning*, 2nd. ed. Chicago: American Health Information Management Association.

Sultz, H., & Young, K. (2009). *Health Care USA: Understanding its Organization and Delivery*, 6th ed. Sudbury, MA: Jones & Bartlett.

Wagner, L. (2008, August). News Currents: Advancing Excellence Extends Its Run. *Provider*, p. 12.

Wunderlich, G., & Kohler, P. (2001). *Improving the Quality of Long-Term Care.* Washington, DC: National Academies Press.

Index

Exhibits, figures, and tables are indicated with exh, *f*, and *t* following the page number.

A

AAC (Activity Assistant, Certified), 220
AAHSA (American Association of Homes and Services for the Aging), 315
AARP, 102, 183, 288, 295
Abuse, 58–59
Academic medical centers, 26
Access, 67–76
  to care, 110–113
  current indicators of, 74–76, 75–76*t*
  dimensions of, 70–71
  elderly population and, 111
  framework of, 68–70, 69–70*f*
  long-term care policy and, 188
  low income and, 112–113
  measurement of, 72–74
  minorities and, 111–112
  persons with AIDS and, 113
  in rural areas, 112
  types of, 71–72
Accountability, 132
Accreditation, 32–33
Accreditation organizations, 318
ACS (American College of Surgeons), 32
Activities of daily living (ADL), 166, 284
Activity Assistant, Certified (AAC), 220
Activity Director, Certified (ADC), 220
Activity professionals, 221
Acuity, 167
Acute conditions, 159
ADA (American Dietetic Association), 219
ADL (Activities of daily living), 166, 284
Administrative costs, 57–58
Administrative information systems, 223–224
Administrative professionals, 213–215
Administrators, long-term care, 213, 215
Adolescents, 167–168
Adult day care, 171
  providers, 203–204

Adult foster care (AFC) homes, 206
Advance directives, 34–35
Advancing Excellence in America's Nursing Homes, 316–317
Aesthetics of nursing home design, 247–248
AFDC (Aid to Families with Dependent Children), 100–101
Agency for Healthcare Research and Quality (AHRQ), 83, 116, 313
Aging-in-place, 210, 222
Aging of workforce, 139
AHA. *See* American Hospital Association
AHCA/NCAL (American Health Care Association/National Center for Assisted Living), 315
AHQA (American Health Quality Association), 317
AIDS. *See* HIV/AIDS
Aid to Families with Dependent Children (AFDC), 100–101
Aligning Forces for Quality, 318
Alliance for Quality Nursing Home Care, 316
Allocative tools, 98
Allopathic medicine, 216
All-payer system, 60
Alzheimer's disease, 209–210
AMA (American Medical Association), 26, 32, 83, 102
American Association of Health Plans, 84
American Association of Homes and Services for the Aging (AAHSA), 315
American Association of Retired Persons. *See now* AARP
American College of Physicians, 32
American College of Surgeons (ACS), 32
American Dietetic Association (ADA), 219
American Health Care Association, 102
American Health Care Association/National Center for Assisted Living (AHCA/NCAL), 315
American Health Quality Association (AHQA), 317